Critical Care Nursing in Resource Limited Environments

All hospitals have critically ill patients, and their management depends upon the resources available. In many low income countries, critically ill patients may be admitted to a critical care unit; however, many are nursed on wards due to a lack of critical care beds or simply die before they reach the hospital.

This book provides guidance on the unique situations for nurses working in these challenging environments, while considering ethical decision-making, providing appropriate services, and the types of patients admitted. Topics covered include:

- working in a resource limited environment;
- cultural awareness and international agendas;
- provision and access to healthcare services;
- ethical considerations in the context of resource limited environments;
- best practice and knowledge regarding rehabilitation, pain management, managing a major incident;
- relevant research concerning resource limited environments.

Critical Care Nursing in Resource Limited Environments prepares readers to consider how best to utilise their skills and deliver safe patient care within a resource limited context. Each easy-to-read chapter provides core knowledge and relevant research, as well as useful ideas and solutions, with further reading sections to signpost readers to key international resources. This text provides practical ideas for nurses working in critical care and defence nursing, and acute areas in resource limited environments. It can also be used to support educational courses and pre-deployment training for nurses hoping to work in Global Health.

Chris Carter is a Major in Queen Alexandra's Royal Army Nursing Corps, where he has had roles as a practitioner and as an educator. He is currently a nurse lecturer at the Defence School of Healthcare Education, Department of Healthcare Education, Birmingham City University, UK. Major Carter chairs the Royal College of Nursing Defence Nursing Forum.

Critical Care Nursing in Resource Limited Environments

Chris Carter

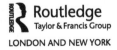

Routledge
Taylor & Francis Group

LONDON AND NEW YORK

First published 2019
by Routledge
2 Park Square, Milton Park, Abingdon, Oxon OX14 4RN

and by Routledge
52 Vanderbilt Avenue, New York, NY 10017

Routledge is an imprint of the Taylor & Francis Group, an informa business

British Library Cataloguing-in-Publication Data
A catalogue record for this book is available from the British Library

Library of Congress Cataloging-in-Publication Data
A catalog record has been requested for this book

ISBN: 978-1-138-09350-8 (hbk)
ISBN: 978-1-138-09351-5 (pbk)
ISBN: 978-1-315-10677-9 (ebk)

Typeset in Sabon
by Swales & Willis Ltd, Exeter, Devon, UK

Contents

Acknowledgments

When James Orbinski collected the Nobel Peace Prize in 1999 he famously said, 'We are not sure that words can always save lives, but we know that silence can certainly kill'. With few resources available to help prepare critical care nurses to work in resource limited environments, it is hoped the words in this book will assist nurses deliver the best standard of care, wherever they are in the world. This work has been inspired by the many civilian and military critical care nurses and healthcare professionals who I have had the opportunity to work alongside and meet. This book is dedicated to those who work in resource limited environments.

Reference

Orbinski J. (2008). An imperfect offering: dispatches from the medical frontline. London: Rider Books.

Introduction

1

Most of the world's population lives in low-income countries and approximately 1 billion people will never have access to a trained healthcare professional (*Lancet* Commission, 2016). In many countries, healthcare systems are fragile, with limited workforce, financing and resources, yet in many of these countries critical care services have developed over time. With limited additional professional support, nurses are often the backbone of these services. They provide expert care not only to critically ill patients and to their families within their critical care units but are often called upon to support nurses and doctors on wards and emergency departments. Respected by their peers and other professionals, just a small number of critical care nurses often have a hospital-wide impact, and investment in them has shown to have a ripple effect throughout the hospital (Towney & Ojara, 2008). However, critical care nurses and services are often not recognised for the impact and potential impact they have.

There is now increasing recognition that surgery and critical care has been the 'neglected stepchild of global health' and with changing epidemiological trends, the burden of non-communicable diseases and injuries, there is a need for critical care (Meara & Greenberg, 2015; Dean, 2016; *Lancet* Commission, 2016). This provides critical care nurses with opportunities and a responsibility to share knowledge with peers in other countries and to be recognised for this contribution to improving the health of communities.

When considering working in a resource limited environment, it must be recognised the environment is different to what you know, and additional training and preparation will be required. We work in high-tech environments and our education programmes and clinical experiences are unlikely to prepare us for the situations or conditions you are likely to see (Castledine, 2010). While there are several courses available, most do not focus specifically on the nursing of a critically ill patient and gaining experience to become confident and be of value is difficult. This book allows you, the experienced nurse, to translate your skills and experiences into a different environment, but also helps you recognise areas you may need to undertake further study or experience in. Each section focuses on a specific area of critical care nursing, and can be used as a resource in practice, as it provides useful references and suggestions that may help you when faced with a situation or disease you are not familiar with. In conjunction with short courses, reflection and discussion with experienced nurses this resource will be a valuable guide in preparing to provide critical care in resource limited environments.

References

Castledine G. (2010). Humanitarian nursing aid. British Journal of Nursing. 19. 3. 203.

Dean 2016. Take a walk on the wild side. Nursing Standard. 30. 28. 64.

Lancet Commission. (2016). The *Lancet* Commission on Global Safe Surgery. Available at: www.lancetglobalsurgery.org/.

Meara JG. Greenberg SLM. (2015). Global surgery as an equal partner in health: no longer the neglected stepchild. The Lancet Global Health. 3. S1–2.

Towney RM. Ojara S. (2008). Practice of intensive care in rural Africa: an assessment of data from Northern Uganda. African Health Sciences. 8. 1. 61–64.

2 | Global health and United Nations Sustainable Development Goals

Global health is a relatively new 'buzz' phrase in the international community and means different things to different people and organisations (Webb & Giles-Vernick, 2013). Global health is defined as the 'sharing of knowledge, resources and experience across cultures, societies, and international boarders' (Merry, 2012). The origins of global health are complex and unique to each country. When choosing to work internationally, taking time to understand the history of the provision and response to health will give you a greater understanding of how healthcare is provided and used, and the view towards international health agendas.

To improve the health of individuals and populations, global health focuses on partnerships and it is important that the next generation of healthcare workers understands the 'worlds in which their projects would operate' (Webb & Giles-Vernick, 2013 p. 1). Countries may have been affected by wars, colonialism, the transition to independence, geopolitics, the Cold War and epidemics including HIV and Ebola. In consequence, global health principles have been applied in response to these, and there is no one solution which can be applied to every country. In this chapter, we explore how decisions made in the past have contributed to our current thinking and international response to global health (Webb & Giles-Vernick, 2013).

The impact of colonialism

The history of tropical medicine is based on colonialism, when Europeans found their own experiences and knowledge was limited with dealing with many infectious diseases seen in the tropics (Webb & Giles-Vernick, 2013). This lead to the investment of resources to understand and control major diseases and the establishment of many schools and institutes in European countries.

In many low resource settings, the need to provide healthcare resulted in nurse education and healthcare systems being modelled on their colonial leaders' (Taylor, 2017). During the transition from colonialism to independence countries faced the challenge of how to upscale healthcare services which were designed for the colonial elite (WHO, 2018b). Today, many of these challenges continue with most healthcare facilities based in cities but most of the population living in rural communities. Primary healthcare attracted significant funding and development which has resulted in positive changes; however, many secondary care services did not develop concurrently, resulting in the varied provision of a range of healthcare services including critical care.

Policy

The World Health Organization was formed in 1948 with a primary role to direct and co-ordinate international health within the United Nations (UN) system (WHO, 2018b). A range of initiatives to combat disease have been tried by a variety of organisations and failed (WHO, 2018a). These activities tended to be disease-specific programmes, which allowed for donors not to get involved in political and economic priorities and provided technical solutions to provide results quickly (Webb & Giles-Vernick, 2013). The response to these failings resulted in countries requesting that the WHO take a greater role in co-ordinating a collaborative response. In recent years, there has been an explosion in the number of philanthropic and non-governmental organisations (NGOs), each with a different focus and view on global health, which at times has resulted in overlapping and a fragmenting of healthcare (WHO, 2018c).

Cold War and geo-politics

Between 1949 and 1956, the Soviet Union and other communist countries withdrew from the UN and WHO, resulting in a greater American influence globally (Webb & Giles-Vernick, 2013). The ideological war between the East and West was played out in many low-income countries (WHO, 2018a). At the height of the Cold War it was acknowledged that many of the grants and loans would not achieve their desired goals, yet the funds continued to secure political allegiances. The long-standing effect of epidemics, political instability and ethnic conflicts have driven out foreign investment and prevented new areas of development in many countries (Little & Green, 2009).

The end of the Cold War marked a change in the provision of aid to low-income countries, with a greater focus on independence. In the 1980s, the HIV epidemic became a real threat for the world and governments became increasingly concerned about the impact. The USA acknowledged the HIV pandemic as a geo-political threat that could destabilise African states by impacting on their economies. This fear became a driver for an international response to HIV and attracted significant donor funding.

Views of healthcare workers

A lack of transparency in healthcare delivery can influence the views of healthcare workers and those accessing healthcare. For example, in Egypt, the largest iatrogenic transmission of blood-borne pathogens resulting in a significant increase in hepatitis C and hepatitis B cases was due to the re-use of needles during a mass immunisation programme. The subsequent lack of acknowledgement by the government resulted in a significant proportion of the public not trusting the healthcare system or healthcare workers (Moulin, 2013).

In many countries, doctors may be shielded from patients' views and concerns behind scientific expertise, jargon and technology. Doctors may be expatriates and tend to be held in high esteem, with prestige, resulting in some patients being unwilling to challenge them (Moulin, 2013; Livingston, 2012). In contrast, nurses tend to be local nationals, who cannot hide behind jargon and may not have the status in their communities enjoyed by medics. Nursing is also more accessible, visible and public, meaning evaluation of nursing care is an easier target for those dissatisfied with healthcare (Livingston, 2012). This can result in nurses being blamed and becoming easy targets for deficiencies in the healthcare system.

Access to healthcare workers and outbreaks

Often both doctors and nurses struggle to provide services within very fragile healthcare systems which can become overwhelmed. Prior to the Ebola outbreak in Sierra Leone in 2014, there were just 70 surgeons and 68 nurse specialists providing care to 5.8 million people through 23 public hospitals (Brown et al., 2015). Following the outbreak, the number of healthcare workers reduced, because they fled, died or could not come to work as they were afraid or looking after relatives. While the immediate outbreak was contained and managed, the long-term recovery from this disaster will take years, due to the loss and void left by experienced healthcare workers (Holmer et al., 2015). In addition, globally there is a shortage of healthcare workers; the WHO estimate there could be a shortage of 12.9 million healthcare workers by 2035 (WHO, 2013). With nurses forming the largest part of the healthcare workforce in many countries, the shortfall in nurses will have a significant impact on how universal access to health coverage (UHC) and the SDGs will be achieved (International Perspectives, 2016). In consequence, the demand for healthcare services will continue to increase and with fewer 'trained' healthcare professionals, global health agendas need to be realistic with the current and future workforce and resources available.

Global health today

Today, the world is better connected and recent epidemics including Ebola, Middle East respiratory syndrome coronavirus, severe acute respiratory syndrome (SARS) and Zika virus have demonstrated that national healthcare systems, governments and international organisations need to work collaboratively to respond to global health issues. Until the Millennium Development Goals (MDGs), healthcare campaigns tended to be isolated, and not connected or linked to other areas of development, for example reducing gender inequality or recognising the true value of global partnerships.

The MDG marked a historic 15-year approach of 'global mobilisation' to achieve a set of social priorities worldwide (Sachs, 2016). The acceptance, international adoption of and commitment to a set of moral and practical, non-legally binding principles was rare and demonstrated an international commitment to change (Sachs, 2016). Critics felt there needed to be a wider focus as the MDGs only focused on LICs and LMICs and the role of HIC was to provide support, financial and technological assistance. This was felt to be one sided and there was no recognition of factors which affect healthcare globally, for example over half of the 1 billion people affected by poverty now live in middle-income countries and these countries have the financial and technological ability to address poverty (Sachs, 2016).

Building on the successes and responding to lessons learnt from the MDGs, the UN replaced this programme with the Sustainable Development Goals (SDG) (Figure 2.1) in 2015. The SDGs outlined 17 new ambitious goals and 156 associated targets, which were far more wide-reaching and took account of the inter-dependency between health, financial security, education and environmental damage. In addition, the SDGs are relevant to all countries regardless of status. Agreed by 193 world leaders and, if achieved, it is hoped by 2030 there would be an end to extreme poverty, inequality and climate change (Bradbury-Jones & Clark, 2017). Described as 'easy to understand, ambitious and achievable', the SDGs have had to compromise to make them easy to communicate (Brende & Hoie, 2015). Waage *et al.* (2015) outlined that the SDGs have three layers, reflecting their impact on an individual's well-being, infrastructure and environment. Health-related goals have been identified as forming part of people's overall well-being. Concerns regarding health have been voiced, as three MDG health goals were merged into one SDG under one defining goal. This has been referred to as a 'shopping list' and opponents are concerned one goal with many standards will not be seen as a priority (Brende & Hoie, 2015). Buse and Hawkes (2015) suggested the move to the SDG requires a significant paradigm shift with a need for leadership across sectors (health, legal, social, political and economic), with a change in focus from treatment to prevention, civic engagement and social accountability and responsibility for health.

The nursing profession was felt to be slow to respond to the opportunities offered by the MDG and this was deemed to be a potential missed opportunity to showcase the unique roles nurses play in promoting health, and preventing disease and disability (Benton & Shaffer, 2016). Nurses are the backbone of healthcare services globally and play a vital role in meeting many of the SDGs and it is recognised that universal access to healthcare will be won or lost by nurses (All-Party Parliamentary Group on Global Health, 2016). In 2017, the International Council of Nurses launched a campaign, 'Nurses: A voice to lead – Achieving the Sustainable Development Goals'. The aim of this campaign is to raise awareness amongst the nurses, the public and policy makers to what the SDGs are and why they matter. Recognising the evidence on the vital role nurses play in healthcare, the Nursing Now campaign was launched by the WHO and ICN (Nursing Now, 2018) to raise the status and profile of nursing and respond to the changing healthcare challenges we will all face.

For nurses choosing to work internationally, the opportunity to inform, shape and develop the future through capacity building partnerships is vast. However, it should

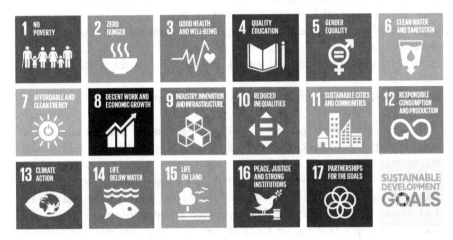

Figure 2.1 United Nations Sustainable Development Goals

be recognised that the opportunity is not solely limited to this type of work; opportunities must include sharing experiences through professional publications, research and education roles (Sachs, 2016; Benton & Ferguson, 2016). This will have the long-term impact on peers, policy makers and the public, to demonstrate the unique contribution nurses make in meeting the SDGs and patient care.

This book focuses on critical care conditions; and critical care services needs to fit within the wider healthcare system. When choosing to work in a particular country, understanding the healthcare infrastructure will help prepare you to understand how nurses and other healthcare workers are employed and services provided. Areas you may want to research include the following:

- What has the World Bank classified the country as?
- What is life expectancy?
- How did the country meet the MDG/SDGs relating to health?
- Review the WHO Health Systems Framework (2017a) and consider the following:
  o How much of the country's GDP is allocated on healthcare?
  o How is healthcare delivered and funded (consider primary healthcare, chronic disease management and rehabilitation)?
  o Whether nurses and midwives are registered?
  o How are nurses regulated?
  o What strategic leadership roles do nurses undertake? Is there a chief nursing officer?

- Look at the WHO country profile for life expectancy, communicable and non-communicable diseases and other metrics including maternal and child health.
- What is the culture, national religion?
- Do nurses have a Code of Conduct to follow in practice? Are there any other guidelines available, e.g. standards for medicines management, continuing professional development?
- What is the educational standard of nurses during pre-registration and at post-registration?
- How many nurses, midwives, doctors are there for the population?

Exploring these concepts before you travel will provide a useful background to the wider delivery of healthcare in the country you are choosing to work in and how well information and data are collected and shared.

In summary, each country and region will have their own healthcare priorities; healthcare can no longer be seen in isolation, and the WHO (WHO 2017b) has called for health to feature in all policies. The SDGs provide an opportunity to 'reimagine global health' and to re-position health centrally on the wider national and international agenda (Buse & Hawkes, 2015).

Understanding the country's history, how healthcare has been developed and delivered and the views of the public towards healthcare workers will help provide context and a deeper understanding of the potential challenges you may face. This will help prepare you for your role, and no matter how small you may consider your contribution when working internationally, you are going to play a vital role in helping the country and healthcare system to meet their national and international goals.

References

All-Party Parliamentary Group on Global Health. (2016). Triple impact. How developing nursing will improve health, promote gender equality and support economic growth. Available at: www.appgglobalhealth.org.uk/.../i/.../DIGITAL%20APPG%20Triple%20 Impact.pdf.

Benton DC. Ferguson SL. (2016). Windows to the future: can the United Nations Sustainable Development Goals provide opportunities for nursing? Nursing Economics. 34. 2. 101–103.

Benton D. Shaffer F. (2016). How the nursing profession can contribute to the sustainable development goals. Nursing Management. 23. 7. 29–34.

Bradbury-Jones C. Clark M. (2017). Globalisation and global health: issues for nursing. Nursing Standard. 31. 39. 54–62.

Brende B. Hoie B. (2015).Towards evidence-based, quantitative Sustainable Development Goals for 2030. The Lancet 385. 206–208.

Brown C. Arkell P. Rokadiya S. (2015). Ebola virus disease: the 'Black Swan' in West Africa. Tropical Doctor. 45. 1. 2–5.

Buse K. Hawkes S. (2015). Health in the sustainable development goals: ready for a paradigm shift? Globalization and Health. 11. 13. DOI: doi.org/10.1186/s12992-015-0098-8.

Holmer H. Lantz A. Kunjumen T. Finlayson S et al. (2015). Global distribution of surgeons, anaesthesiologists, and obstetricians. DOI: http://dx.doi.org/10.1016/S2214-109X(14)70349-3.

International Council of Nurses. (2017). Nurses: A voice to lead – Achieving the Sustainable Development Goals. Available at: www.icn.ch/publications/2017-nursing-a-voice-to-lead-achieving-the-sustainable-development-goals/2017-nursing-a-voice-to-lead-achieving-the-sustainable-development-goals.html.

International Perspectives. (2016). Nursing input strengthens WHO global strategy for health human resources. International Nursing Review. 153. DOI: https://doi.org/10.1111/inr.12277.

Little AW. Green A. (2009). Successful globalisation, education and sustainable development. International Journal of Educational Development. 29. 164–174.

Livingston J. (2012). Improvising medicine: an African oncology ward in an emerging cancer epidemic. London: Duke University Press.

Merry L. (2012). Global health for nursing . . . and the nursing for global health. The Canadian Journal of Nursing Research. 44. 4. 20–35.

Moulin AM. (2013). Chapter 6: Defenceless bodies and violent afflictions in a global world. In: Giles-Vernick T. Webb JLA (eds). Global health in Africa: historical perspectives on disease control. Athens, OH: Ohio University Press.

Nursing Now. (2018). Nursing Now. Available at: www.nursingnow.org/.

Sachs JD. (2016). From Millennium Development Goals to Sustainable Development Goals. The Lancet. 379. 2206–2211.

Taylor A. (2017). Getting it right: culturally safe approaches to health partnership work in low to middle income countries. Nurse Education in Practice. 24. 49–54.

Waage J. Yap C. Bell S et al. (2015). Governing the UN Sustainable Development Goals: interactions, infrastructures and institutions. The Lancet. 3. E251–252.

Webb JLA. Giles-Vernick T. (2013). Introduction. In: Giles-Vernick T. Webb JLA (eds). Global health in Africa: historical perspectives on disease control. Athens, OH: Ohio University Press.

World Health Organization. (2013). A universal truth: no health without a workforce. Available at: www.who.int/workforcealliance/knowledge/resources/GHWA-a_universal_truth_report.pdf?ua=1.

World Health Organization. (2017a). Health in all Policies – Health in all SDGs: call for action on climate change. Available at www.euro.who.int/en/health-topics/environment-and-health/Climate-change/news/news/2016/10/ministers-endorse-joint-statement-on-climate-change-and-health-at-high-level-meeting-of-small-countries/health-in-all-policies-health-in-all-sdgs-call-for-action-on-climate-change.

World Health Organization. (2017b). The WHO Health Systems Framework. Available at www.wpro.who.int/health_services/health_systems_framework/en/.

World Health Organization. (2018a). Consensus during the Cold War: back to Alma-Ata. Bulletin of the World Health Organization. 86. 10. October 2008. 737–816.

World Health Organization. (2018b). About WHO. Available at: http://who.int/about/en/.

World Health Organization. (2018c). Public health in the 21st century: optimism in the midst of unprecedented challenges. Director General Speech. 3 April 2007. Available at: www.who.int/dg/speeches/detail/public-health-in-the-21st-century-optimism-in-the-midst-of-unprecedented-challenges.

United Nations. (2015). Sustainable development goals. Available at: https://sustainabledevelopment.un.org/?menu=1300.

3 | Surgical care

In 1980, the Director-General of the World Health Organization identified surgery as an essential part of primary healthcare and challenged the global community to address the inequalities in surgical care (Mahler, 1980). This was largely ignored and for the next 30 years surgical care remained the neglected stepchild in healthcare. Only recently has the international community acknowledged the need to provide universal access to safe surgery (Ng-Kamstra et al., 2016; Akenroye et al., 2013).

Today, the provision of safe surgical care is variable, with an estimated 4.8 billion of the world's population not having access to surgery and ongoing surgical care (Alkire et al., 2015). Within low resource settings often preventable and treatable surgical conditions such as fractures, appendicitis, strangulated hernia or childbirth result in permanent disability or death. Those that make it to a surgical facility are still not safe due to a lack of staff, and those available may not be appropriately trained or have the resources to treat them safely. For the first time in history, people are more likely to die from a surgically treatable condition rather than an infectious disease, representing a global crisis (Lifebox, 2018). However, many of the specialities involved in surgical care are underdeveloped and under-resourced, and with most resources focusing on the immediate intraoperative period (Kinnear et al., 2013), with variations in care during the pre-, post-operative and rehabilitation periods. The following case studies demonstrate the complexities in providing universal access to surgical care.

Case study 1: Accessing surgical care

Ugboma et al. (2014) describe the care of a 35-year-old female trader who had a 6-day journey involving local remedies, a private clinic consultation, and travelling to a public hospital before receiving surgical care for a ruptured ectopic pregnancy. The patient initially sought treatment from a traditional healer. As her condition continued to deteriorate the generalised symptoms of early gestation, including malaise, weakness, nausea and vomiting, made it difficult to diagnose an ectopic pregnancy. When she developed a low-grade pyrexia caused by blood in the pelvis, these symptoms were attributed to malaria. She then passed dark-coloured loose stool suggesting an upper gastro-intestinal bleed, further making diagnosis difficult.

Delays in performing confirmatory investigations were cited due to the patient having to pay for them and she had limited health insurance. In addition, an incomplete history and examination resulted in a delay in diagnosing an ectopic pregnancy. There was then a delay before surgery could be performed due to limited resources and unavailability of the surgical team. The challenges raised in this scenario are complex and touch on cultural issues towards traditional versus Western medical approaches, access to emergency healthcare services, training of healthcare workers and the provision of surgical care.

Case study 2: 'You can't fix it without data' (Weiser *et al.*, 2015)

A retrospective cohort study of perioperative deaths of surgery within a tertiary referral hospital (Lillie *et al.*, 2015), found the surgical pathway within the hospital had several areas of vulnerability, including:

- a delay in booking operating theatres, resulting in a delay in surgery and a lack of blood for transfusion;
- communication breakdown, including a failure to consult cases with senior colleagues;
- failure to recognise and respond to the deteriorating patient;
- few intensive care beds, limited equipment and resources, coupled with no dedicated intensive care physicians, which lead to delays in escalating care;
- suboptimal nursing care on the ward due to few staff.

Lillie *et al.* (2015) compared their data with a previous study published in 1987 (Heywood *et al.*, 1989) and concluded they were unable to show a decrease in the total perioperative mortality rate. Lillie *et al.* (2015) cited limitations in the study including gathering standardised data, inconsistencies in record-keeping and a lack of reliability with records, for example records were missing or nurses told auditors of patients who had died but who were not listed in mortuary records.

This case study highlights the realities of surgical care within a hospital and the challenges in collecting perioperative statistics. Weiser *et al.* (2015) commented that the lack of data potentially demonstrates the lack of interest amongst Ministries of Health and international bodies to encourage comprehensive data collection. In consequence, without data to identify the need and measure the impact of interventions, the allocation of resources and funding will remain sporadic and not focused to areas where they are most needed.

Case study 3: Surgical workload in critical care

Studies have shown most reasons for admission to critical care are due to surgery, demonstrating the high burden of surgical disease in LICs or LMICs (Towney & Ojara, 2008; Tomlinson *et al.*, 2013). Tomlinson *et al.* (2013) found most patients admitted to a tertiary referral hospital in Malawi were due to trauma (58.3%), surgery (39.3%) and obstetrics/gynaecology (32.9%). Mortality was highest amongst patients who sustained a head injury (57.1%). Similar findings were obtained in a regional referral hospital in Uganda. Ttendo *et al.* (2016) found 49.3% of admissions were due to surgery, obstetrics/gynaecology (22.3%) and medical/paediatric (27.4%). The authors further identified most patients were young (median age 22 years), which reflected the younger population with a lower life expectancy than seen in HIC. In addition, Ttendo *et al.* noted due to limited access to rural healthcare, this resulted in many patients being admitted with advanced stages of diseases, and the majority of patients died within the first 23 hours of admission (46.9%). These papers demonstrate the difference in case mix, ages and outcomes of patients admitted to critical care units in low-income countries compared to HICs.

Case study 4: Stoma care in LICs or LMICs

The formation of a stoma involves complex surgery and is often undertaken in tertiary centres. Following surgery individuals are often unable to afford disposable commercial stoma products (Buckley *et al.*, 2012). Many individuals improvise ostomy devices and use pieces of plastic or jar lids to secure plastic food bags or gloves in place over the stoma, then elastic garters, leather, cloth are wrapped around the body to hold the stoma bag in place. While many of these are noted to be effective, the prevalence of skin excoriation is significant (Razon-Gonzalez, 2011). Once discharged from hospital the ongoing care for these patients will likely be provided by primary healthcare nurses and doctors who may be unfamiliar with stoma care. With limited access to specialist knowledge and support groups this leads to isolation. This scenario demonstrates the need for the whole surgical care pathway to be understood, including the long-term consequences of a surgical intervention.

There remains little information available on adults and children requiring improvised ostomy devices and evidence tends to focus on the surgical intervention. As outlined in case study 1, the surgical pathway for both acute and emergency surgery is complex and not only the domain of the hospital setting. Healthcare workers at every stage of the patient journey, from referral to ongoing care, need to have access to current information and resources. However, deciding what is a priority when there are so many competing priorities within an already limited environment is a significant issue for policy planners and governments.

Lancet Commission on Safe Surgery

Recognising the inequalities in access to surgical care globally, the Global Safe Surgery Campaign was launched in January 2014. The findings of a worldwide review of surgical and anaesthetic care in low-income and low-middle-income countries outlined a vision for 'universal access to safe, affordable surgical and anaesthetic care when needed' (Global Safe Surgery, 2018). The campaign recognised that for over 20 years, global health had focused on individual disease and the scale-up of hospital services including surgery had been neglected. The campaign has set goals to be achieved by

2030 and requires donors, governments and healthcare workers to work towards the recommendations (Global Safe Surgery, 2018):

- Access to timely essential surgery;

  o Minimum 80% coverage of essential surgical and anaesthetic services per country;

- Specialist surgical workforce;

  o 100% of countries with at least 20 surgeons, anaesthetists, obstetricians per 100,000 population;

- Surgical workforce;

  o In stages, develop tracking of surgical volume:
    o 80% of countries by 2020;
    o 100% of countries by 2030. With the aim of a minimum of 5000 procedures per 100,000;

- Perioperative mortality rate (PMOR);

  o In stages, identify PMOR:
    o 80% of countries by 2020; this will allow evaluation of global data and setting of national targets to be achieved by 2030;
    o 100% of countries by 2030 tracking POMR;

- Protection against impoverished expenditure;

  o 100% protection against poverty caused by out-of-pocket payments;

- Protection against catastrophic expenditure;

  o 100% protection against extreme poverty caused by out-of-pocket payments for surgical and anaesthetic care.

Finally, for many countries, surgical systems are unlikely to meet the population need by 2030 (Uribe-Leitz et al., 2015) unless there is a significant scale-up in resources, healthcare workers and research. Critical care nursing is an essential but small part of the surgical patient pathway; however, with an estimated 70% of admissions to critical care requiring post-operative care (WHO, 2003) nurses have an important part to play in improving the outcome of surgical care. In this chapter we have explored the complexities in providing surgical care through a series of case studies to demonstrate the complexity in accessing and providing safe surgery.

References

Akenroye OO. Adebona OT. Akenroye AT. (2013). Surgical Care in the Developing World-Strategies and Framework for Improvement. Journal of Public Health in Africa. 4. 2. DOI: https://doi.org/10.4081/jphia.2013.e20.

Alkire, BC. Raykar N. Shrime MG *et al.* (2015). Global access to surgical care: a modelling study. Lancet. 3. 6. E316–323.

Buckley BS. Razon-Gonzalez JP. Lopez MC. (2012). The review: the people that the ostomy industry forgot. British Journal of General Practice. Oct. 544–545.

Global Safe Surgery. (2018). Global surgery 2030: report summary. Available at: http://docs.wixstatic.com/ugd/346076_713dd3f8bb594739810d84c1928ef61a.pdf.

Heywood AJ. Wilson IH. Sinclair JR. (1989). Peri-operative mortality in Zambia. Annals of the Royal College of Surgeons of England. 72. 354–358.

Kinnear JA. Bould MD. Ismailova F. Measures E. (2013). A new partnership for anaesthesia training in Zambia: reflections on the first year. Canadian Journal of Anesthesia. DOI: 10.1007/s12630-013-9905-y.

Lifebox. (2018). Safe Surgery. Available at www.lifebox.org/safe-surgery/.

Lillie E. Holmes CJ. O'Donohoe EA *et al.* (2015). Avoidable perioperative mortality at the University Teaching Hospital, Lusaka, Zambia: a retrospective cohort study. Canadian Journal of Anesthesia. 62. 12. 1259–1267.

Mahler H. (1980). Surgery and health for all. Available at: www.who.int/surgery/strategies/Mahler1980speech.pdf?ua=1.

Ng-Kamstra J. Greenberg SLM. Abdullah F *et al.* (2016). Global surgery 2030: a roadmap for high income country actors. BMJ Global Health. 1. E000011. DOI: 10.1136/bmjgh-2015-000011.

Razon-Gonzalez EV. Gonzalez JP. Lopez MP. Roxas MF. (2011). Commercial versus modified appliance in patients with intestinal stomas [abstract]. Annals of Oncology. 22. (Suppl. 5): v125.

Tomlinson J. Haac B. Kadyaudzu C *et al.* (2013). The burden of surgical diseases on critical care services at a tertiary referral hospital in sub-Saharan Africa. Tropical Doctor. 43. 1. 27–29.

Towney RM. Ojara S. (2008). Practice of intensive care in rural Africa: an assessment of data from Northern Uganda. African Health Sciences. 8. 1. 61–64.

Ttendo SS. Was A. Preston MA *et al.* (2016). Retrospective descriptive study of an intensive care unit at a Ugandan Regional Referral Hospital. World Journal of Surgery. 40. 2847–2856.

Ugboma HAA. Oputa VOA. Ugboma EW. (2014). Ruptured ectopic pregnancy: the long and tortuous journey to theatre. Tropical Doctor. 44. 3. 173–175.

Uribe-Leitz T. Esquivel MM. Molina G *et al.* (2015). Projections for achieving the Lancet Commission recommended surgical rate of 5000 operations per 100,000 population by region-specific rate estimates. World Journal of Surgery. 39. 21. 2168–2172.

Weiser TG. Makasa EM. Gelb AW. (2015). Improving perioperative outcomes in low-resource countries: It can't be fixed without data. Canadian Journal of Anesthesia. 62. 12. 1239–1243.

World Health Organization. (2003). Chapter 15: Anaesthetic infrastructure and supplies. In Surgical Care at the District Hospital. Geneva: World Health Organization.

4 | Choosing to work internationally

There are many opportunities for nurses to work internationally, with Non-Governmental Organisations (NGOs), to join the military or work with other organisations such as international assistance teams. These experiences provide nurses with an opportunity to work in an unfamiliar environment, experiencing a new culture, gain an appreciation of conditions not seen in their practice, learn about global health, ethics, professionalism, health systems and policy. The experience can also bring personal benefits for the individual too, for example the experience may give you a new perspective on your own life or get innovative ideas for the future (Crisp, 2017).

The benefits and the impact of working internationally is acknowledged as having a positive impact on practice when individuals return home (Simms, 2016; Carter, 2015; Carter & Snell, 2016). In 2015, 96% of 339 volunteers who had been working in a low resource setting self-reported or demonstrated improved clinical and leadership skills (Haines, 2016). In addition, working internationally helps develop resourcefulness, cultural competence and resilience, which are all key skills nurses need regardless of where they work (Crisp, 2007).

Often the terms 'resource limited' and 'low resource setting' can be used interchangeably; however, it is worth recognising they often have different meanings to different organisations. You may have the skills but lack the resources, for example, due to the physical situation (during times of conflict), being in a remote area (dealing with a medical emergency onboard an aircraft), living and working in a low-income country or in a disaster or the immediate aftermath (Iserson, 2016). Within this book, the focus is on nursing in an LIC or LMIC, where you will have limited access to resources and professionals. Working in this environment will provide unique experiences and challenges and how you respond will be determined by your previous experiences and how well prepared you are.

Working in any resource limited environment will require you to adapt to the new situation quickly; nurses often practise in controlled situations, with additional resources and immediate access to specialist staff. In practice, you may find yourself on your own or with few resources available as often healthcare services are fragile and function with limited trained healthcare professionals. In consequence, it is widely accepted that your current role may not adequately prepare you with the necessary judgement and skills for your role abroad (Hodgetts, 2012; Cox & Briggs, 2004). When planning to work abroad, you need to think about the organisation and role you are planning to undertake. Often following an immediate humanitarian disaster there is constant media coverage; however, the opportunities and roles available are much more varied, ranging from immediate disaster response, to capacity building and sustainable development programmes to help improve livelihoods, health, policy or education (Royal College of Nursing, 2017).

When choosing to work abroad it is important to consider the roles available and match your skills and experience to the right organisation. It takes confidence to work abroad, especially if you are going to work in a conflict or humanitarian situation. Many NGOs vary in their work, for example Médecins Sans Frontières (MSF) and the Voluntary Service Overseas (VSO) have contrasting approaches to projects. MSF is independent and tends to focus on the immediate response to a crisis, whereas VSO works on long-term projects with placements with host organisations (Royal College of Nursing, 2017).

It is important to research the organisation you chose to work with; NGOs can be based on faith or a political view with an expectation volunteers participate in daily worship or take a political viewpoint (Royal College of Nursing, 2017). Understanding the type of organisation you plan to work with and your own values, motivation and goals can help you choose the correct organisation.

In recent years, there has been a focus on greater collaboration between NGOs and military organisations (termed CIMIC). For example, following the Ebola outbreak in Sierra Leone, the UK Defence Medical Services shared pre-departure training and resources to deal with the humanitarian response. However, working with military organisations can be viewed as a blurring of lines by some NGOs as it risks their security and neutrality. Even within the NGO community, different mandates and expectations between organisations can cause conflict over expectations and roles, which risks the goals of the project. Understanding other organisations that you may be working alongside is an important part of the pre-departure process.

Working abroad will require you to respond to conditions not normally seen in your home country, which will test your leadership, resilience and resourcefulness. To help you prepare, the following guidance can help you consider the type of organisation, role and the practicalities of working internationally.

- Choosing an organisation:

  o Does the organisation you are working for require you to have any additional training prior to departure? For example, some organisations require you to have tropical medicine courses or experience of working in a low resource setting.

    ▪ How long will it take to achieve all the courses and where will the training take place?
    ▪ Who will pay for this?

  o How long do you plan to be away for?

○ What about your commitments at home? For example, how will you meet your financial commitments while you are away? How will your family take you not being around or not having frequent regular contact?

- Consider any cultural sensitivities, for example what are you expected to wear? Can men treat women and vice versa? There may be different attitudes to what you agree with, for example views towards women, LGBT people, minority groups, which you may not agree with.
- Language. Not everywhere will speak English; therefore, you may need to consider if you don't speak another language it may limit your working opportunities in some countries and environments. Some groups may speak in local dialects or languages, which may hinder your role in delivering healthcare.
- Professional perspective:

  ○ Do you need to register as a nurse with the country you are planning to work in?
  ○ How will you maintain your home registration while you are away? With limited access to the internet if your registration requires renewing, how will you do this?

- Professional indemnity. Who will provide professional indemnity? Ideally the organisation you are working with should provide this; however, it is work considering.
- What are your plans when you return home? You need to consider your long-term nursing career. While there are many benefits and opportunities when working internationally, you may want to consider how this meets your short-, medium- and long-term career aspirations.
- You may want to talk to others who have worked in that country. Often talking to someone who has worked in that country or done a similar role can provide you with more information than you could find on the internet and give you some handy practical tips. Box 4.1 provides some ideas of useful tips.
- Safety. Look at your government and international websites for information on safety. Consider how you are going to look after yourself while away.

  ○ Upload copies of any important documents to the Cloud, so that if you lose any critical documents you can access copies of the documents.

    ▪ Many places are dangerous and there is a risk of serious incident and death. Incidents may include exposure to tropical diseases, dangers of war, hospitals being targeted, unexploded ordnance, violence, abduction and rape –these are all potential risks you may face. It is important to consider what security and support will be available by your organisation. Often road traffic collisions are the highest cause of injury.

  ○ How will you communicate in-country, e.g. mobile phones?
  ○ How will you have access to communications with people outside of the country, e.g. internet access, satellite phones, or will there be restrictions dues to security?

    o   Health considerations:
- Do you need to take malaria prophylaxis?
- Do you need to have any vaccinations?
- Do you need a personal first aid kit?
- Sun protection?

– Be careful with your personal belongings, for example cash, valuables like laptops, phones.

(Royal College of Nursing, 2017)

Box 4.1 Practical critical care resources

– Head torch (including spare batteries).
– Pocket book with relevant useful information (paediatric observations, emergency calculations, conversion from mmHg to kPa, normal ranges, etc).
– Stethoscope.
– Pens and a notebook.
– Fob watch.
– Pen torches – take a few.
– Permanent markers – useful for writing on IV bags when you have added a drug if there are no additive labels available or you are dating a giving set, etc.
– Padlocks.
– Pocket alcohol hand gel bottles.
– Non-latex/powdered gloves.
– Scrub uniforms.
– Comfortable shoes.
– Goggles.
– 'Bum bag' to keep key documents and essential equipment together and on your person.

Professional and ethical issues

First, expect things to be different; you are going to experience a different culture, healthcare system and expectations towards medicine. You need to expect there are going to be different professional perspectives and potential ethical challenges. Nurses work in the real world and need to make ethical decisions while delivering care. Working in resource limited environments provides unique ethical challenges (Matheson & Hawley, 2010). The situation could determine the type of professional issue you may face. These may include the following:

- Dealing with child soldiers and prisoners of war or captured persons.
- Theft and crime towards patients or healthcare facilities.

- Treating children, which can be emotive and deciding who to admit can be challenging, particularly if it is undertaken by junior staff.
- Making complex treatment decisions when you have limited blood and blood products, or surgical sets.
- Critical care is political, as you will need to co-ordinate human and other resources daily to manage patients. Limited critical care resources could result in a potential 'competition' for a bed; this may be uncomfortable particularly if the decision is to admit an important person who may not require critical care, but the care is deemed better due to a higher nurse to patient ratio.
- Working with multi-national staff with differences in opinion with regards to care delivery and management.
- If there are no 'step-down' or high-dependency beds, when is it appropriate to discharge a patient, with little follow-up?
- How appropriate is it to perform complex surgery, when there may be limited access to dressings, to manage complex wounds, undertake future skin grafts or provision of basics such as stoma bags? In addition, following complex surgery and critical care illness there may be limited rehabilitation opportunities including prosthetics, physiotherapy services.
- Dealing with end-of-life decisions and withdrawal of treatment, for example when dealing with brain death and decisions to stop ventilation. These variations in cultural perspectives may cause conflict.
- Medication challenges:
  o You may not have access to the internet, computer or resources to check medications.
  o There may be no paediatric liquid medications and you may see people crushing tablets and capsules and adding water.
  o Drugs may come in different names, strengths and routes of administration.
  o Instructions may not be in English.
  o Drugs may be counterfeit, therefore not effective.
- Lack of patient safety, guidelines, policies to support care. The WHO (2008) estimated in low resource settings adverse events occur in 4–16 of all hospitalised patients.
- You are likely to have more responsibility than you do back home and have to make decisions and clinical judgements in isolation.

(One Nurse at a Time, 2015; Royal College of Nursing, 2017)

It is important to remain within your scope of practice. To help you prepare, the organisation you are working for should provide you with a set of terms of reference or a job description, so you can understand what will be expected of you. You may find talking to others who have worked in that country or reading their blogs can provide you with up-to-date information and real-world perspectives, and provide top tips to take or consider. There are also a variety of global tools and resources available, which may help you prepare for your role, for example:

- The Sphere Project provides humanitarian protocols and guidance for working in disaster situations.
- The World Health Organization provides a variety of resources to be used in clinical practice.
- The International Council of Nurses provides resources and has a code of ethics for nurses.

Dealing with a professional or ethical issue can be challenging, as the views may be very different to what you are used to or believe is right or wrong. Understanding the context in which you are practising can help you prepare; for example, you may also need to deal with complex hierarchies, where nurses may feel powerless to challenge doctors or escalate their concerns (Thornton, 2017; Royal College of Nursing, 2017). If you do not understand the issues facing healthcare staff, this may result in unrealistic expectations and 'exporting' of our practices and views which are unrealistic (Tingle, 2012). The process of understanding the diverse values, beliefs and behaviours forms part of cultural competence. Poor cultural competence can lead to poor communication, negative experiences, misunderstanding and compliance amongst both healthcare workers and patients (Benbenishty *et al.*, 2017).

Looking after yourself

It is important to look after yourself before, during and after your trip. Therefore, you need to prepare both emotionally and mentally before you go (Royal College of Nursing, 2017). You are going to experience a different culture, healthcare system and expectations towards medicine, and it is not unusual to be overwhelmed at first. You may have travelled for several days, crossed time zones and be expected to work immediately on arrival. Your working days may be 12–14 hours. This will be tiring and cause stress on your body.

There is likely to be lots of work to do and prioritising what needs to be done can be difficult. Writing a to-do list and prioritising tasks which need to take place and those that can wait can be helpful. You are likely to have some good and bad days, and identifying your achievements and positive aspects of your trip can help when you are having a difficult day. There are various apps and organisations which can also be helpful, for example Headspace is a mindfulness app that is endorsed by various NGOs. Your organisation may also have support mechanisms in place if you are really struggling. Other tips to look after yourself include the following:

- Give yourself time to settle in and understand your unfamiliar environment.
- It is important to make sure you eat, hydrate and rest. When you can take a lunchbreak, the short time away from work can be refreshing and help you re-focus. Before you go find out, what the food will be like. If food is expensive, you may be served things you don't like. Therefore, you may want to take snacks or dry foods with you to help.
- Don't work longer than nine hours per day.
- Take one day off per week.

- Make time for social interaction.
- If you are allowed, bring some reminders of home, e.g. pictures of family.
- If safe to do so, go for a walk to help clear your head, or go to the gym.
- Make sure you take your medication regularly.

(Royal College of Nursing, 2017)

When you return home, you may experience 'reverse culture shock' and feel numb, frustrated with Western views and priorities. It is important to participate in the debriefing provided by your organisation and having a strong support network, accommodation and plan for when you come home can help (Royal College of Nursing, 2017).

It is important to look out for signs of post-traumatic stress disorder (PTSD) which may include flashbacks, nightmares, repetitive distressing images and physical signs, e.g. pain, sweating, nausea, vomiting (NHS, 2018). It is important to seek help.

Working abroad is a life-changing experience, which will hopefully leave you with many good memories and lasting friendships. In this chapter, we have explored the importance of being adequately prepared, informed and trained from your role.

References

Benbenishty J. Gutysz-Wojnicka A. Harth I. *et al*. (2017). The migrant crisis and the importance of developing cultural competence in the intensive care unit. Nursing in Critical Care. 22. 5. 263–264.

Carter C. (2015). Opportunity to make a difference. Nursing Standard. 29. 52. 64–65.

Carter C. Snell D. (2016). Nursing the critically ill surgical patient in Zambia. British Journal of Nursing. 25. 20. 1123–1128.

Cox E. Briggs S. (2004). Disaster nursing: new frontiers for critical care. Critical Care Nurse. 24. 3. 16–22.

Crisp N. (2007). Global Health Partnerships – the UK contribution to health in developing countries. London: COI.

Crisp N. (2017). Foreword. In: Working internationally: a guide to humanitarian and development work for nurses and midwives. London: Royal College of Nursing. Publication Code: 005 960.

Haines A. (2016). Why health partnerships are good for global health. BMJ Blogs. 11 Jul7 2016. Available at http://blogs.bmj.com/bmj/2016/07/11/andy-haines-why-health-partnerships-are-good-for-global-health/.

Hodgetts TJ. (2012). The future character of military medicine. Journal of the Royal Army Medical Corps. 158. 3. 271–278.

Iserson KV. (2016). Improvised medicine: providing care in extreme environments. 2nd Edition. New York: McGraw Hill Education.

Matheson JIDM. Hawley A. (2010). Making sense of disaster medicine: a hands on guide for medics. London: Hodder Arnold.

National Health Service. (2018). Post-Traumatic Stress Disorder. Available at: www.nhs.uk/conditions/post-traumatic-stress-disorder-ptsd/symptoms/.

One Nurse at a Time. (2015).The role of the nurse in the developing world or how do I fit it? Available at: http://onenurseatatime.org/education/humanitarian-nursing-102/.

Royal College of Nursing. (2017). Working internationally: a guide to humanitarian and development work for nurses and midwives. Available at: www.rcn.org.uk/professional-development/publications/pub-005960.

Simms B. (2016). Sending our professionals overseas is one of the best things the NHS can do. Available at: www.hsj.co.uk/leadership/sending-our-professionals-overseas-is-one-of-the-best-things-the-nhs-can-do/7005839.article.

Thornton J. (2017). Working with nurses in Myanmar opened my eyes. Nursing Standard. 31. 38. 26–28.

Tingle J. (2012). Patient safety in the developing world: new frontiers. British Journal of Nursing. 21. 4. 256–257.

World Health Organization. (2008). Patient safety in African Health Services: issues and Solutions. Report of the Regional Director. Available at: http://apps.who.int/iris/handle/10665/19987.

5 | Project management

Theory of change

Theory of change (ToC) is a methodology for planning and participation used by not-for-profit organisations and governments to promote social change. ToC are used by philanthropic, Non-Governmental Organisations (NGOs) and government organisations when planning projects. ToC involves identifying the steps of an intervention and how it will achieve the goals of improving people's lives (Brown, 2016). Other models include Logical Frameworks (also referred to as LogFrames). Although different, both the ToC and Logical Frameworks aim to provide a structure to projects and how they will lead to results (Bullen, 2014). There are various models and terminology for theories of change, most involve identifying inputs, activities, outputs, outcomes and impact (Figure 5.1). The process involves identifying long-term goals and begins by 'backward' mapping and connecting pre-conditions or requirements needed to achieve the goal. Identifying assumptions and interventions your project will need to achieve and developing indictors to measure and evaluate outcomes. This process is developed in a log frame which contains a matrix of outputs and a narrative explaining the stages (Center for Theory of Change, 2017; Tropical Health & Education Trust (THET), 2018a).

To develop a ToC it requires good understanding of the situation, which can be difficult when first establishing a project. To understand the situation, this may involve visits and completing a needs assessment. The needs assessment may follow standardised tools, for example the WHO (2019a) equipment lists for essential equipment, anaesthetic supplies and needs assessment. This provides baseline data and initial information that can be used to identify the specific issues. It is recommended needs assessments are completed with local partners to understand the environment and context in which they work. Considerable time is required to develop and evaluate the use of ToC, which can be challenging when working with limited resources and short funding timeframes (THET, 2018a). The ToC model provides an overall picture of the problem, the environment and context. To show the interdependent and interlinking in finding solutions, links to other variables which may affect the change are also included; these may be external to the project. It provides a logical structure to the process for change and how it will be happen. The ToC model is presented as a diagram with an accompanying narrative to explain each stage. (Brown, 2016)

Monitoring and evaluation

The term 'M&E' is used by many NGOs and international organisations including the World Bank and the United Nations to determine the impact of programmes and provide accountability to donors. M&E is developed as part of the ToC model and provides evidence to raise awareness and promote debate about the efficiency of public programmes and projects (World Bank, 2013). M&E promotes accountability, as many donor projects are publicly funded and ultimate accountability to governments who provide international development funding needs to be justified. M&E involves strategic support and collaboration with governments, organisations and healthcare workers where the project is going to take place; this provides the basis for sustainability and acceptance of the data. The World Bank (2013) requires M&E to use data to analyse the difference in outcomes with or without the project.

At local level, M&E is an ongoing process to allow the project team to check they are meeting targets, provide evidence to motivate and celebrate successes with teams, support the evidence for change, provide accountability to stakeholders and funders and identify strong and weak areas (Burn & Ritman, 2013). The principles of good M&E should be: independent, intentional, transparent, ethical, impartial, high quality, timely and, finally, used (United Nations, 2006). Good M&E practices involves the following:

- Designing and agreeing the M&E activities at the start of the project. M&E activities are identified and agreed during the project planning stages of the project.
- M&E should involve all stakeholders involved in the project. This provides good project governance as strategic and organisational partners understand their role within the project and who is responsible for collecting what data and when.
- Data should be collected at key stages throughout the project in order to inform decisions to keep the project on track and support the overall project evaluation.
- Depending on the initial needs assessment completed, this may provide baseline data for subsequent M&E to be compared against. If standardised templates and reports are used, this may allow for the data to be compared to other sources and projects.
- M&E results should be shared with stakeholders and include recommendations.

A partnership project between the Kambia Appeal and Kambia District Health Management Team in Sierra Leone to upskill healthcare workers (THET, 2018b), used both qualitative and quantitative M&E approaches to monitor change:

- Mini-evaluations of the project. This included visits led by the UK partners in conjunction with local healthcare workers.
- Assessment. Pre- and post-testing of knowledge and skills after education and training of trainer events.
- Observation in practice. Conducted by ward nurses, standardised data collection forms provided consistency and standardisation.

- Volunteer pre- and post-self-assessments to identify what they had learnt and experienced. Post-trip reports provided information on activities undertaken, including successes and challenges.
- Regular audits of notes and practice, with results being shared at all levels.
- Recognising the importance of personal evaluations and comments to identify issues and concerns early.

The Kambia partnership (THET, 2018b) identified a series of challenges relating to M&E, which included the following:

- Maintaining momentum when there is a high turnover of volunteers.
- Once competency charts and observations in practice were completed, they lost value as the activity was deemed completed and resulted in limited change in ongoing practice.
- When strengthening data systems, the health indicators are likely to be worse, as the data becomes more accurate.
- Data collection tended to focus on immediate results and only at local level. The importance of sharing the data widely including those managing services at organisational, regional and national levels ensures the information can be used for future planning.
- Additional challenges to M&E include poor or inconsistent pay, demotivation and high turnover of staff, which will then impact on the long-term sustainability of any projects (Burn & Ritman, 2013).

While it may not be possible to address all these factors within partnerships and programmes, identifying these factors and challenges during the ToC process can help the partnership to recognise the impact of their project. In addition, reviewing and recognising new factors influencing M&E provides valuable information which can be used in future ToC models (THET, 2017).

Evidence-based practice

The International Council of Nurses (ICN) (2016) acknowledged that evidence-based practice and nursing research is essential to provide quality and cost-effective healthcare. Sharing ideas and promoting the nursing research agenda through publications allows it to be visible and accessible to those who deliver nursing care (ICN, 2016). In recent years, there has been a paradigm shift from HIC conducting research and health programmes to now including local healthcare workers helping to design, implement and evaluate programmes (Webb & Giles-Vernick, 2013). While LICs and LMICs have been viewed as the 'laboratory for human research and experimentation' (Webb & Giles-Vernick, 2013), research must be appropriate and ethical. Access to local staff with research skills may be limited and some staff may have academic titles but have limited research and scientific experiences (Zerem, 2013). However, including local nurses in research activities helps build the nations' research capacity and development opportunities for nurses.

Research and audit may form part of M&E processes and can be used to strengthen health data systems and identify problems. To effectively use the data there must be a willingness to accept these problems and have the leadership capable and motivated to change (Hirst & Jeffrey, 2013). There are examples of research that encompasses these elements, for example the QUARITE trial demonstrated a 15% reduction in maternal mortality and was the first randomised control trial to incorporate education and audit on a large scale (Dumont et al., 2013). It was recognised as a comprehensive approach to using changing practice and M&E to include audit, leadership development, training in obstetric emergency care and outreach programmes.

The challenge to providing quality healthcare in low resource settings includes a significant shortage of healthcare workers, imbalanced skill mix and uneven distribution of healthcare workers (WHO, 2018). Those providing direct care often have difficulty accessing current, appropriate information and opportunities to conduct research and publish their ideas and undertake continuing professional development (CPD).

The increased use of the internet has allowed many publications and resources to become more accessible. To improve access to critical healthcare information, the WHO HINARI project has facilitated over 140 publishers to provide free access to journals in resource poor countries. In recent years, improved access to the internet has meant there is also an increasing move towards open-access journals, for example NursingPlus Open.

The United Nations (UN) (2011) acknowledged access to information and the internet is deemed a basic human right, yet in many countries internet connections remain expensive and access to databases such as HINARI are only available in institutions while on courses. In consequence, this means unless nurses are on a course with access to both the internet and databases they do not have access to current information. Limited internet means downloading documents can be time-consuming and challenging. In addition, many journals are not accessible as users need to pay to access the journals (Deonandan et al., 2017).

This may result in nurses and other healthcare workers accessing information from various sources such as Wikipedia. In both high- and low-income countries studies have shown doctors and medical students use Wikipedia to answer clinical questions (Park et al., 2016). Wikipedia is easy to access and it is likely many healthcare workers globally use it as a source of information to make clinical decisions. While it could be argued Wikipedia lacks credibility, is not evidence-based and can be changed by anyone (Rasberry, 2014), it has been proposed Wikipedia could reach millions of people and already has many health-related pages, which could be expanded and validated (Bould et al., 2014). This provides a potential practical solution to the immediate access to information, there is still the need for support for local nurses to publish their work in peer-reviewed journals.

With limited national journals many nurses and doctors are forced to publish in Western journals; in addition, this may be the only way to increase their research profile and attract international donor funding for projects. Most nursing journals are published in English, yet only 5% of the world population speaks English, making it difficult when authors are preparing submissions (Rezaei-Adaryani, 2012). For nurses who do not use English as their first language manuscripts may get rejected due to poor grammar or an inability to afford the translation into English.

Mentorship for novice authors is often limited or non-existent. With limited support within hospitals and Schools of Nursing to help prepare manuscripts many promising ideas and evidence is not getting published and ultimately shared. The *Lancet* Commission on Global Safe Surgery made recommendations for journal editors and publishers to improve access to relevant knowledge, authorship to properly reflect contributions from low-income countries, strengthen the quality of research conducted, educate researchers, promote global agendas and aid development of manuscripts (Ng-Kamstra *et al.*, 2016). However, in practice 'local level' support remains limited.

Within medicine the African Journal of Emergency Medicine (AFEM) recognises the need to 'improve the quality and quantity' of publication and developed a formalised mentorship programme. The 'author assist' programme used a peer-to-peer service of experienced volunteer assistants to help authors develop their work. Bruijns *et al.* (2017) reported through this programme that out of 47 (43%) original articles initially rejected, 28 (60%) took this opportunity to work with the 'author-assist' programme, resulting in 14 (50%) manuscripts re-submitted and 12 (86%) being accepted for publication. In consequence, peer mentorship schemes for nurses will increase the body of evidence available within a specific context (Klopper & Uys, 2013). This will help other practitioners to put the 'evidence into practice', bridge the theory–practice gap and contribute to scaling up quality health systems (WHO, 2019b).

'Train the trainer' programmes

Many projects involve increasing the number of skilled healthcare workers through training and education (Burn & Ritman, 2013). Within all projects the wider issues facing the education of healthcare workers will need to be considered, for example, projects may support the increase in the number of nurses being trained, but this needs to be delivered within the current provision of teaching staff. With few nurse tutors, they often manage high workloads and may have limited access to peer support, CPD opportunities and time to research and develop novel teaching strategies. This can result in the content on nursing programmes being outdated, with a reliance on literature and materials that have been unchanged for years and focus on rote learning (British Council, 2016; Livingston, 2012).

Often educational resources, for example textbooks and journals, are donated to libraries and while they provide an insight into current thinking, using high-income country resources is unrealistic as pathologies and conditions seen in low resource settings are not covered in these resources (Martey & Hudson, 1999; British Council, 2016). Nurses often work with limited resources and have greater responsibilities than those from HIC, therefore they need to develop specialist skills to be able to bridge theory to practice and find solutions to their problems (Van Wyk, 2002). In addition, treatment strategies may not reflect current thinking; for example, in Botswana, cancer care specialists reported reviewing medical journals from the late 1960s, to review the

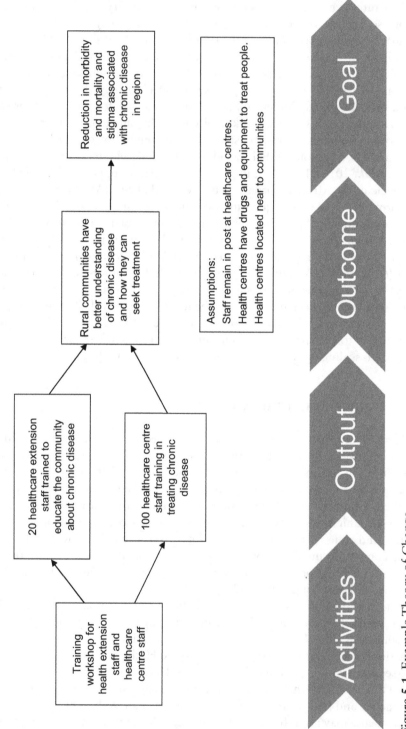

Figure 5.1 Example Theory of Change

THET, 2018a

literature, debate and determine the best evidence as they were using drugs and treatments from this era (Livingston, 2012, p. 33).

Critical care patients require specialist nursing care, and nurses need to complete specialist post-registration courses to help them provide holistic evidence-based care. Some LIC and LMIC organisations have provided 'short-courses' in critical care lasting from one to two weeks. While these short-term courses have upskilled the workforce, the World Federation of Critical Care Nurses (WFCCN, 2005) mandates 'innovative strategies need to be implemented to address the deficit of qualified critical care nurses, rather than resorting to short training courses to resolve the problem'. Critical care nurses are often the largest part of the critical care workforce and often called upon to share their skills with other healthcare workers. This 'ripple effect' results in a wider impact across the whole healthcare system, as knowledge, skills and experiences are shared at patient care level. Education and healthcare are inextricably linked and understanding how nurses are trained and access post-registration courses will help you understand how nursing care is delivered.

As a nurse you may be involved in developing and delivering 'training of trainer' programmes. This provides an opportunity to share ideas and resources to update curriculums, provide CPD opportunities and support the longer-term sustainability of projects. It is important you do not make assumptions about what is right or wrong in a new culture and go about making changes (Norton & Marks-Maran, 2014). Depending on your teaching experience you need to think carefully about how you are going to deliver and evaluate courses, as you may be used to having more resources and using different teaching styles. To help you prepare the following points may help:

- Language:
    o Will you need a translator?
    o Will your slides/resources need to be translated? Translation of slides may take time, so you will need to be organised and share these in advance.

- How will the environment affect you and the students?
    o For example, teaching in a classroom in elevated temperatures.

- What resources and tools do you have available?
    o You may want to use PowerPoint, but there may be intermittent power or no projector.
    o You may want to use simulation/skills but have limited equipment.
    o You may not be able to use a flip-chart as paper is too expensive and not available.
    o You may need to use chalkboards to teach.
    o Without access to resources, it may not be possible to provide students with a comprehensive reading list as they will need to be able to access the texts. You should consider how you are planning to do this.

- Paper and photocopying can be expensive, so if you want students to have handouts how will you share these? Using students' memory sticks may expose your computer to viruses.

- Newer computers may not have connections to projectors, therefore you will need to check connectors before you start teaching. If you need to buy a cable this may be expensive or not available.
- When developing ToT programmes it is important to involve local nurses and leaders in the process and to confirm the content is culturally appropriate and meets the context in which the students work.
- Didactic lectures are often the mainstay of teaching methods used; the use of case studies, presentations and group work may be one way to introduce student participation and are often well received.
- Accessing the internet can be challenging, making your preparation or providing references difficult. Internet connections can be slow and expensive. Accessing journals requires people to pay subscription fees which are often too expensive and with variable internet connectivity you may not be able to download articles. If you want students to read resources and have access to the information following the session, how do you plan to give this to them?
- It is important to understand who will be attending your courses. Healthcare workers may not attend training sessions unless they are paid per diem (also termed 'sitting allowances'). Those that attend may agree to the content, but it may not result in a change in practice (Royal College of Nursing, 2017).

For ToT programmes to be effective in improving the knowledge of healthcare workers and ultimately the health of the nation, the programme must form part of a strategic plan. The strategic long-term goals of a project are identified through the ToC and the training programme should form part of this change and the M&E process.

In summary, International projects often involve an element of training programmes. Establishing and sustaining programmes with limited resources is a challenge for trainers, and something you will need to consider if you are involved in these activities. When working internationally we are often involved in the delivery of projects; however, understanding the project's ToC and M&E plan will help you understand your role in more detail, the long-term goals and why certain activities have been chosen.

References

Bould MD. Hladkowicz ES. Pigford A-AE *et al.* (2014). References that anyone can edit: review of Wikipedia citations in peer reviewed health science literature. British Medical Journal. 38. G1585.

British Council (2016). Concept Note: Strategic Partnerships for Higher Education Innovation and Reform (SPHEIR) open call for partnership proposals. 20 September 2016. Available at: www.spheir.org.uk/sites/default/files/call_for_spheir_partnership_proposals_concept_note.pdf.

Brown AM. (2016). What is this thing called 'Theory of Change'? Available at: www.annmurraybrown.com/single-post/2016/03/09/What-is-this-thing-called-Theory-of-Change.

Bruijns SR. Banner M. Jacquet GA. (2017). Improving publication quality and quantity for acute care authors from low and middle income settings. Annals of Emergency Medicine. 69. 4. 462–468.

Bullen PB. (2014). Theory of Change vs logical framework – what's the difference? Available at: www.tools4dev.org/resources/theory-of-change-vs-logical-framework-whats-the-difference-in-practice/.

Burn E. Ritman D. (2013). Project monitoring. Tropical Health & Education Trust. Available at: www.thet.org/wp-content/uploads/2017/09/121204EB-Project-Monitoring-Workshop-Resource.pdf.

Center for Theory of Change. (2017). How does theory of change work? Available at: www.theoryofchange.org.

Deonandan R. Sangwa N. Kanters S. Nsanzimana S. (2017). Writing skills enhancement for public health professionals in Rwanda. Advances in Medical Education and Practice. 8. 253–256.

Dumont A. Fraser WD. Fournier P et al. (2013). Quality of care, risk management, and technology in obstetrics to reduce hospital-based maternal mortality in Senegal and Mali (QUARITE): a cluster randomised trial. The Lancet. 382. 9887. 146–157.

Hirst J. Jeffrey H. (2013). Education, audit and outreach to prevent maternal mortality. The Lancet. 382. 108–110.

International Council of Nurses (2016). Nursing research: a tool for action. Available at: www.old.icn.ch/publications/2012-closing-the-gap-from-evidence-to-action/.

Klopper H. Uys L (eds). (2013). The state of nursing and nurse education in Africa. A country-by-country review. Indianapolis, IN: Sigma Theta Tau International Honour Society of Nursing.

Livingston J. (2012). Chapter 2: Neoplastic Africa. In Improvising medicine: An African Oncology Ward in an Emerging Cancer Epidemic. Durham, NC: Duke University Press.

Martey JO. Hudson CN. (1999). Training specialists in the developing world: ten years on, a success story for West Africa. British Journal of Obstetrics and Gynaecology. 106. 91–94.

Ng-Kamstra KS. Greenberg SLM. Abdullah F et al. (2016). Global Surgery 2030: a roadmap for high income country actors. British Medical Journal Global Health. 1. E000011.

Norton D. Marks-Maran D. (2014). Developing cultural sensitivities and awareness in overseas nursing. Nursing Standard. 28. 44. 39–43.

Park E. Masupe T. Joseph J et al. (2016). Information needs of Botswana healthcare workers and perceptions of Wikipedia. International Journal of Medical Informatics. 95. 8–16.

Rasberry L. (2014). Citing Wikipedia. British Medical Journal. 348. DOI: https://doi.org/10.1136/bmj.g1819.

Rezaei-Adaryani M. (2012). Nursing and health policy perspectives. International Nursing Review. 4.

Royal College of Nursing. (2017). Working internationally: a guide to humanitarian and development work for nurses and midwives. London: Royal College of Nursing.

Tropical Health & Education Trust. (2017). Monitoring, evaluation and learning. Health Partnership Symposium, 1 March 2017, London.

Tropical Health & Education Trust. (2018a). Project planning: theory of change. London: THET.

Tropical Health & Education Trust. (2018b). Monitoring change in a health partnership project. London: THET.

United Nations. (2006). The Evaluation of Policy of UNDP. Available at: http://web.undp.org/evaluation/policy.shtml.

United Nations. (2011). Promotion and protection of all human rights, civil, political, economic, social and cultural rights, including the right to development. Human Rights Council. A/HRC/17/27. Available at: https://www2.ohchr.org/english/bodies/hrcouncil/docs/17session/A.HRC.17.27_en.pdf.

Van Wyk N. (2002). Development of critical thinking skills through distance learning in developing countries. Available at: www.hsag.co.za/index.php/HSAG/article/viewFile/642/691.

Webb JLA. Giles-Vernick T. (2013). Introduction. In: Giles-Vernick T. Webb JLA (eds). Global Health in Africa: historical perspectives in disease control. Athens, OH: Ohio University Press.

WFCCN. 2005. Position Statement on the Provision of Critical Care Nursing Education – Declaration of Madrid, 2005. Available at: http://wfccn.org/declarations/.

World Bank. (2013). Monitoring and evaluation for better development results. Available at: www.worldbank.org/en/news/feature/2013/02/14/monitoring-and-evaluation-for-better-development-results.

World Health Organization. (2018). Education and training. Available at: www.who.int/hrh/education/en/.

World Health Organization. (2019a). Emergency and essential surgical care: equipment lists and needs assessment. Available at: www.who.int/surgery/publications/immesc_equipt_needsmaneg/en/.

World Health Organization. (2019b). Putting evidence into practice in low-resource settings. Available at: www.who.int/bulletin/volumes/83/12/editorial11205html/en/.

Zerem E. (2013). Right criteria for academia in Bosnia and Herzegovina. The Lancet. 382. 128.

6 Critical care in resource limited environments

This chapter explores the provision of critical care services in resource limited environments. The World Health Organization (2004) defines a critical care unit as 'an advanced and highly specialised care provided to medical and surgical patients whose conditions are life threatening and require comprehensive care and constant monitoring. It is usually administered in a specially equipped unit of a healthcare facility'. Critically ill patients can be classified into three groups (Adhikari *et al.*, 2010):

1. Those with acute organ dysfunction.
2. Those who have undergone major surgery and are monitored to detect any deterioration.
3. Those who have not responded to critical care and are receiving end-of-life care.

Within the low- and middle-incomes countries often many critically ill patients do not reach critical care units due to a lack of critical care beds or they simply die before they reach the hospital (Dart *et al.*, 2017). The appropriateness of providing critical care services has been widely debated. Often sophisticated tertiary referral hospitals co-exist with inadequate primary healthcare and limited healthcare infrastructures making it difficult for patients to access care (Li *et al.*, 2013). Critical care requires intensive resourcing in terms of personnel, equipment, resources and financing. Critics argue critical care services may not significantly decrease overall mortality and the development of these services is unrealistic. With limited resources and funding available the focus should be on investment in prevention programmes such as mass immunisation projects and primary healthcare services (Basnet *et al.*, 2011).

Conversely, it is recognised all hospitals have critically ill patients and the debate should not be about 'is intensive care appropriate?' but rather 'what is appropriate?' (Watters *et al.*, 2004). The recent *Lancet* Commission on Global Safe Surgery included the development of critical care as an essential aspect of improving outcomes from surgery (Meara *et al.*, 2014). In addition, most of the population in low-income settings are young (less than 60 years old), therefore providing critical care services may save the life of a patient who otherwise would have died from an avoidable or preventable cause in a ward (WHO, 2016). Survivors may then be able to return to their communities and contribute to society and their economies (Krishnamoorthy *et al.*, 2014, Firth & Ttendo, 2012).

When working in a critical care unit in a resource limited environment it is important to understand what is appropriate. On assessment, the unit may appear severely limited by our standards but may be well equipped by local and national standards (van Wijhe, 2017). Understanding the limitations and opportunities will help you make appropriate decisions, which are not guided by Western standards. The basic requirements for a critical care unit must include adequate human resources, medical equipment, for example ventilators, suction units, and sufficient resources and drugs to provide a comprehensive service to the population at risk.

Staffing

To manage an effective critical care unit, there needs to be an identified medical and nursing lead for the unit. To provide direct care, there must be appropriately trained nursing and medical staff to meet the needs of patients 24 hours a day. There should be an adequate number of nurses on duty to meet the patient dependency. All critical care patients must have access to a registered nurse with a post-registration critical care nursing qualification, with the minimum of one qualified critical care nurse on duty for each shift.

Nurses are essential to effective critical care services, as of any service, and often spend the most time with patients. The success of any intensive care unit is based on motivated and trained critical care nurses (Giannou *et al.*, 2013). Investing in critical care nurses often results in a hospital-wide impact as they are often called upon to work outside of the critical care units and review or provide advice to other healthcare professionals concerned about patients; this results in a sharing of knowledge and skills (Towney & Ojara, 2008; Basnet *et al.*, 2011).

The role of the nurse in a resource limited environment critical care unit can be broad, with a lack of locally trained medical doctors and other professionals, e.g. physiotherapists, leading to 'task-sharing', whereby nurses undertake additional skills traditionally performed by other professionals. As outlined above, the type of patient admitted to critical care is likely to be different to high-income settings, and nurses may need to look after both adults and children. Insufficient numbers of nurses may mean nurses look after three to four ventilated patients. However, when compared to the wards, where nurse to patient ratios can be as low as 1 nurse to 40–60 patients, this is a significant escalation in patient care (Carter & Snell, 2016).

The role of the nurse is to provide effective nursing care by:

- providing patient-centred evidence-based care;
- observing and being proactive in patients' management, so that any deterioration or changes can be immediately identified and acted on;
- being able to cope with unpredictable events;

- being able to explain all nursing procedures to patients and provide emotional support to patients and their relatives;
- providing detailed information to other members of the healthcare team;
- maintaining and respecting patient dignity and confidentiality.

To achieve these goals, nurses must receive specialist training and opportunities for continuing professional development.

Critical care unit

The critical care environment should be a dedicated area within the hospital, with agreed admission and discharge guidelines (Boxes 6.1 and 6.2). The unit should have an admission book and agreed protocols and guidelines for the provision of care, for example, ventilator care bundles, transfer standards. These standards should be agreed by key stakeholders and monitored for compliance.

There must be sufficient space between each bed area to prevent cross-contamination and ensure there is sufficient space for extra equipment. In addition, dedicated side rooms for the provision of infectious cases and those requiring barrier nursing, e.g. burns patients, should be available. Walls should be washable, floors smooth and curved at the edges to meet the walls, so dirt cannot be trapped. A cleaning rota should be developed and monitored.

Units must have:

- continuous supply of electricity. Power failures without back-up generators are a significant patient safety risk making it difficult to provide continuous ventilation, infusions and renal replacement therapy. During a power failure, sufficient staff need to be immediately available to respond and manually ventilate patients as any disruption in treatment may be associated with increased mortality (Iniabasi & Kalu, 2012);
- access to clean water;
- dedicated nurses station including a working telephone, with the ability to phone outside of the hospital;
- designated clean and dirty (sluice) utility rooms;
- store room near to the unit;
- designated refrigerator for medicines;
- lockable controlled drugs cabinet;
- lockable cupboards for drugs;
- kitchen area to store and prepare patient feeds;
- office space for the nurse in charge;
- relatives' waiting area;
- unit library and resource area where electro-medical manuals and other professional resources can be stored and accessed by staff;
- an educational resource board;
- ward clerk/desk area for storing notes.

Each bed-space must have:

- sufficient access around the bed, with access to the head in case of an airway emergency;
- a continuous supply of oxygen either piped or cylinder immediately available at every bed-space, with emergency back-up cylinders available. Nursing staff need to be vigilant when using cylinders to monitor when they are nearly empty and ensure they are changed. If using oxygen concentrations during a power failure these may fail, potentially leading to hypoxia and death;
- height-adjustable bed with bedrails;
- curtains or screens between each bed-space for privacy;
- good lighting;
- sufficient number of plug sockets around the bed-space;
- monitoring and leads. Pulse oximetry probes and ECG leads are delicate, may become damaged and are often difficult to replace, resulting in many working monitors not being used;
- ventilator;
- suction unit with appropriately sized suction catheters;
- appropriate number of infusion and syringe pumps to deliver medications;
- enteral feeding pump;
- charting trolley and area to keep patient notes;
- intravenous drips stand;
- sharps box;
- appropriately sized bag, valve mask and Waters circuit in case of an emergency;
- fire blanket;
- emergency torch;
- any other equipment necessary for specific patient groups, e.g. syringes, needles, etc.

Additional equipment and resources:

- glucometer and test strips;
- urinalysis test strips;
- pH test strips for checking position of NG tubes;
- weighing scales;
- arterial blood gas analyser, test strips and reagents;
- adult/paediatric emergency trolley, including:

  o emergency drugs;
  o emergency oxygen (with appropriate connect to attach oxygen tubing);
  o emergency airway equipment (including difficult airway equipment);
  o manual defibrillator with ability to perform DC cardioversion and external pacing;

- emergency torches and spare batteries;
- transfer bag;

- portable X-ray;
- ultrasound machine;
- computers to access laboratory results and educational resources.

Equipment care

The World Health Organization (2008) states:

> Every patient has the right to be treated using the safest technology available in health facilities. This implies freedom from unnecessary or potential harm associated with healthcare. All health professionals and institutions have obligations to provide safe and quality healthcare and to avoid unintentional harm to patients.

Electro-medical equipment is an essential to the running of a safe critical care unit. Each bed-space should have appropriate equipment; however, limited equipment, sometimes shared between patients, increases the risk of suboptimal monitoring or risk of infection. Within a resource limited environment, the ideal equipment would (McNicholas & Henning, 2011):

- be light, compact and portable so it could be used in a variety of situations and moved locations if required;
- work at different climatic temperatures;
- have adequate battery back-up;
- require minimal calibration;
- have all staff trained in its use and have access to the user manual.

Specific challenges you may face when working in resource limited environments may include the following:

- Being unfamiliar with equipment, which may be different from HIC hospitals.
- HIC may donate equipment; while this may be useful initially, it may not be the best equipment for the environment and without user manuals or training of electro-medical engineering staff it makes it difficult for staff to use and engineers to maintain the equipment.
- Battery back-up may be affected by the extremes of heat and overcharging.
- Poor electrical safety or varying types of plug sockets or voltage may affect the equipment.
- Lack of consumables, for example oropharyngeal airways, ventilator tubing, means equipment is cleaned and then re-used on another patient. This may increase the risk of spreading hospital-acquired infections if incorrectly decontaminated or may result in a lack of basic monitoring, e.g. pulse oximetry when ventilating.
- When equipment breaks or requires servicing, there are often insufficient biomedical engineers available or skilled to service the delicate specialist equipment. In one country in sub-Saharan Africa an estimated 35–50% of medical equipment is out

of service, compared to the less than 1% in HIC (Tropical Health & Education Trust, 2013, 2015).

- Often when equipment breaks it cannot be repaired due to a lack of parts, resulting in the equipment being dumped.
- Ad hoc planning, weak procurement and regulatory systems affect equipment planning.
- Budget problems for operating and maintaining equipment lead to equipment not being used.
- Some equipment may be 'locked away' by senior staff to ensure it does not get damaged.

Although electro-medical resources may be limited, Table 6.1 provides an overview of essential devices required to manage the variety of potential patients admitted to a critical care unit (Low & Harris, 2015). When using some point of care (POC) tests, including glucometers and arterial blood gas analysers, cartridges, test strips and reagents required to undertake daily tests may not be available or calibrated, potentially causing incorrect readings. In addition, some tests may be recorded in different measurements, for example arterial blood gases may be recorded in kPa or mmHg. As an international nurse you may need to convert these results until you are familiar with the normal ranges.

Table 6.1 Point of care testing equipment

Device	Example of use	Serial monitoring
Glucometers	Diagnosis of cause of collapse	In management of diabetic ketoacidosis (DKA)
I-Stat	Diagnosis acute renal failure and coronary syndromes	CO_2 control in a ventilated patient with traumatic brain injury (TBI)
Hemocue	Decision to administer blood, often used in the pre-hospital environment	Major haemorrhage
CoaguChek	Checking INR on patient with intra-cerebral bleed	Not required
Hemochron Jr	Patients on intravenous heparin requiring regular anticoagulation monitoring	Patients with an arterial or central venous catheter in situ
Urine test strips	Diagnosis of pre-eclampsia	Ketones in DKA
Pulse oximetry	Monitoring of oxygen therapy	Continuous monitoring when providing anaesthesia or mechanical ventilation in ICU

In the absence of fully functioning laboratory and/or point of care testing, this results in delayed reporting of results which may be critical to a patient's condition. In consequence, care may be provided empirically, for example dextrose solutions may be given if there are any signs of hypoglycaemia (Bisanzo *et al.*, 2016), or when weaning a patient from ventilation, care is based on clinical judgement and experience, which can lead to variations in treatment strategies.

A lack of functioning medical equipment is one of the main challenges facing healthcare professionals daily (Tropical Health & Education Trust, 2017). When working in an unfamiliar environment you must be competent to use any equipment. The Tropical Health and Education Trust (THET) (2013) has outlined a series of recommendations for training users:

- How to use the equipment safely and properly.
- How to understand the user manual.
- What to do if you suspect a problem.
- How to care for the equipment (user care and maintenance).
- Training should be 'hands-on' so healthcare workers become comfortable and familiar with the device.

Some equipment may be donated from HIC. There are international standards for donating medical equipment to the low-income countries and some organisations, for example Lifebox, who provide pulse oximetry to support safe surgery, provide equipment, training and peer support to effectively support the implementation of equipment.

When working internationally, as part of your induction you should familiarise yourself with the equipment you are going to use and complete the necessary training to ensure you can use it safely.

In summary, critical care services in low resource settings will continue to evolve and develop, and can contribute to improving the health of the nation and wider hospital services. Nurses are essential for any critical care service and play a key role in the development and delivery of services. Services are likely to be very different to critical care units in HICs; understanding the type of patients admitted, outcomes and resources available will help you to ensure appropriate decisions can be made.

Box 6.1   Types of patients that may require admission to critical care for continuous monitoring and observation (WHO, 2016)

- Cranial neurosurgery.
- Head injuries with airway obstruction.
- Intubated patients, including tracheostomy.
- Major trauma – post-operatively.
- Abdominal surgery for a condition neglected for more than 24 hours.
- Chest drain in the first 24 hours.

(continued)

(continued)

- Ventilation difficulties.
- Airway difficulties, potential or established, e.g. post-thyroidectomy, removal of a large goitre.
- Unstable pulse or blood pressure, high or low.
- Anuria or oliguria.
- Severe pre-eclampsia or eclampsia.
- Surgical sepsis.
- Complications during anaesthesia or surgery, especially unexpected haemorrhage.
- Hypothermia.
- Hypoxia.
- Neonates, after any surgery.
- Medical conditions, e.g. organophosphate poisoning.

Box 6.2   The following conditions should be met before discharge from critical care (WHO, 2016)

- Conscious.
- Good airway, extubated and stable for several hours after extubation.
- Breathing comfortably.
- Stable blood pressure and urine output.
- Haemoglobin >6 g/dl or blood transfusion in progress.
- Minimal nasogastric drainage with the presence of bowel sounds; abdomen not distended.
- Afebrile.
- Looks better, sitting up, not confused.

References

Adhikari NK. Fowler RA. Bhagwanjee S. Rubenfeld GD. (2010). Critical care 1: critical care and the global burden of critical illness in adults. The Lancet. DOI: https://doi.org/10.1016/S0140-6736(10)60446-1.

Basnet S. Adhikari N. Koirala J. (2011). Challenges in setting up paediatric and neonatal intensive care units in a resource-limited country. Pediatrics. 128. E-986-992.

Bisanzo M. Gema F. Wangola R (2016). Chapter 127: Malaria. In: Wallis LA. Reynolds TA (eds). AFEM Handbook of acute and emergency care. Oxford: Oxford University Press.

Carter C. Snell D. (2016). Nursing the critically ill surgical patient in Zambia. British Journal of Nursing. 10. 25. 20. 1123–1128.

Dart PJ. Kinnear J. Bould MD *et al.* (2017). An evaluation of inpatient morbidity and critical care provision in Zambia. Anaesthesia. 72. 172–180.

Firth P. Ttendo S. (2012). Intensive care in low-income countries – a critical need. New England Journal of Medicine. 367. 21. 1974–1975.

Giannou C. Baldan M. Molde A. (2013). War surgery: Working with limited resources in armed conflict and other situations of violence. Volume 2. Available at: https://shop.icrc.org/la-chirurgie-de-guerre-travailler-avec-des-ressources-limitees-dans-les-conflits-armes-et-autres-situations-de-violence-volume-416.html.

Iniabasi I. Kalu QN. (2012). Intensive care admissions and outcomes at the University of Calabar Teaching Hospital, Nigeria. Journal of Critical Care. 27. 1. 105. E1–E105.e4.

Krishnamoorthy V. Vavilala MS. Mock CN. (2014). The need for ventilators in the developing world: an opportunity to improve care and save lives. Journal of Global Health. 4. 1. 010303.

Li PKT. Burdmann EA. Mehta RL for World Kidney Day Steering Committee. (2013). Acute kidney injury: global health alert. Advances in Chronic Kidney Disease. 20. 2. 114–7. DOI: 10.1053/j.ackd.2012.12.003.

Low A. Harris T. (2015). Chapter 14: Near Patient Testing and Imaging. In: Low A. Hulme J (eds). ABC of Transfer and Retrieval Medicine. Hoboken, NJ: Wiley Blackwell. BMJ Books.

McNicholas J. Henning J. (2011). Major Military Trauma: Decision Making in the ICU. Journal of the Royal Army Medical Corps. 157. S284–S288.

Meara JG. Hagander L. Leather AJM. (2014). Surgery and global health: a Lancet Commission. The Lancet. 383. 12–13.

Towney RM. Ojara S. (2008). Practice of intensive care in rural Africa: an assessment of data from Northern Uganda. African Health Sciences. 8. 1. 61–64.

Tropical Health & Education Trust. (2013). A toolkit for medical equipment donations to low-resource settings: making it work. Available at: www.thet.org/wp-content/uploads/2017/08/THET_MakingItWork_Toolkit_Final_Online.pdf.

Tropical Health & Education Trust. (2015). Biomedical engineering training needs. Available at: www.thet.org/our-work/zambia-programme/medical-equipment-maintenance-in-zambia.

Tropical Health & Education Trust. (2017). Managing the lifecycle of medical equipment. Available at: www.thet.org/wp-content/uploads/2017/08/THET_Managing_the_medical_equipment_lifecycle_LOW-RES.pdf.

Van Wijhe M. (2017). Anaesthesia: An assessment mission in the Congo. In: Kushner AL (ed.). Operation crisis: surgical care in the developing world during conflict and disaster. Baltimore, MD: John Hopkins University Press.

Watters DAK. Wilson IH. Leaver RJ. Bagshawe A. (2004). Care of the critically ill patient in the tropics and sub-tropics. 2nd Edition. Oxford: Macmillan.

World Health Organization. (2004). A glossary of terms for community healthcare and services for older persons. Kobe, Japan: WHO Centre for Health Development. Available at: www.who.int/kobe_centre/ageing/ahp_vol5_glossary.pdf.

World Health Organization. (2008). Patient safety in African Health Services: Issues and Solutions. Report of the Regional Director. Available at: http://apps.who.int/iris/handle/10665/19987.

World Health Organization. (2016). Best Practice Safety Protocol: Intensive Care. Available at: www.who.int/surgery/publications/s16373e.pdf?ua=1.

7 Military critical care

In times of conflict and disaster, military medical units may be deployed to provide critical care services to an identified population at risk. Military organisations aim to provide the same standard of care as expected in their own country, therefore the type of care provided is likely to be different to those provided by local or Non-Governmental Organisations (NGOs) and local national healthcare facilities.

Within military medicine, critical care has evolved in terms of its evidence base, technology and resources required in response to recent conflicts and injury patterns (McNicholas & Henning, 2011). Each conflict has its own unique signature pattern and resources will be dependent on the threat and injury patterns seen. Many deployed Medical Treatment Facilities (MTFs) are located in isolated and austere environments, which requires the facility and its staff to be as self-sufficient as possible. Where the MTF is located, for example in a desert, on a ship away from shore or onboard an aircraft, will determine the challenges for staff, patients and care provided (Box 7.1).

North Atlantic Treaty Organization (NATO) countries escalate treatment from point of injury to definitive care; this paradigm is described in stages from Role 1 to 4 (Box 7.2). As the casualty moves through the operational patient care pathway, at each stage more resources and expertise are available. Patients may need to move over large geographical distances or varying terrain, therefore patients may be moved by specialist teams in helicopters or special battlefield ambulances.

Box 7.1 Considerations when providing deployed critical care in different situations

Providing critical care on a naval ship (Risdall et al., 2011)

- No dedicated hospital facility onboard, space and size of the facility is restricted by the area available to the team.
- Lack of space to store medical supplies.
- Differences in power voltage.
- Patients can arrive either via helicopter or boat. Moving the patients off these platforms and through the ship to the medical facility may be difficult. This may involve lifts, ladders and hatchways.

- All equipment will need to be secured to prevent movement.
- Re-supply of essential medical supplies may be challenging, for example blood has shelf life of 35 days. In addition, ensuring blood is kept at the correct temperature throughout the entire chain may be resource intensive.
- Evacuation of patients to definitive surgery may be delayed, resulting in patients remaining in the facility for longer periods, until tactically safe or other ships or helicopters can ensure the patient can be evacuated.

Providing critical care during aeromedical transfer (Turner et al., 2009)

- Healthcare professionals being awake for a prolonged period and crossing time zones results in fatigue and increases the risk of potential error.
- Cramped and limited environment.
- Limited access to running water.
- Noise and vibrations.

Providing nursing care in tents (Whitcomb et al., 2008)

- There may be no piped oxygen, suction or power.
- Running water may be limited.
- Cleaning of canvas if there is a spillage.
- Extremes of temperature and limited ability to control temperature.
- Difficulty in maintaining dignity and privacy.
- Nursing patients on narrow stretchers may prevent re-positioning and pressure area care; no backrests to perform the ventilator care bundle or neurological protection.
- Performing CPR on a stretcher.

Box 7.2   NATO roles of care (Remick & Bailey, 2017)

Role 1   Battlefield First Aid (UK)/Combat Casualty Care (USA) to provide immediate lifesaving care
Triage

Role 2   Triage, resuscitation, treatment and holding of patients so they can return to duty
Emergency surgery, critical care and essential post-operative management

Role 3   Specialist diagnostic radiography, surgical and medical capabilities
Preventative medicine, mental health teams, dentists
Ability to hold patients, so they can return to duty

Role 4   Definitive care often provided in the patient's home country. Specialities include reconstructive surgery, rehabilitation and convalescence

Resources

Resources will always be the challenge in any deployed setting. With limited re-supply of resources and the fragility of the cold chain in maintaining blood and drugs at the right temperature this can pose many problems. While the technology available has significantly advanced, certain advances, for example renal replacement therapy or advanced haemodynamic monitoring, in a remote environment are currently limited or not possible (Nesbitt *et al.*, 2011). Arguably, recent operations have allowed for innovation and development of technology which is more robust and able to work within these environments. Advances in transfusion practices, including the use of Rotational Thromboelastometry (ROTEM) and platelet apheresis to provide goal directed transfusion practices, have revolutionised transfusion practices and helped conserve blood stocks and prevent unnecessary transfusions (Coull, 2013).

Care of local nationals

Most countries are signatories of the Geneva Convention, which requires them to provide lifesaving life, limb or eyesight surgery. It is recognised clinical care for local nationals must be appropriate and meet the technology and ongoing care available locally (Ramasamy *et al.*, 2010). The ongoing care of patients must be considered during the planning phase of operations and shared with healthcare professionals. However, the realities of providing high-income standards of care in a low-income country, which has never had that level of care or been able to continue to provide that level of care, will cause potential professional and personal dilemmas.

In conflict, it is likely outside of the military MTFs critical care services will be non-existent or considerably different. The International Committee of the Red Cross War Surgery Manual recognises critical care may not consist of highly sophisticated equipment, but may include cohorting sick patients together and providing good nursing care by increasing the patient to nurse ratio from 20 or 30 to 1 to 4 to 1 (Giannou *et al.*, 2013). Therefore, deciding when it is appropriate to discharge a local national to an NGO or local hospitals with complex injuries, knowing they have limited facilities, can be a professional and ethical issue facing military healthcare professionals (Lockley *et al.*, 2004).

Wanting to do more

When looking after local national patients, it can be emotive, and decisions to change treatment parameters and provide more when faced with someone with a potentially reversible condition that could be easily treated is a considerable challenge for clinicians. Senior commanders and politicians may encourage 'hearts and minds' programmes to build relations with local communities; however, in reality this may be difficult, particularly when treating more complex or non-life-threatening conditions. When clinicians provide treatment not part of the medical rules of engagement, this is termed 'mission creep'. This describes the gradual change to the original mission or plan and can affect both military and NGOs, demonstrated in the following vignette of UK Defence Medical Services (DMS) in Bosnia-Herzegovina.

Over a three-year period, emergency department admissions at a multi-national military field hospital deployed to Sipovo, Bosnia-Herzegovina; data identified there was an increase in civilian admissions during that time (Kenward *et al.*, 2004). This lead to dependence amongst the local community, which created a complicated exit strategy when the operation was completed as the local population had become reliant on these services. Civilians perceived the standard of care was better than what was available in their local hospitals, which were gradually being rebuilt. This posed enormous challenges both for the military and the local agencies to capacity build local services. In consequence, military medical services often engage with local services and NGOs particularly when planning the ongoing care of local nationals (Bricknell & Cameron, 2013). This not only provides sustainability for countries recovering from conflict or disasters but also helps to re-establish local healthcare services.

Working with Non-Governmental Organisations (NGOs)

Often both military and NGOs will be working in the same space and there needs to be communication, but tensions may exist. NGOs aim to be neutral, impartial and apolitical, whereas by the very the nature of military organisations they are neither neutral nor apolitical. Some NGOs will not employ military healthcare staff including reservists to support their missions or will require them to have a significant period away from the military.

NGOs can determine their own mandate and mission which is guided by their own values and beliefs. They may also decide not to work collaboratively with other NGOs, as they may be competing or trying to attract more donor funding and be independent and not reliant on others (Bricknell & Cameron, 2013). From a military perspective, operations tend to be short and often withdraw once the political mandate has been achieved. In the post-conflict period, there needs to be an integrated approach between countries and the 'myriad' of humanitarian organisations (Sullivan *et al.*, 2011).

Depending on the situation in recent years, there has been greater collaboration between military and civilian organisations including local authorities, government agencies, NGOs or international governments, resulting in joint training and operations (Ankersen, 2008). Humanitarian operations have demonstrated this joint approach can be powerful. In 2014–2015 the Ebola virus outbreak in West Africa was a disaster and a global risk. As part of the UK response, in conjunction with the Department for International Development (DFID), the UK DMS worked with several NGOs to provide an Ebola Treatment Facility in Sierra Leone (Davies *et al.*, 2015).

Skills of healthcare professionals

As outlined in Chapter 2, the skills of the healthcare professionals in any resource limited environment are different than what they would expect in a high-income country.

Recent UK operations in Afghanistan recognised that one six-week deployment provided the equivalent exposure to penetrating trauma similar to a three-year trauma experience in the UK National Health Service (Ramasamy *et al.*, 2010). Changes to healthcare systems and training of healthcare professionals in Western countries means often military healthcare professionals require significant training, competencies and exposure to the types of conditions seen on operations (Beaumont & Allan, 2012). While treatments have advanced, they may not be able to be used within the deployed environment and there is a requirement to teach older and simpler skills which are still appropriate but have been replaced in back home (Ramasamy *et al.*, 2010). This highlights the importance of appropriate training and understanding of the realities of deployed healthcare, so that appropriate decisions can be made.

For military critical care nurses responding to the changing challenges and threats will always be a requirement of the military nurse. Professor Sir Michael Howard (2015) famously said 'No matter how clearly one thinks, it is impossible to anticipate precisely the character of future conflict. The key is to not be so far off the mark that it becomes impossible to adjust once that character is revealed'. While the future may be uncertain, history has shown many advances and innovations in critical care have been influenced by military experiences or being close to conflicts (Murray, 2011).

References

Ankersen C. (2008). Chapter 1: Introduction: interrogating civil-military co-operation. In: Ankersen C. (ed.). Civil-military cooperation in post-conflict operations: emerging theory and practice. Cass Military Studies. London: Routledge.

Beaumont SP. Allan HT. (2012). Supporting deployed operations: are military nurses gaining the relevant experience from MDHUs to be competent in deployed operations. Journal of Clinical Nursing. DOI: https://doi.org/10.1111/j.1365-2702.2012.04315.x.

Bricknell MCM. Cameron E. (2013). Military medical engagement with the civilian health sector. Medical Corps International Forum. 4. 34–37.

Coull A. (2013). In-flight and defence nursing forum 'Sharing Best Practice' conference. In: Carter C. Cumming J., Royal College of Nursing Critical Care. Journal of the Royal Army Medical Corps. 159. 4. 320–322.

Davies BC. Bowley D. Roper K. (2015). Response to the Ebola crisis in Sierra Leone. Nursing Standard. 29. 26. 37–41.

Giannou C. Baldan M. Molde A. (2013). War surgery: Working with limited resources in armed conflict and other situations of violence. Volume 2. Available at: https://shop.icrc.org/la-chirurgie-de-guerre-travailler-avec-des-ressources-limitees-dans-les-conflits-armes-et-autres-situations-de-violence-volume-416.html.

Howard M. (2015). Ministry of Defence. Strategic Trends Programme: Future Character of Conflict. London: HMSO.

Kenward G. Jain TNM. Nicholson K. (2004). Mission Creep: an analysis off accident and emergency room activity in a military facility in Bosnia-Herzegovina. Journal of the Royal Army Medical Corps. 150. 20–23.

Lockley D. Nordmann G. Field J. Clough D. Henning J. (2004). The deployment of an intensive care facility with a military field hospital to the 2003 conflict in Iraq. Resuscitation. 62. 3. 261–265.

McNicholas JJK. Henning JD. (2011). Major military trauma: decision making in the ICU. Journal of the Royal Army Medical Corps. 157. 3 Suppl. 1. S284–S288.

Murray MJ. (2011). Review: The influence of armed conflict on the development of critical care medicine. Military Medicine. 176. 6. 674–678.

Nesbitt I. Almond MK. Freshwater DA. (2011). Renal replacement in the deployed setting. Journal of the Royal Army Medical Corps. 157. 2. 179–181.

Ramasamy A. Hinsley DE. Edwards DS. Stewart MPM. Midwinter M. (2010). Skill sets and competencies for the modern military surgeon: lessons from UK military operations in Southern Afghanistan. Injury – International Journal of the Care of the Injured. 41. 453–459.

Remick KN. Bailey JA. (2017). US military joint trauma system and roles of care. In: Kushner AL. Operation crisis: surgical care in the developing world during conflict and disaster. Baltimore, MD: Johns Hopkins University Press.

Risdall JE. Heames RM. Hill G. (2011). Role 2 Afloat. Journal of the Royal Army Medical Corps. 157. 4. 362–364.

Sullivan R. McQuinn B. Purushotham A. (2011). How are we going to rebuild public health in Libya? Journal of the Royal Society of Medicine. 104. 490–492.

Turner S. Ruth M. Tipping R. (2009). Critical care air support teams and deployed intensive care. Journal of the Royal Army Medical Corps. 155. 2. 171–174.

Whitcomb JJ. Newell KJ. (2008). Skill set requirements for nurses deployed with an expeditionary medical unit based on lessons learnt. Critical Care Nursing Clinics of North America. 20. 1. 13–22.

8 Infection prevention control considerations

Healthcare associated infections (HCAIs) are viewed as the most frequent adverse event threatening patient safety globally (Allegranzi *et al.*, 2011). Critically ill patients often develop multi-organ failure that requires complex invasive monitoring and treatments; these factors increase the infection risk and challenge the healthcare team (Albarran & Scholes, 2018). In LICs and LMICs, the incidence of HCAI in critical care units is significantly higher than HIC, with infections ranging from 4.4% to 89.9% (Ulu-Kilic *et al.*, 2013; WHO, 2008). Surveillance and reporting of HCAIs is difficult as not all countries have effective national systems in place. The WHO identified only 23 (16%) out of 147 LICs had effective national surveillance systems for monitoring HCAIs (WHO, 2010).

Critically ill patients are at significant risk of developing an HCAI, due to:

- poor hand hygiene due to limited access to continuous running water or alcohol hand gel;
- increased antimicrobial resistance due to a lack of microbiology services;
- effects of malnutrition;
- limited access to sterilised equipment;
- mechanical ventilation;
- use of open suction catheters;
- invasive lines, e.g. central venous catheters or peripheral cannula;
- urinary catheters;
- wounds, e.g. surgical site infections, pressure sores
- re-use of single-use items.

Standard precautions

Standard precautions, previously termed 'universal precautions', aim to reduce the risk of blood-borne pathogens and other pathogens from recognised and unrecognised sources (WHO, 2007). The principles of standard precautions include:

- hand hygiene;
  - ○ hand washing (40–60 seconds): wet hands, apply soap, rub all surfaces, rinse hands and dry thoroughly with a single towel. Use towel to turn off faucet (Figure 8.1);
  - ○ hand rub (20–30 seconds): apply enough product to cover all areas of hands, rub hands until dry (Figure 8.1).
- appropriate use of gloves;
- facial protection (eyes, nose and mouth);
- gowns;
- prevention of needle-stick injuries and correct disposal of sharps;
- respiratory hygiene and cough etiquette;
- effective environmental cleaning;
- correct management and disposal of patient linen;
- correct disposal of clinical waste;
- cleaning and decontamination of patient care equipment.

Additional personal protective equipment (PPE) may be required in specific situations, for example nursing a patient with a viral haemorrhagic fever (Chapter 25) or influenza (Chapter 27).

Access to running water and hand hygiene

Hand hygiene is a major component of standard precautions and one of the most effective methods of prevention of transmission of HCAIs. However, access to continuous running water is a problem for many hospitals. A study of 430 hospitals in 19 LICs and LMICs identified that 34% did not have continuous running water (Chawla *et al.*, 2016). This impacts on healthcare workers' ability to maintain basic hand hygiene and increases the risk of exposing the patients and staff to hospital-acquired infections and unsanitary conditions. A lack of running water may impact on hospitals' ability to clean and sterilise instruments, resulting in a delay in surgery and further patient deterioration. If running water, soap and disposable hand towels are limited or intermittent, this makes it difficult to maintain hand hygiene practices; as a solution, some units store water in special containers.

Use of gloves

Single-use examination gloves can be either sterile or non-sterile. They are made from natural rubber latex or synthetic non-latex materials, for example vinyl, nitrile and neoprene (WHO, 2009). Healthcare workers, regardless of setting, may inappropriately use and have an over-reliance on using gloves in clinical practice. Gloves do

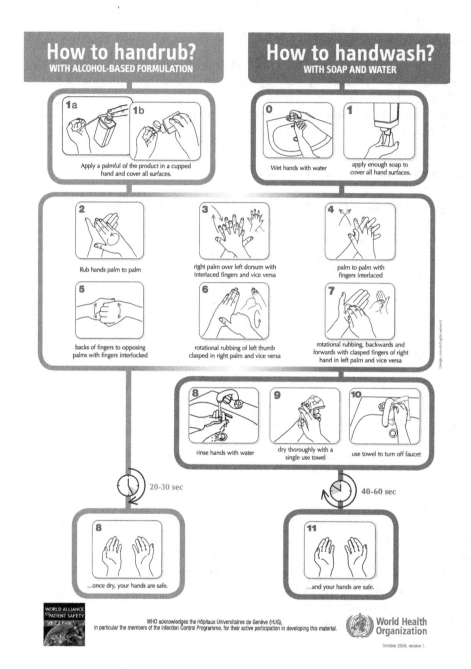

Figure 8.1 How to use hand rub and handwash

Reproduced with kind permission from the World Health Organization.

not provide absolute protection and do not replace hand washing and hand rubs. Unnecessary use of gloves is a waste of resources and may result in missed hand hygiene opportunities (WHO, 2006).

In LICs and LMICs, often gloves are latex and powdered, which increases the risk of latex allergy and dermatitis. The use of powder may be used if gloves are re-processed. The re-processing causes the glove to stick together, and the powder allows the glove to be worn. The WHO (2009) identified that the reprocessing of gloves should be avoided as the integrity of the glove is reduced due to an increased risk of tears. The loss of integrity provides a false confidence and exposes both the patient and healthcare worker to potential infection. The WHO also identified the importance of appropriate disposal of clinical waste and reported illegal recovery and recycling of discarded gloves from hospital dumping areas. Often illegal practices, with uncontrolled or regulated practices, adds a potential additional healthcare risk.

Antimicrobial resistance

The WHO (2018b) defines antimicrobial resistance (AMR) as 'the ability of a microorganism to stop an antimicrobial from working against it'. This results in treatments becoming ineffective. AMR is present in every country and is a real issue, due to overuse and inappropriate and uncontrolled use of antibiotics, which has led to increased resistance (Figure 8.2). Resistance has been found in TB, HIV, influenza and malaria. Patients with these conditions often require admission to critical care either as a primary cause or as a complication.

AMR in healthcare is complex and involves production, distribution, prescription, dispensing and administration of the antibiotic (Ayukekbong et al., 2017). Factors exacerbating and affecting the quality of antibiotics may include poor drug quality, counterfeit drugs, high ambient temperatures and humidity, poor storage (Ayukekbong et al., 2017). Further challenges may include easy access to purchasing antibiotics from vendors with little experience or knowledge of complications, dosage or indications. Patients may expect to be prescribed antibiotics as they believe it will cure them. Doctors may prescribe broad-spectrum antibiotics, due to limited access to microbiology services. This results in overuse of antibiotics and early de-escalation may not happen due to a lack of microbiology information. The Centers for Disease Control and Prevention (2017) identifies four actions to prevent the spread of AMR:

- Preventing infection by following standard precautions, effective hand hygiene, immunisations and good food preparation.
- Surveillance to identify trends and sources of infection.
- Improving antimicrobial prescribing and stewardship. Avoiding unnecessary and inappropriate use of antibiotics; in critical care, this can be achieved by effective daily microbiology rounds which review the patient's condition, microbiology and antibiotics, and amending or stopping antibiotics as appropriate.
- Developing new drugs and diagnostic tests to respond to AMR.

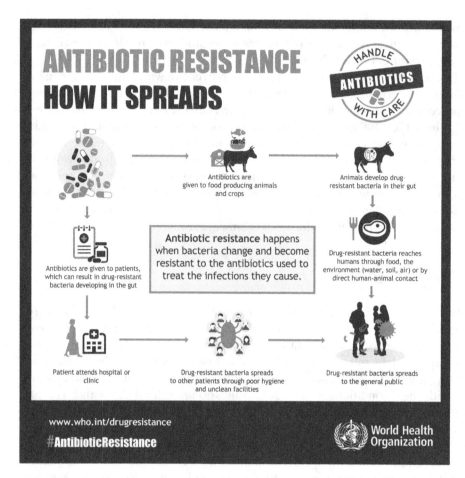

Figure 8.2 Antibiotic resistance: how it spreads

Reproduced with kind permission from the World Health Organization.

Sterilising and re-using equipment

Within resource limited environments, sterilisation departments may not be central-ised, with each unit being responsible for sterilising instruments. Re-use of medical equipment is controversial due to the risk of cross-contamination due to inadequate cleaning, disinfection and sterilisation, which may lead to cross-transmission of dis-eases (Iserson, 2016). Unfortunately, this is a reality for many resource limited settings and many single-patient-use items such as airways, oxygen masks and ventilator tubing are reused, by employing a process of washing and immersing equipment in various solutions including chlorine and glutaraldehyde. This practice is not uncom-mon within critical care units (Association of Surgeons of Great Britain and Ireland (ASGBI), 2014).

Extreme care must be taken when using sterilising instruments; solutions including glutaraldehyde may be effective but can cause allergic reactions to the skin and respiratory problems (Box 8.1) (ASGBI, 2014).

Box 8.1 Considerations when using glutaraldehyde (ASGBI, 2014)

- Wear gloves, a mask and eye protection whenever handling instruments that have been soaked in glutaraldehyde.
- Ideally, an extractor hood should be over the glutaraldehyde tank. If there is no extractor hood, make sure the tank is placed in a large space with plenty of good ventilation.
- Always check how long instruments should be submerged to kill bacteria and viruses.
- Instruments must be rinsed in sterile water before use on any patient.
- If anyone has a sensitisation, they should not work near glutaraldehyde.
- Explore the potential of using other products which may be safer, for example peracetic acid, which is non-toxic, but expensive.

While the re-use of the single-use items is controversial and less than ideal, it is recognised as necessary to provide lifesaving care. Other aspects of medical equipment may need to be improvised, for example the ICRC War Surgery manual (Giannou & Baldan, 2010) identifies in extreme circumstances the following items may be used:

- sterilised mosquito netting for hernia repair;
- recycling used surgical gloves, washed in hypochlorite solution, rinsed, dried, powdered and autoclaved;
- cotton thread or fishing tackle for sutures;
- any sterile tube as a chest drain (Foley catheter, naso-gastric tube, IV giving set);
- chest drainage bottle made from jerry cans or plastic water bottles and fixing the tubing with tape to prevent the end rising above the level of normal saline;
- urinary catheters used as naso-gastric or tracheal suction catheter.

Needle-stick injuries

All healthcare workers who use or are exposed to needles are at risk of a needle-stick injury. Accidental exposure to blood-borne diseases is common, and the cost of follow-up is an estimated $3000 per needle-stick even if no infection occurs (Habib *et al.*, 2011; International Council of Nurses, 2009a). Nurses suffer the most needle-stick injuries, with an average of 1–4 sharps injuries per year, exposing them to over 20 different blood-borne infections (International Council of Nurses, 2009b). Unfortunately, unsafe sharps practices are common, and globally there remains a lack of policy and regulations to protect healthcare workers from exposure (WHO, 2017).

Poor sharps practices may include having to re-use needles and syringes, no retractable finger pricking devices for use when checking blood glucose levels, no safety needles, poor sharps safety, e.g. limited sharps boxes or having to use improvised sharps boxes, bending needles or re-capping/re-sheathing needles. These practices pose significant risks for both patients and healthcare workers. The WHO (2018a) estimated approximately 1.7 million people were infected with hepatitis B virus, approximately 315,000 with hepatitis C virus and an estimated 33,800 with HIV through unsafe injections by healthcare workers.

The International Council of Nurses (2009a) has identified a series of standards relating to nurses' rights and how to protect yourself and others (Box 8.2). These include:

- a comprehensive national policy on occupational health;
- establishment of occupational health services;
- access to health surveillance, ideally during working hours and at no cost to the healthcare worker concerned;
- medical confidentiality of health surveillance;
- financial compensation for those exposed;
- participation in all aspects of protection provision.

Box 8.2   Sharps safety (Ross & Furrows, 2014)

- Sharps containers must be a suitable size for the needs of the department.
- Only approved sharps containers should be used.
- Sharps containers must be correctly assembled, with the lid securely attached all the way around.
- Sharps containers should be clearly labelled and kept off the floor. Ideally at waist height. Containers must be out of the reach of children/members of the public.
- Sharps containers should be signed and dated by the person assembling the container. Details of the ward/hospital should also be identified.
- When the container is to no longer be used, the person locking the container should sign and date the label.
- Do not overfill sharps containers. Containers may have a 'fill level'.

Organisations should have a policy and guidance on what to do in the event of a needle-stick injury. Principles include the following:

- Encourage the site to bleed. Do not suck, scrub or squeeze it. Wash the area under running water. Cover puncture site with a waterproof dressing.

- Irrigate splashes to nose, skin and mouth with running water; do not swallow.
- Irrigate eyes with clean water or saline.
- Report the incident immediately.
- Immediately seek medical advice to commence post-exposure prophylaxis.

(Centers for Disease Control and Prevention, 2016; Ross & Furrows, 2014)

Care bundles

A care bundle is a 'set of treatment goals [usually three to seven] that when grouped and achieved together over a finite time span are believed to promote optimum outcomes' (Dellinger & Townsend, 2013). Examples of care bundles used in critical care which aim to reduce HCAI include:

- ventilator care bundle (Chapter 14);
- central venous catheter insertion and maintenance care bundle (Chapter 17).

Care bundles are only effective if all the elements are completed consistently. To check compliance audit and observations of practice should take place and the results shared with staff.

Environmental considerations

Depending on the environment, extremes of temperature will affect:

- electro-medical equipment and consumables, resulting in equipment degrading/ failing faster than expected;
- battery life, which may be reduced;
- equipment, which may not function in extremes of temperature and overheat increasing risk of fire or explosion;
- storage of drugs and blood products, which may be compromised;
- maintaining a clean environment in wet or sandy environments;
- healthcare workers wearing personal protective equipment (PPE) becoming dehydrated or collapsing due to heat illness;
- providing care in elevated temperatures, e.g. working in the heat of the day or performing CPR in a hot climate with no air conditioning;
- the clinical environment being unfit for its role, for example in a disaster working in a makeshift hospital or a tented facility;
- lack of access to cleaning materials to perform adequate decontamination of equipment or basic environmental cleaning;
- laundry facilities, which may be unable to process linen and ensure correct temperatures are reached to prevent cross-contamination;
- staff having limited access to laundry facilities for uniforms to be cleaned between shifts or if they become soiled.

HCAI are a significant risk for critically ill patients; healthcare staff have a vital role in maintaining best practice with the resources available to prevent the spread of infections. Allegranzi *et al.* (2011) argue HCAI must be included in the WHO list of major diseases contributing to the global burden of disease and the UN SDGs. Infection prevention in a resource limited environment will be challenging, and nurses are faced with practices, for example reusing equipment, or trying to challenge practices which are deemed appropriate by others; equally, finding sustainable alternative solutions with few resources will also be a challenge for the most experienced practitioner.

References

Albarran J. Scholes J. (2018). Virtual issue on infection control. Nursing in Critical Care Virtual Edition.

Allegranzi B. Nejad SB. Combescure C *et al.* (2011). Burden of endemic health-care associated infection in developing countries: systematic review and meta-analysis. The Lancet. 377. 228–241.

Association of Surgeons of Great Britain and Ireland. (2014). Theatre skills for staff in poorly resourced countries. Issues in Professional Practice. Available at: www.asgbi.org.uk/publications/issues-in-professional-practice?term=issues+in+professional+practice.

Ayukekbong JA. Ntemgwa M. Atabe AN. (2017). The threat of antimicrobial resistance in developing countries: causes and control strategies. Antimicrobial Resistance & Infection Control. 6. 47. DOI: https://doi.org/10.1186/s13756-017-0208-x.

Centers for Disease Control and Prevention. (2016). Emergency sharps information. Available at: www.cdc.gov/niosh/topics/bbp/emergnedl.html.

Centers for Disease Control and Prevention. (2017). About anti-microbial resistance. Available at: www.cdc.gov/drugresistance/about.html.

Chawla SS. Gupta S. Onchiri FM *et al.* (2016). Water accessibility at hospitals in low- and middle-income countries: implications for improving access to safe surgical care. Journal of Surgical Research, DOI: 10.1016/j.jss.2016.06.040.

Dellinger RP. Townsend SR. (2013). Point: are the best patient outcomes achieved when ICU bundles are rigorously adhered to? Yes. Chest. 144. 2. 372–374.

Giannou C. Baldan M. (2010). War surgery: Working with limited resources in armed conflict and other situations of violence. Volume 1. Geneva: International Committee of the Red Cross.

Habib H. Ahmed Khan E. Aziz A. (2011). Prevalence and factors associated with needle stick injuries among registered nurses in public sector tertiary care hospitals of Pakistan. International Journal of Collaborative Research on Internal Medicine & Public Health. 3. 2. 124–130.

Iserson KV. (2016). Improvised medicine: providing care in extreme environments. 2nd Edition. New York: McGraw Hill Education.

International Council of Nurses. (2009a). Nursing Matters: ICN on preventing needle-stick injuries. Geneva: ICN.

International Council of Nurses. (2009b). Nursing Matters: ICN on selecting safer needle devices. Available at: www.icn.ch/sites/default/files/inline-files/D05_Patient_Safety.pdf.

Ross S. Furrows S. (2014). Rapid infection control nursing. Chichester, West Sussex: Wiley Blackwell, pp. 33–34.

Ulu-Kilic A. Ahmed SS. Alp E. Doğanay M. (2013). Challenge of intensive care unit-acquired infections and Acinetobacter baumannii in developing countries. OA Critical Care. 1.1. 2–5.

World Health Organization. (2006). The first global patient safety challenge: clean care is safer care. Available at: www.who.int/gpsc/tools/Infsheet6.pdf.

World Health Organization. (2007). Standard precautions in healthcare. Available at: www.who.int/csr/resources/publications/EPR_AM2_E7.pdf.

World Health Organisation. (2008). Patient safety in African health services: issues and solutions. Report of the Regional Director. Available at: http://apps.who.int/iris/handle/10665/19987.

World Health Organization. (2009). Glove use information leaflet. Available at: www.who.int/gpsc/5may/Glove_Use_Information_Leaflet.pdf.

World Health Organization. (2010). The burden of health care-associated infection worldwide a summary. Available at: www.who.int/gpsc/country_work/burden_hcai/en/.

World Health Organization. (2017). Occupational health: needle stick injuries. Available at: www.who.int/occupational_health/topics/needinjuries/en/index1.html.

World Health Organization. (2018a). WHO calls for worldwide use of 'smart' syringes. Available at: www.who.int/mediacentre/news/releases/2015/injection-safety/en/.

World Health Organization. (2018b). Antimicrobial resistance. Available at: www.who.int/antimicrobial-resistance/en/.

9 Managing a major incident in critical care

A major incident (MI) is defined as an incident 'where the number, type and severity of live casualties, or location requires special response measures' (Smith & Zakariah, 2016a). An MI can be classified as simple when the infrastructure, e.g. roads, bridges, remains intact, whereas a compound MI occurs when there is a breakdown of infrastructure. A compensated MI is defined when medical resources can deal with the incident compared to uncompensated when services are overwhelmed; this is termed a disaster (Carter, 2014). MIs may not only be caused by a pre-hospital incident; but other incidents may include pandemic influenza (Chapter 27), a family involved in an explosion resulting in several children with severe burns all requiring critical care (Chapters 35 and 38) or a power failure within the hospital causing a critical loss of electricity.

Triage

During an MI, the hospital will need to adapt, prioritise and compromise to meet the needs of the incident (Sinclair, 2017). Challenges for the hospital may include re-focusing services to meet the needs of the major incident as it may already be chaotic and overwhelmed even before the incident (Carlson *et al.*, 2017). To prioritise patient need, triage is used to identify those in need of immediate care. Triage needs to be fast, reliable, reproducible, and easy to use and teach (Smith, 2012). Triage is a dynamic process, and at each stage of the patient pathway they should be triaged, for example at the scene and on arrival to hospital (Sinclair, 2017).

With limited pre-hospital emergency services, often patients will 'self-triage', meaning those that are too sick often die at the scene or die before reaching the hospital. Those who are not in immediate danger following the incident may deteriorate on the way to the hospital and arrive critically ill. There are various triage categories and codes used by different organisations and countries to triage patients. The commonest system used is either the treatment ('T') or priority ('P') triage system (Smith, 2012):

- Red (T1 or P1): Casualties who are in immediate danger and require immediate treatment, for example catastrophic haemorrhage.

- Yellow (T2 or P2): Casualties who are not in immediate danger, but are likely to require surgery within two to four hours, for example casualties with complicated fractures.
- Green (T3 or P3): Casualties with minor injuries who will eventually require hospital treatment, for example simple fractures, lacerations.
- Blue (T4 Expectant/no priority)/Black (Dead): A patient who is dead or their injuries are so severe they are unlikely to survive and cannot be saved with the limited resources available.

T4 Expectant category

The term 'expectant' is given to casualties whose survival due to the severity of injuries is unlikely, to the level of available care. (Carlson *et al.*, 2017; Ministry of Defence, 2012). The T4 Expectant is the category that is the most ethically and emotionally challenging triage category. The decision to use the T4 category is normally made by the senior medical officer and not used routinely. If used, palliative care and pain relief must be provided. Some organisations do not use the expectant category and only use the 'dead' category.

Triage sieve and cards

The triage code is used within a triage sieve (Table 9.1) to filter and identify the sickest casualties. If emergency medical services have already undertaken triage, patients may arrive with a label, stating their triage category (Pictures 9.1, 9.2), any treatment given and a unique patient identification number, which can be used for casualty tracking. All healthcare workers need to be able to use the triage tool used within the emergency department, as staff may be allocated to triage patients at the entrance to the hospital to help identify the patients requiring immediate care and help with the flow into the hospital.

Often casualties will present at the nearest hospital for treatment, even though the hospital may not have the full range of services or resources to deal with the influx. For hospitals responding to an influx of casualties, resources will be needed to safeguard and maintain services for other patients with long-term conditions, for example dialysis, cancer and those already admitted to the hospital who will need ongoing care (Amatya, 2017). Once an MI is declared, the hospital will need to rapidly expand and reorganise its capabilities (Smith & Zakariah, 2016b). A unified approach to MI planning follows the CSCATTT principles; this includes Command, Safety, Communication, Assessment, Triage, Treatment, and Transport. Figure 9.1 outlines an MI plan for a hospital.

Critical care nurses may be required to support the care of patients in emergency departments and help with post-operative care; re-directing critical care staff helps meet the short-term needs of other departments. The wider impact on the critical care will mean the unit will be unable to prepare to receive casualties either post-operatively

Table 9.1 MI plan for a hospital

Command	– Decide who is in command. – Close the gates and entrances, to channel patients through a single entrance. – Call in additional staff.
Safety	– Ensure personnel have access to appropriate personal protective equipment (PPE). – Ensure security of staff – what is the cause of the incident?
Communication	– Compile a list of all patients admitted to the facility. – Allocate staff to manage enquiries about patients.
Assessment	– Information may come from a variety of sources including social media (e.g. Twitter, Facebook), as well as radio and television. This information may be conflicting, e.g. official versus eye-witness reports of those arriving at the hospital. – Ongoing assessment of the incident and the hospital response to re-allocate resources as appropriate and ensure the response is effective.

Triage	– Allocate staff to triage patients.
	– As patients arrive:
	   o Triage (Priority 1 (immediate), 2 (urgent), 3 (walking wounded).
	   o Number all patients on arrival – ideally use a triage tag.
	   o Channel patients to the appropriate treatment area.
	– Apply surgical triage and prepare theatre list.
	– Assemble all bodies in a practical area for management by police.

Treatment	– Only request diagnostically significant investigations. – Ensure T3 patients are monitored and re-assessed if any deteriorate; re-triage and allocate to the appropriate area. – Ensure documentation including treatment given and valuables. – Start surgery as soon as possible and ensure appropriate post-operative care.
Transport	– Prepare ward for admissions and channel all stabilised patients to wards. – Consider if appropriate transferring patients from critical care to wards or other hospitals to create capacity.

Source: Smith & Zakariah, 2016b

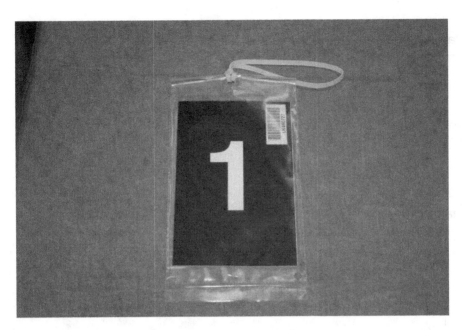

Picture 9.1 Example triage card attached to a patient

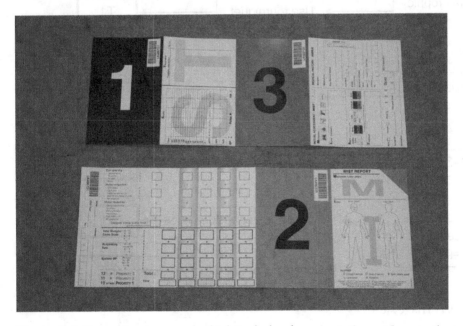

Picture 9.2 Example triage card which includes documentation, unique patient identification number. If the casualty's condition changes, the triage category is changed and displayed

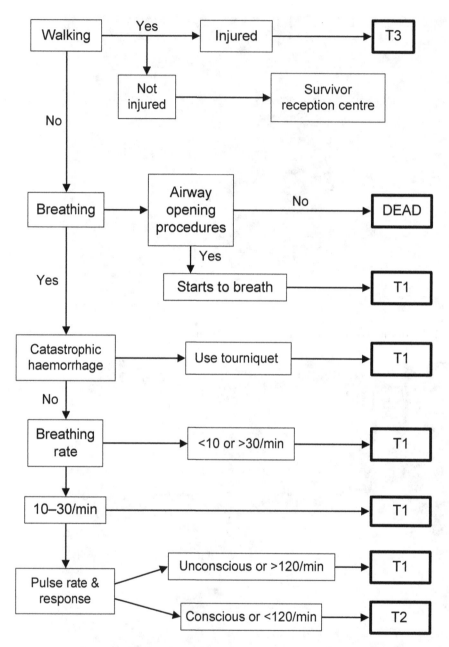

Figure 9.1 Triage sieve

Ministry of Defence, 2012

or directly from the emergency room. Also, critical care units may be unable to create capacity for new patients and respond to in-hospital emergencies and potential admissions, for example in-hospital cardiac arrests, acute deterioration of ward patients or an obstetric emergency requiring a caesarean section may require critical care resources.

All hospitals and departments must have an MI plan which includes training of staff. The plan should include identification of surge capacity which can be used to accommodate patients, action cards with key information for staff, determining what additional equipment and resources are required/available (Smith & Zakariah, 2016b). In the hospital setting, triage may consist of identifying patients who can be moved to other wards or discharged home. While no formal 'model' will be available to achieve this, good clinical judgement by experienced healthcare professionals will need to be utilised and may also include up-skilling families and community teams to help with the patients' ongoing needs.

While the immediate response to the MI will be dealt with quickly, the ongoing impact to the hospital may last from days to weeks. Patients admitted will require ongoing care, which may include return trips to theatres, ward and rehabilitation care. In consequence, the hospital may not return to normal services for hours, days and weeks after the incident.

Disaster management

Any MI will put additional pressures on an already stretched healthcare system; depending on the incident, this may tip the balance, resulting in services being no longer able to function, leading to a disaster. The WHO defines a disaster as 'a serious disruption of the functioning of a community or a society causing widespread human, material, economic or environmental losses which exceed the ability of the affected community or society to cope using its own resources' (WHO, 2017). The United Nations Office for Disaster Risk Reduction (2015) reported 90% of disasters have been caused by weather-related events and are increasing.

Many of the MI principles including triage, and CSCATTT principles and hospital disaster/MI plan, can be used. During a disaster or conflict, it is unlikely critical care services will be appropriate, as services may have been destroyed or become overwhelmed; however, the skills of critical care nurses and doctors are likely to be invaluable in other areas of the hospital. Governments may request assistance from other countries and international organisations; however, to mobilise these resources may take time and be influenced by political views. The Ebola outbreak in 2014 was a large-scale, gradual onset natural disaster; initially, the political and international response was slow (Shepherd-Barron, 2015). In consequence, healthcare workers needed to continue providing care until additional resources were made available; this put considerable strain on an already stretched healthcare system and healthcare workers.

During a disaster, it may be appropriate to cohort seriously ill patients in one part of the hospital and provide good nursing care (ICRC, 2013). Following the Pakistan earthquake in 2005, within 24 hours renal dialysis and critical care were provided in the basement of a destroyed hospital (Ryan, 2010). This was in direct response to the needs assessment which identified many civilians had been crushed and entrapped, causing crush syndrome and renal impairment. The capability of the care will depend on the resources available; however, any slight increase in nurse to patient ratios may allow for increased monitoring, administration of oxygen, analgesia and fluids and observation for any signs of deterioration.

During the Ebola outbreak in West Africa, critical care focused on avoiding and correcting hypovolaemia, correction of electrolyte and metabolic abnormalities and provision of oxygen, ventilation, vasopressors and renal replacement therapy (Leligdowicz *et al.*, 2016). With few staff and a highly contagious disease, there was restricted continuous monitoring, with physiological observations being recorded daily, and care focused on aggressive oral and occasional intravenous fluid resuscitation. As the number of cases reduced and the number of healthcare personnel available increased, greater assessment and monitoring was possible. Monitoring included vital signs monitoring, urine output, gastro-intestinal and fluid balance monitoring. Over time, the ability to provide oxygen, non-invasive ventilation, aggressive volume resuscitation, enteral feeding, renal replacement therapy was possible (Leligdowicz *et al.*, 2016). During this outbreak, the role of critical care nurses evolved and spanned both providing care but also training other healthcare professionals in fundamental critical care skills.

Conflict and disaster provide a unique situation causing a breakdown in infrastructure; social structures and the hospital and staff are at risk of attack (Attar & Gupta, 2017). Healthcare staff may be required to undertake other tasks to keep the hospital operational; this may include building and repairing the facility. These effects and other degrading factors, for example limited sleep, extremes of temperature and staff having to administer themselves in this environment, will be challenging (Attar & Gupta, 2017). As outlined in Chapter 4, it is important to look after each other and yourself in these stressful environments.

In summary, MIs and disasters are tragic events, which require healthcare systems to respond. Hospitals need to develop effective planning, training and resources to develop strong response systems to not only meet the needs of the incident but also meet the ongoing health needs of the population at risk. While the international community may be able to provide elements of the response system, it is often the local healthcare providers who are faced with the immediate and ongoing response and provide most of the care in these situations. Critical care nurses have a skill set that can be transferrable to other areas of the hospital and situations.

References

Amatya KS. (2017). Chapter 1: Surgical care after the April 2015 Nepal Earthquake. In: Kushner A (ed.). Operation crisis: surgical care in the developing world during conflict and disaster. Baltimore, MD: Johns Hopkins University Press.

Attar S. Gupta S. (2017). Chapter 2: A health system destroyed. In: Kushner A (ed.). Operation Crisis: surgical care in the developing world during conflict and disaster. Baltimore, MD: Johns Hopkins University Press.

Carlson LC. Kamara TB. Kingham TP. (2017). Chapter 5: Triage and training. A mass casualty incident exercise in Sierra Leone. In: Kushner A (ed). Operation Crisis: surgical care in the developing world during conflict and disaster. Baltimore, MD: Johns Hopkins University Press.

Carter C. (2014). Managing a major incident in the critical care unit. Nursing Standard. 28. 31. 39–44.

International Committee for the Red Cross. (2013). War surgery: working with resource limited resources in armed conflict and other situations of violence. Volume 2. Available at: www.icrc.org/en/publication/4105-war-surgery-working-limited-resources-armed-conflict-and-other-situations-violence.

Leligdowicz A. Fischer WA. Uyeki TM *et al*. (2016). Ebola virus disease and critical illness. Critical Care. 20. 217. DOI: https://doi.org/10.1186/s13054-016-1325-2.

Ministry of Defence. (2012). Chapter 30: triage in tactical combat casualty care. pp. 671–707. In Salomone JP. Pons PT (eds). Pre-hospital trauma life support. Military Edition. 7th Edition. Maryland Heights, MO: Elsevier Mosby Jems.

United Nations Office for Disaster Risk Reduction. (2015). The human cost of weather related disasters. Available at: www.unisdr.org/2015/docs/climatechange/COP21_WeatherDisastersReport_2015_FINAL.pdf.

Ryan J. (2010). Chapter 7: Surgery in disasters. In: Matheson JIDM. Hawley A (eds). Making sense of disaster: a hands-on guide for medics. London: Hodder Arnold.

Shepherd-Barron J. (2015). Ebola: most unnatural disaster. The Lancet Global Health Blog. Available at: http://globalhealth.thelancet.com/2015/03/24/ebola-most-unnatural-disasters.

Sinclair M. (2017). Chapter 3: A surgeon's day in South Sudan. In: Kushner A (ed.). Operation Crisis: surgical care in the developing world during conflict and disaster. Baltimore, MD: Johns Hopkins University Press.

Smith W. (2012). Triage in mass situations. African Journal of Emergency Medicine. 30. 11. 413–415.

Smith W. Zakariah AN. (2016a). Chapter 351: General principles of disaster medicine. In: Wallis LS. Reynolds TA (eds). AFEM Handbook of Acute and Emergency Care. Oxford: Oxford University Press.

Smith W. Zakariah AN (2016b). Chapter 354: Hospital disaster response. In: Wallis LS. Reynolds TA (eds). (2016). AFEM handbook of acute and emergency care. Oxford: Oxford University Press.

World Health Organization. (2017). Humanitarian health action. Definitions: emergencies. Available at: www.who.int/hac/about/definitions/en/.

<table>
<tr><td>

10

</td><td>

Assessment of the critically ill patient

</td></tr>
</table>

Critical care nursing is not just a list of skills or tasks provided to critically ill patients. Nurses provide continuous observation and care to the patient and detect any deterioration. To achieve this, a thorough patient assessment should be completed to identify nursing needs and provide structured care. This chapter focuses on the recognition of the deteriorating patient and the assessment of the critically ill patient. The assessment principles can be applied in any situation, for example in the emergency department, on a ward or in a critical care unit.

Recognition of the deteriorating patient

Recognition of the acutely ill patient may be difficult, due to the number of trained staff, a limited number of nurses and low nurse to patient ratios, limited education and resources, e.g. oxygen, pulse oximetry, sphygmomanometers to monitor and manage patients. Often the number of critically ill patients requiring critical care services exceeds demands. Dart *et al.* (2017) conducted a point prevalence study of morbidity in acute admissions to identify demand for critical care services in a university teaching hospital in sub-Saharan Africa. Dart *et al.* (2017) used the UK National Early Warning Scoring Tool (NEWS) and included HIV testing on adult patients on admissions to filter, medical and surgical admission wards over 48 hours. The study found 71% of patients tested were HIV positive, which was higher than expected, and 45% had objective evidence of a 'requirement for a critical care review and potential or probable admission to an intensive care unit'. In consequence, an acutely ill patient may be initially managed on a ward, until a critical care bed becomes available.

Without an Early Warning Score (EWS) often recognition of the acutely ill patient may be based on the nurses' knowledge, intuition and skill of observation. If available, using an EWS in resource limited environments may be limited due to tools not being appropriate or sensitive enough to detect deterioration within the patient population, a lack of equipment to complete full sets of observations and limited staff to respond to deterioration. In Uganda, Kruisselbrink *et al.* (2016) outline the use of a Modified Early Warning Scoring (MEWS) tool (Table 10.1), which has been developed specifically

Table 10.1 Modified Early Warning Scoring tool

	3	2	1	0	1	2	3
Systolic blood pressure (mmHg)	<70	71–80	81–100	101–199			
Pulse rate (beats per minute)		<40	41–50	51–100	101–110	111–129	>130
Respiratory rate (breaths per minute)		<9	9–14	15–20	21–29	>30	
Temperature (°C)		<35		35–38.4		>38.5	
AVPU Score				Alert	V	P	U

AVPU: A alert; V responding to voice; P responding to pain; U unresponsive

Source: Kruisselbrink *et al.*, 2016

for sub-Saharan Africa. As found with other studies, Kruisselbrink *et al.* (2016) found patients with high MEWS exceeded the physical critical care capacity within the hospital, but concluded developing and using resources such as the MEWS allowed:

- grouping of unstable patients together to enable closer observation and monitoring (including pooling of resources). In some hospitals, this area is termed an 'acute bay', whereby patients identified at risk of deterioration are nursed nearest the nurses' station, to increase observation and have access to oxygen and suction equipment;
- initiating individual and realistic treatments for the deteriorating patient, including oxygen for hypoxia and intravenous crystalloid for hypotension;
- the MEWS to be used as a triage tool to identify the sickest patients, which allowed treatment to either avert admission to critical care or death or initiate admission to critical care.

EWS tools assist healthcare workers in identifying the deteriorating patient. However, in practice, there can be an over-reliance on the tools used, or they are not effectively used because full sets of observations are not recorded, and the frequency of observations may decline over time. Reasons for this are complex but may include low nurse to patient ratios on the wards, and lack of diagnostic tools, resources and staff to respond to the deteriorating patient (Asiimwe *et al.*, 2014).

Critical care nurses may be called up to review an unwell patient in the emergency department or in a ward setting. As outlined in Chapter 6, appropriate critical care admission guidelines will help identify suitable patients who may benefit from critical care interventions. Before transferring a critically ill patient, they must be stabilised first; recommendations are outlined in Box 10.1. Prioritising care using the Airway, Breathing, Circulation, Disability (neurological) and Exposure approach provides structure and identification of potentially life-threatening conditions and prioritises care.

**Box 10.1   Core standards to be completed
prior to admission to critical care
(Mwewa & Mweemba, 2010)**

To be completed before admission to critical care:

- Secure airway; all patients in respiratory distress should be intubated before transfer to ICU.
- Baseline procedures, e.g. intravenous cannulas, naso-gastric tube insertion, intercostal drainage tube insertion, urethral catheterisation.
- Stat doses of drugs should always be given and signed for.
- All patients who are unconscious should have their blood glucose level checked to rule out hypoglycaemia.
- Patients with head injuries must have Glasgow Coma Scale completed and pupil size and reaction assessed and recorded.
- Critical care nurses should be informed in advance about the patient and include a detailed handover.

Assessment of the critically ill patient

A patient assessment must be completed immediately following handover, on admission or if you have any concerns with the patient's condition. Assessment includes safety checks of emergency equipment, infusions, ventilator, monitor settings and patient checks (see Table 10.2).

Table 10.2 Considerations when assessing a critically ill patient

Emergency equipment	Oxygen and suction are immediately available at every bed-space. Check each bed-space has a spare oxygen cylinder, either three-quarters full or full. Portable, battery-operated suction should also be available within the unit.
Bed-space layout	Each bed-space should have:
	– equipment which may be used frequently or in an emergency, e.g. syringes, needles, gauze. Ideally, this equipment should be kept covered (in drawers or boxes);
	– an appropriately sized sharps box. This should be kept off the floor and out of reach of children or confused patients.

Table 10.2 Continued

First steps	Ensure your personal safety – wear appropriate PPE.
	Introduce yourself to the patient (remember even though your patient may be semi-conscious or unconscious they may still be able to hear, so talk and explain all procedures and interventions to reassure your patient).
	Look at the patient in general – your first impressions are important. Do they look uncomfortable, breathing fast, sweaty?
Alarm checks	Check the monitor and ventilator alarm limits are appropriate and not silenced.
	It is important appropriate alarms are set so that nurses and healthcare workers do not become desensitised to the alarms and fail to respond to an emergency.
	Transducers:
	– Zero arterial and central venous catheter transducer sets
	– Check transducer pressure bag is set to 300mmHg
	– Check pressure bag fluid is 0.9% Sodium Chloride
	– Transducer table in line with the phlebostatic axis (4th intercostal space, mid axillary line)
Patient safety checks	Does the patient have a name band on? Is the information correct (check against the patient's medical notes, drug chart/observation charts)?
	Any allergies are clearly documented in the patient's notes and drug chart.
	Ventilator connected to an uninterrupted power supply.
	Intravenous infusions are correct (check against drug chart).
Airway	Is the airway patent?
	Any signs of a partial or fully occluded airway?
	– Is the patient talking in full sentences?
	– Signs of obstruction (choking)?
	– Noisy breathing, (stridor, gurgling or wheeze)?
	Does the patient have an airway adjunct in place?
	What type and is it effective?
	– oropharyngeal airway (OP)
	– nasopharyngeal airway (NP)
	– laryngeal Mask Airway (LMA)
	– endo-tracheal tube (ETT)
	– tracheostomy tube (TT)
	ETT specific checks:
	– Date of grade of intubation and/or any complications?
	– Size at ETT
	– Length at teeth
	– Is the tube secure?

Table 10.2 Continued

- Any signs of pressure damage from the ties, e.g. corners of mouth?
- Last time suctioning performed?
- If available:

  o ETT cuff pressure
  o EtCO$_2$

TT specific checks:

- Bedside emergency TT kit available?
- Size of TT?
- Type of tube?

  o Does it have an inner tube?
  o When was the inner tune last checked/changed/cleaned?

- Is the TT secure?
- Any signs of pressure damage from the ties?
- TT dressing clean and intact?
- Last time suctioned?
- If available:

  o TT cuff pressure
  o If ventilated EtCO$_2$

Breathing

Is the chest moving ok?
Assess respiratory rate, rhythm and depth.
Is the patient on supplementary oxygen?

- How much oxygen is the patient on?
- What type of oxygen delivery system is being used, e.g. venturi mask, non-re-breath mask, ventilated?
- Are you using an oxygen cylinder? If so, how much is left? Are spares available on the unit?

Assess oxygen saturations.
Assess arterial blood gases.
Respiratory effort:

- Any signs of distress?
- Accessory muscle use?
- 'See-saw' breathing?

Auscultate chest.
Is the patient ventilated?

- If so, what mode of ventilation used? Is it effective?

Tracheal sections?

- When were they last suctioned?
- What was the colour, type and consistency of secretions?
- Is a sputum specimen required? When was one last sent and what where the results?

Table 10.2 Continued

Any forms of humidification?

- Nebulisers (frequency and type)
- Humidification circuit
- Heat, moist exchange (HME) filters

Does the patient have a chest drain?

- Reason for insertion?
- Date inserted?
- Size and type?
- Swinging, draining and bubbling?
- Dressing intact?

Circulation   Is the patient clammy, cold or warm to touch?
Pulse rate, rhythm and strength (compare central versus peripheral)
Cardiac monitoring?

- Cardiac rhythm (Chapter 15)
- Alarm limits appropriate

Blood pressure:

- Arterial/non-invasive
- Non-invasive – appropriate sized cuff, time cycle for readings?
- Mean arterial pressure (MAP)

Central venous pressure measurements. Within appropriate parameters?
Any cardiac drugs in progress?

- Anti-arrhythmic, e.g. digoxin, amiodarone
- Vaso-active drugs, e.g. adrenaline

Measure central and peripheral perfusion pressure.
Core temperature.
Neurovascular observations:

- Pedal pulses present
- Peripheral perfusion
- Colour, warmth, sensitivity

Urine output >0.5ml/kg/hr
Any sources of fluid loss?

- Wounds
- Surgical drains
- Naso-gastric aspirates
- Bowels
- Burns
- Insensible losses

IV fluids in progress?

- Type
- Speed

Table 10.2 Continued

Skin turgor
Fluid balance (previous 24 hours)
Vascular access:

- Type
- Location
- Size
- Date inserted
- Line patent?
- Dressing intact
- Signs of infection?

Assess blood results (Tables 10.3–10.5). Reference ranges may vary between laboratories and hospital and are shown as a guide:

- When last taken?
- White cell count
- Haemoglobin level
- Clotting
- Urea and creatinine
- Potassium
- Magnesium
- Phosphate
- Blood glucose levels

Does the patient require bloods, Cross Match or Group and Save?

Disability (neurological assessment)	Examine pupils (size, equality and reaction to light)? Assess Glasgow Coma Scale and/or Alert, Voice, Pain, Unresponsive.

Glasgow Coma Scale	
Eyes	4 Spontaneous
	3 To voice
	2 To pain
	1 None
Verbal response	5 Orientated
	4 Confused
	3 Inappropriate words
	2 Incomprehensible sounds
	1 None
Motor response	6 Obeys commands
	5 Localises to pain
	4 Withdraws
	3 Abnormal flexion
	2 Abnormal extension
	1 None

Table 10.2 Continued

Pain assessment? (Chapter 19)

– Use of an appropriate tool?

Sedation assessment?

– Use of an appropriate tool?
– Is the patient:

  o combative?
  o very agitated?
  o restless?
  o calm and alert?
  o drowsy?
  o lightly sedated – responds to voice?
  o moderately sedated – movement or opening eyes to voice?
  o deeply sedated – no response to voice, but movement or eye opening to physical stimulation?
  o unrousable – no response to voice or physical stimulation?

– Any analgesic and sedation drugs: continuous infusion, regular or as required?

  o Are they working?
  o Do these infusions need to be increased or decreased?
  o Last time a sedation hold was completed?

History of seizures?

– Reason for seizures?
– When was last seizure?
– Any medication given?

Blood glucose level (including last time checked).

Exposure	Any rashes or other wounds? Any signs of abdominal distension? Bowel sounds present? Bowels last opened? Nutritional status – oral fluids, enteral feeding, etc. Are the calves swollen or tender? Deep vein thrombosis prophylaxis? Peripheral oedema Skin/colour mucosa Assess pressure areas. When was the patient last turned? Assess the patient's eyes: – Assess eyelid closure – Assess each eye using a bright light for signs and symptoms of infection or disease, e.g. redness, discharge, conjunctival swelling, haziness or cloudiness of the cornea, patches or spots on the cornea

Table 10.2 Continued

	Assess the patient's mouth:
	- Are they dry?
	- Signs of infection?
	- Last time eye and mouth care performed?
	- Do you need to give eye and mouth care?
Finally!	Have a look at the charts:
	- Observation chart: trends, the frequency of observations recorded
	- Medical notes and specific information/plan?
	- Drug chart: any allergies?
	Any spiritual/religious needs?
	Communication aids required, e.g. glasses, language?
	Next of kin/family aware of admission and current condition?
	Next of kin details checked and correct?
	Document your findings and make an appropriate nursing plan.

Sources: Birmingham City University, 2017; Marsden & Davies, 2016; Resuscitation Council (UK), 2016

Table 10.3 Biochemistry normal ranges

Test	Range
Albumin	36–47g/L
Alkaline phosphatase (ALP)	25–115u/L
Aspartate aminotransferase (AST)	10–35u/L
Amylase	0.4–174ukat/L, 200u/L
Bilirubin (total)	3.5–17umol/l
Calcium	2.20–2.67mmol/L
Chloride	100–106mmol/L
Creatine kinase	0.94–2.89ukat/L 0.51–2.3ukat/L
Creatine	60–120umol/L Male: 24–194u/L Female: 24–170u/L
Glucose	4–6mmol/L
Potassium	3.5–5mmol/L
Sodium	135–145mmol/L
Magnesium	0.75–1.2mmol/L
Urea	2.5–6.7mmol/L

Table 10.4 Haematology normal ranges

Test	Range
Red blood cells	Male: 4.5–6.5 × 10^{12}/L Female: 3.8–5.3 × 10^{12}/L
White cell count	4–11 × 10^9/L
Haemoglobin (Hb)	Male: 13–18g/dl Female: 11.5–16.5g/dl
Haematocrit	Male: 0.42–0.53l/L Female: 0.32–0.45l/L
Lymphocytes	1.5–4.0 × 10^9/L
Monocytes	0.02–0.08 × 10^9
Neutrophils	3.5–7.5 × 10^9/L
Platelets	150–400 × 10^9/L
Erythrocyte sedimentation rate (ESR)	Male: 1–10mm/hour Female: 3–15mm/hour

Table 10.5 Coagulation normal ranges

Test	Range
International normalized ratio (INR)	2.0–3.0
Activated partial thromboplastin time (aPTT)	30–50sec
Prothrombin time (PT)	16–18sec
Fibrinogen	2–4glL
D-Dimer	<1.37nmmol/L

Sources: Peate, 2009; Skinner, 2005

References

Asiimwe SB. Okello S. Moore CC. (2014). Frequency of vital sign monitoring and its association with mortality among adults with severe sepsis admitted to a general medical ward in Uganda. PLOS One. 9. 2. E89879.

Birmingham City University. (2017). Critical care nursing in Sub-Saharan Africa: An educational resource. Birmingham City University.

Dart PJ. Kinnear J. Bould MD et al. (2017). An evaluation of inpatient morbidity and critical care provision in Zambia. Anaesthesia. 72. 2. 172–180.

Kruisselbrink R. Kwizera A. Crowther M *et al.* (2016). Modified Early Warning Score (MEWS) identifies critical illness among ward patients in a resource restricted setting in Kampala, Uganda: a prospective observational study. PLOS One. 11. 3. 1–13.

Marsden J. Davies R. (2016). How to care for a patient's eyes in critical care settings. Nursing Standard. 31. 16–18. 42–45.

Mwewa B. Mweemba P. (2010). Knowledge and utilization of ICU admission criteria and guidelines, Lusaka, Zambia. Medical Journal of Zambia. 37. 3. 143–152.

Peate I. (2009). Nursing care and the activities of daily living. Chichester: John Wiley & Sons Inc.

Resuscitation Council (UK). (2016). Advanced life support. 7th Edition. London

Skinner S. (2005). Understanding clinical investigations: a quick reference manual. 2nd Edition. Edinburgh: Bailièrre Tindall (Elsevier).

11 Medicines management and useful calculations

In critical care, nurses often administer multiple high-risk medicines via bolus or infusions (e.g. potassium and vasopressor drugs) simultaneously to a critically ill patient. In this chapter, the practicalities of drug administration in resource limited environments including medication errors, useful/commonly used drug calculations and potential complications including anaphylaxis will be outlined.

Medication errors

Unsafe medication practices and errors are recognised as leading causes of injury and avoidable harm globally. In 2017, the WHO launched its Third Global Patient Safety Challenge 'Medications without Harm', with the aim of reducing avoidable harm by 50% by 2022 (WHO, 2018). The challenge facing each country differs; patients in low- and low-middle income countries 'experience twice as many disability-adjusted life years lost due to medication-related harm than those in high-income countries' (WHO, 2017) and medication errors are common (Feleke *et al.*, 2015; Rowe *et al.*, 2005; Bull *et al.*, 2017). Medication errors are defined as 'any error in the prescribing, dispensing or administration of a drug' (Feleke *et al.*, 2015). Weak medication systems coupled with human factors as outlined below contribute to medication errors:

- High workloads.
- Exhaustion, including those working night shifts who have had disturbed sleep which leads to performance impairment and exhaustion.
- Few staff to second check drugs.
- Low nurse/patient ratios.
- Lack of training, education and motivation of staff to change practice or understand the rationale for doing things differently.
- Dealing with drugs and patients you are unfamiliar with, e.g. children.
- Errors with drug packaging looking similar or drugs sounding alike.
- Illegible handwritten prescriptions.
- Inaccurate documentation and poor communication at handover.
- Failure to check patient identification.
- Storage of similar drugs in the same area.

- Environmental factors including nurses being interrupted during drug rounds.
- Difficulty in accessing medication resources, e.g. formularies or the internet to check drug dosages; ideally you should have access to local or national IV guides.

(Feleke *et al.*, 2015; Rowe *et al.*, 2005;
Bull *et al.*, 2017; WHO, 2007, 2017)

Preparing to give a medication

To prevent medication errors amongst nurses, you may find the following guidance useful:

- Always use a calculator (make sure you take one (or more) with you).
- Have examples of common formulas used in your clinical area.
- Training of staff.
- Policy and monitoring of prescribing, dispensing and administration of drugs. Medication management requires multi-professional input; therefore a collaborative approach is required to reduce the risk of errors.
- Have access to a local, national formulary in the department.
- If you are in doubt, do not administer the drug and seek advice from the pharmacist or the prescriber.

(Bull *et al.*, 2017; Cavell *et al.*, 2014; Raza *et al.*, 2016;
Feleke *et al.*, 2015; Rowe *et al.*, 2005)

Prior to administration of any drugs (particularly injectable and controlled drugs), they must be double-checked independently, by another practitioner who repeats the calculation independently and then compares answers (Cavell *et al.*, 2014).

Commonly used abbreviations

Kilogram	kg
Gram	g
Milligram	mg
Microgram	should be written as microgram
Nanogram	should be written as nanogram
Litre	L
Millilitre	ml or mL

Units of international units should be written as units or international units

Millimoles	mmol

The following should be avoided:

- Use of fractional doses, e.g. 0.5g to prevent error should be written as 500mg.
- Unnecessary decimal points, e.g. 5mg not 5.0mg.

Converting units of weight and volume

Weight

1kg	= 1000g
1g	= 1000mg
1mg	= 1000micrograms
1microgram	= 1000nanograms

Volume

1L	= 1000ml
1ml	= Weighs 1g
1000ml	= Weighs 1000g or 1kg

Some drug dosages may be calculated on bodyweight or body surface area, e.g. paediatrics.

Calculating oral doses in tablets

Check the amount of drug in each tablet or capsule.

Check the dose on the prescription and that it has the same unit on the medicine label. You may need to convert. Then use the following calculation to work out the number of oral tablets required.

$$\text{Number of tablets} = \frac{\text{Dose}}{\text{Strength of tablet}}$$

Calculating intravenous drug doses

$$\text{Volume required} = \frac{\text{Dose} \times \text{volume of solution in ampoule}}{\text{Amount of drug in ampoule}}$$

Calculating infusion rates for infusion devices

This may be prescribed as either volume or amount of drug per hour or minute.

Volume in ml per hour:

$$\frac{\text{Total volume of infusion (ml)}}{\text{Duration of infusion (hour)}} = \text{ml per hour}$$

Amount of drug in mg per hour:

$$\frac{\text{Total dose in mg}}{\text{Duration of infusion (hour)}} = \text{mg per hour}$$

Syringe pumps, volumetric pumps and gravity giving sets

In resource limited environments, access to syringe pumps and volumetric pumps may be limited. Syringe pumps are used when small doses and volumes of highly concentrated drugs need to be infused at low flow rates. The volume of the fluid is determined by the size of the syringe used. These devices tend to be calibrated for delivery in millilitres per hour. Whereas volumetric pumps deliver fluid from an infusion bag or bottle via an administration set and work by calculating the volume delivered. Large volumes of fluid can be administered this way. Prior to using any infusion devices, nurses need to check they have received appropriate training in the use of these devices, to prevent potential complications and medication errors.

Types of gravity flow infusions include:

- a drug administration set, e.g. 0.9% sodium chloride;
- a blood administration set;
- burettes administration set used to administer paediatric infusions.

Check the administration (giving) set for the number of drops per ml. This is located on the packaging and varies between manufacturers. You will require this information to calculate the drip rates.

$$\text{Number of drops per minute} = \frac{\text{Volume in ml} \times \text{number of drops per ml}}{\text{Intended duration of infusion (in minutes)}}$$

For example, a 1000ml of sodium chloride 0.9% infused over 8 hours.

$$\frac{1000\text{ml} \times 20 \text{ drops per ml}}{480\text{min}} = 42 \text{ drops per minute}$$

Inotropes

Calculating mcg/kg/min

Converting mg to mcg
Drug (mcg) divided by total amount diluted (ml) divided by 60 (time) divided by patient's weight (kg) multiplied by the rate (ml/hr).

For example, 4mg Noradrenaline in 50ml of 5% dextrose running at 3ml/hr. The patient weighs 80kg:

$$4000 \div 50 \div 60 \div 80 \times 3 = 0.05 \text{mcg/kg/min}$$

While there are no internationally agreed standards for medication concentrations in adult critical care, Table 11.1 outlines commonly used concentrations. Using agreed standardised concentrations helps to improve prescribing, forms a critical step in patient safety and efficient use of resources in critical care (Intensive Care Society, 2017).

Table 11.1 Common medication concentrations in adult critical care areas

Drug	Example fluid composition	Concentration	Central (C) or Peripheral (P) administration
Morphine	50mg in 50ml	1mg/ml	C/P
	100mg in 50ml	2mg/ml	C/P
Fentanyl	2.5mg in 50ml	50micrograms/ml	C/P
Alfentanyl	25mg in 50ml	500micrograms/ml	C/P
Remifentanil	2mg in 40ml	50micrograms/ml	C/P
	5mg in 50ml	100micrograms/ml	C/P
Midazolam	50mg in 50ml	1mg/ml	C/P
	100mg in 50ml	2mg/ml	C/P
Clonidine	750micrograms in 50ml	15micrograms/ml	C/P
Dexmedetomidine	200micrograms in 50ml.	4micrograms ml	C/P
	400micrograms in 50ml	8micrograms/ml	C/P
Adrenaline (epinephrine)	4mg in 50ml	80micrograms/ml	C
	8mg in 50ml	160micrograms/ml	C
	16mg in 50ml	320micrograms/ml	C
	8mg in 100ml	80micrograms/ml	C
	16mg in 100ml	160micrograms/ml	C
	32mg in 100ml	320micrograms/ml	C
Noradrenaline (norepinephrine)	4mg in 50ml	80micrograms/ml	C
	8mg in 50ml	160micrograms/ml	C
	16mg in 50ml	320micrograms/ml	C
	8mg in 100ml	80micrograms/ml	C
	16mg in 100ml	160micrograms/ml	C
	32mg in 100ml	320micrograms/ml	C
Dobutamine	250mg in 50ml	5mg/ml	C
	500mg in 100ml	5mg/ml	C
Dopamine	200mg in 50ml	4mg/ml	C
	400mg in 50ml	8mg/ml	C
Vasopressin (argipressin)	20 units in 50ml	0.4units/ml	C/P
Amiodarone (loading dose)	300mg in 50ml	6mg/ml	C
	300mg in 100ml	3mg/ml	C

Table 11.1 Continued

Drug	Example fluid composition	Concentration	Central (C) or Peripheral (P) administration
Amiodarone (continuous infusion)	300mg in 50ml	6mg/ml	C
	600mg in 50ml	12mg/ml	C
	900mg in 50ml	18mg/ml	C
	300mg in 500ml	0.6mg/ml	C
	600mg in 500ml	1.2mg/ml	C
	900mg in 500ml	1.8mg/ml	C
Heparin	20000units in 50ml	1000units/ml	C/P
	25000units in 25ml	1000units/ml	C/P
Magnesium sulphate	20mmol in 50ml	0.4mmol/ml	C
	20mmol in 100ml	0.4mmol/ml	C
	50mmol in 500ml	0.1mmol/ml	C/P
Insulin	50units in 50ml	1 unit/ml	C/P

Source: Intensive Care Society, 2017

Potential complications

Potential complications of intravenous care are outlined in Chapter 17. A serious complication of any administration of drugs is anaphylaxis. Anaphylaxis is defined as a 'severe, life-threatening, generalised or systematic hypersensitivity reaction. Characterised by rapidly developing life-threatening airway and/or breathing and/or circulation problems usually associated with skin and mucosal changes' (Resuscitation Council (UK), 2016. p. 133). The trigger could be food, drugs, stinging insects and latex. In the hospital environment triggers including latex (gloves, masks) and medications including muscle relaxants, antibiotics, nonsteroidal anti-inflammatory drugs, aspirin, and CT contrast are the commonest causes.

The signs and symptoms of anaphylaxis can be associated with other conditions. Differential diagnosis includes life-threatening asthma, hypotension (or normal BP in children) with petechial or purpuric rash caused by septic shock. Non-life-threatening conditions include fainting (vaso-vagal episode), panic attack, breath-holding episode in a child, idiopathic (non-allergic) urticaria and angioedema. Non-life-threatening conditions tend to respond to simple interventions. Life-threatening anaphylaxis is likely if there is:

- sudden onset and progression of symptoms;
- life-threatening airway, breathing and/or circulation problems;
    - airway: airway swelling: throat, tongue swelling, difficulty in breathing, swallowing and the patient feels their throat is closing up;

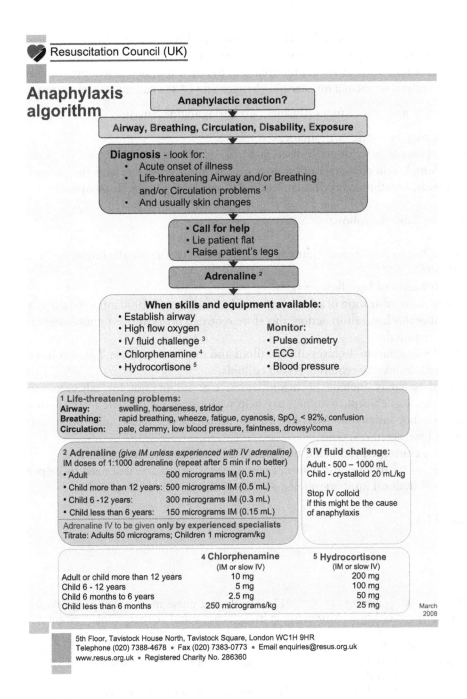

Figure 11.1 Resuscitation Council (UK) anaphylaxis flowchart

Reproduced with kind permission from the Resuscitation Council (UK).

- o breathing: shortness of breath, tachypnoea, wheeze, patient becoming tired, confusion, cyanosis (late sign), respiratory arrest;
- o circulation: signs of shock, tachycardia, hypotension, decreased level of consciousness, ischaemic myocardial changes and ECG changes, cardiac arrest;

- skin and/or mucosal changes (flushing, urticaria, angioedema);
  - o this may be subtle or dramatic;
  - o erythema (patchy or generalised rash);
  - o although skin changes can look serious, without problems with the patient's airway, breathing and circulation do not mean the patient has anaphylaxis.

Treatment includes the following:

- Stop the trigger, e.g. remove latex (gloves, Ambu masks), stop the infusion.
- Positioning.
- Administration of high flow oxygen.
- In adults, administration of adrenaline 0.5ml (500mcg) 1 in 1000 intra-muscularly. Remember this has a short action, therefore repeated doses at five-minute intervals may be required.
- IV fluid resuscitation. Boluses of crystalloid and monitor response. Large volumes of crystalloid may be required. Avoid colloids.
- Other drugs may include bronchodilators, e.g. salbutamol for wheeze; antihistamines, e.g. chlorphenamine, may help with histamine-mediated vasodilation and bronchoconstriction. Steroids, e.g. hydrocortisone, which may prevent or shorten protracted reactions.
- If you are concerned this could be asthma, treat as life-threatening asthma.
- In the event of airway obstruction, early tracheal intubation will need to be performed. If tracheal intubation fails, a surgical airway may be required.

See Figure 11.1.

References

Bull ER. Mason C. Junior FD *et al.* (2017). Developing nurse medication safety training in a health partnership in Mozambique using behavioural science. Globalization and Health. 13. 45. DOI: https://doi.org/10.1186/s12992-017-0265-1.

Cavell G. Nicholls J. Rehman B *et al.* (2014). Good practice for drug calculations: a step-by-step guide for nurses, doctors and all other healthcare professionals. Newbury, Berkshire: Baxter Healthcare Ltd.

Feleke SA. Mulatu MA. Yesmaw YS. (2015). Medication administration error: magnitude and associated factors among nurses in Ethiopia. BMC Nursing. 14. 53. DOI: https://doi.org/10.1186/s12912-015-0099-1.

Intensive Care Society. (2017). Medication concentrations in adult critical care areas. Jan. 2017. Version 2.2. London: Intensive Care Society and Faculty of Intensive Care Medicine.

Raza UZ. Latif S. Naseer A *et al.* (2016). Introducing a structured prescription form improves the quality of handwritten prescriptions in limited resource setting of developing countries. Journal of Evaluation in Clinical Practice. 22. 5. 714–720.

Resuscitation Council (UK). (2016). Chapter 12: Resuscitation in special circumstances. In: Advanced life support. 7th Edition. London: Resuscitation Council (UK).

Rowe AK. De Savigny D. Lanata CF. Victoria CG. (2005). How can we achieve and maintain high-quality performance of healthcare workers in low-resource settings? The Lancet. 366. 1026–1035.

World Health Organization. (2007). Look-alike, sound-alike medication names. Patient Safety Solutions. 1. 1. Available at: www.who.int/patientsafety/solutions/patientsafety/PS-Solution1.pdf.

World Health Organization. (2017). Medication without harm – global patient safety challenge on medication safety. Geneva: The World Health Organization.

World Health Organization. (2018). Medication without harm: WHO's third global patient safety challenge. Available at: www.who.int/patientsafety/medication-safety/en/.

12 In-hospital resuscitation

Critically ill patients are at risk of cardio-respiratory arrest and all hospitals should have approved resuscitation guidelines and training for staff. Hospitals may follow current international or regional resuscitation guidelines and the skills and emergency equipment available may vary, due to:

- limited availability emergency equipment;
- frequency at which equipment is checked;
- equipment may differ from what you have used previously, for example hand-held paddles for manual defibrillation;
- training of staff and in the use of equipment may be limited.

During your induction you should be made aware of the actions in an emergency (calling resuscitation team, location of emergency equipment), training in the resuscitation equipment and protocols used.

Each critical care unit must have an emergency trolley which includes essential emergency equipment (Box 12.1). This list is not exhaustive and may vary depending on the types of patients admitted, for example a critical care unit that accepts paediatric patients must have paediatric resuscitation equipment available.

Box 12.1   Emergency cardiac arrest equipment

- Personal protective equipment.
- Sharps box.
- Defibrillator.
- Depending on the type of defibrillator self-adhesive pads, pads or gel.
- Airway and breathing:

    - Portable oxygen.
    - Portable suction with a rigid suction catheter (Yankeur) and assorted sized tracheal suction catheters.
    - Oxygen mask with reservoir bag (bag, valve mask).

- o   Clear face masks (sizes 3, 4, 5).
- o   Oropharyngeal airways (sizes 2, 3, 4).
- o   Nasopharyngeal airways (sizes 6 and 7).
- o   Laryngeal mask airways.
- o   Lubricating gel.
- o   Oxygen tubing.
- o   Magill forceps.
- o   Stethoscope.
- o   Intubation equipment (as outlined in Chapter 13).

- Circulation:

  - o   ECG electrodes.
  - o   Razor.
  - o   IV cannulas (assorted sizes).
  - o   IV dressings.
  - o   Selection of needles and syringes.
  - o   Tape.
  - o   Gauze.
  - o   Arterial blood gas syringes.
  - o   Intra-osseous device and needles.
  - o   Abbo catheters/central line.
  - o   Saline ampoules.

- Drugs:

  - o   IV fluids (Hartmann's (Ringer's Solution), 5% dextrose. 0.9% sodium chloride).
  - o   IV giving sets.
  - o   Emergency drugs (adrenaline 1 in 10000, atropine, amiodarone) either ampoules or pre-filled syringes.

The sequence of actions after an in-hospital cardiac arrest depends on the following factors (Resuscitation Council (UK), 2016):

- location (clinical/non-clinical; monitored/unmonitored patient);
- skills of the first responders;
- number of responders available;
- equipment available;
- hospital response, e.g. cardiac arrest team.

Critical care nurses may be required to respond to cardiac arrest calls on wards as part of the cardiac arrest team. In consequence, your role will be determined by the situation. In critical care, patients are likely to be monitored, which will allow for clinical deterioration and cardio-respiratory arrest to be identified rapidly (Resuscitation Council (UK), 2016).

Figure 12.1 outlines the initial management of a collapsed patient.

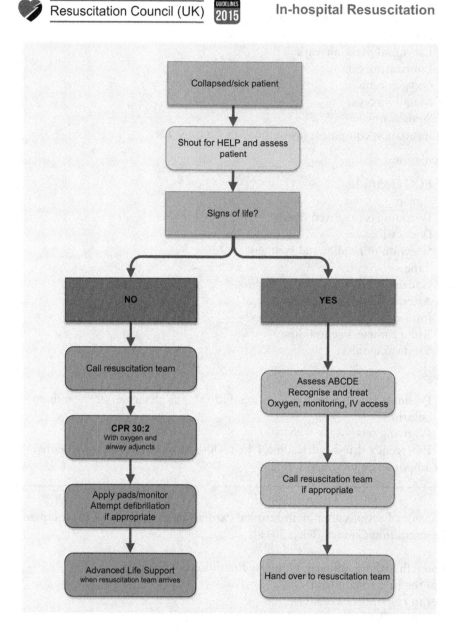

Figure 12.1 In-hospital resuscitation algorithm

Reproduced with the kind permission of the Resuscitation Council (UK).

Step 1: Maintain your personal safety.

- As you approach the patient, put on PPE especially if the patient has a suspected or confirmed infection.
- Be careful of sharps that may be left lying around; any sharps should be immediately disposed of in an approved sharps box.
- Be careful if you need to move an unconscious, collapsed patient.
- Take care if the patient has been exposed to poisoning, e.g. organophosphates that can be absorbed through the skin or respiratory tract.

Step 2: Check for a response.

- Gently shake the patient's shoulders and ask them loudly 'Are you all right?'. This procedure is known as the 'shake and shout'.
- If other staff are immediately available, call for emergency equipment.
- If the patient does not respond:
  - turn the patient onto their back;
  - open the airway using a head, tilt chin lift or jaw thrust if you are concerned about a cervical spine injury;
  - while keeping the airway open:
    - look, listen and feel for breathing and simultaneously check for a carotid pulse (if you are not trained to check for a carotid pulse, look for 'signs of life');
    - take no more than ten seconds;
    - agonal breathing (gasping or occasional breaths) is common in the initial stages of cardiac arrest and should not be confused with normal breathing.

Step 3A: If there are signs of life or a carotid pulse.

- Assess the patient using the A–E approach (Chapter 10) and call for urgent help.
- Do not leave the patient unattended.

Step 3B: If there are no signs of life or no carotid pulse.

- Immediately start cardio-pulmonary resuscitation (CPR):
  - Thirty chest compressions and two ventilations using a bag, valve mask (also known as a self-inflating bag), with reservoir attached to high flow oxygen.
    - Chest compressions should be performed by placing the heel of your hand in the centre of the chest. Place the other hand on top.
    - Ensure high-quality chest compressions by achieving a depth of 5–6 cm and a rate of 100–120 compressions per minute.
    - Allow the chest to fully recoil and minimise any interruptions to chest compressions.
    - You may need to raise or lower the bed height to achieve the best position for chest compressions.

- o Chest compressions can be tiring, therefore the rescuer should be changed regularly (approximately every two minutes).
- o Get a colleague to call the resuscitation team and bring the emergency equipment to the bedside.
- o Work as a team; secure the patient's airway using an oropharyngeal airway, LMA or intubation (Chapter 13). This will depend on the skills of the team and equipment available.
- o If the patient is attached to a mechanical ventilator, increase the oxygen to 100% and set a mandatory mode of ventilation to deliver 10–12 breaths per minute.

- When the defibrillator arrives, do not stop chest compressions; apply the leads/pads around the nurse performing chest compressions.
- Once the defibrillator is attached and switched on, stop chest compressions and assess the rhythm (see below).
- Depending on the rhythm, this will determine the course of action. Shockable rhythms are ventricular fibrillation (VF) and pulseless ventricular tachycardia (VT). Non-shockable rhythms are pulseless electrical activity (PEA) and asystole. The rhythm check should take no longer than five to ten seconds.
- Immediately following defibrillation or confirmation of a non-shockable rhythm chest compressions should immediately commence for two minutes.
- During this time the airway should be secured if not already done. IV or IO access achieved (Chapter 18), prepare or administer any drugs and look for reversible causes of cardiac arrest. Reversible causes include:

- o hypoxia;
- o hypovolaemia;
- o hypo/hyperkalaemia and metabolic disorders;
- o hypothermia;
- o tension pneumothorax;
- o cardiac tamponade;
- o toxins (drugs);
- o thrombosis.

See Figure 12.2.

Step 4: Return of spontaneous circulation (ROSC):

- CPR should only be stopped during a two-minute cycle if there are signs of life, e.g. regular breathing or movement. If a pulse is present, immediately assess the patient using the A–E approach (see Figure 12.3).

Vascular access

Vascular access is outlined in Chapter 18. All cardiac arrest drugs can be given via the IV or IO route. Following administration of any drug, ensure that a large 'flush'/bolus of saline is given after to ensure the drug reaches the central circulatory system.

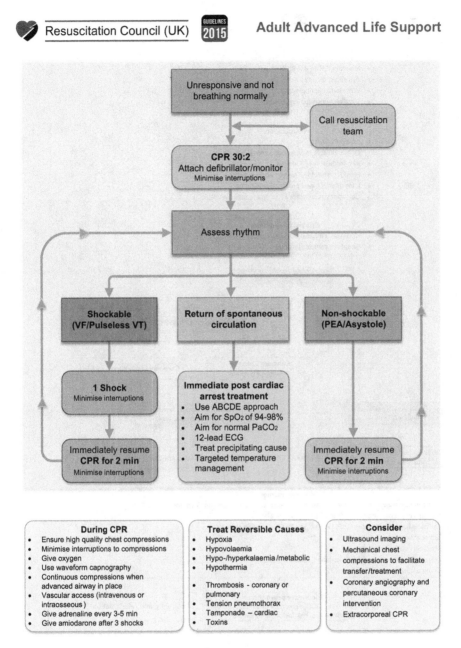

Figure 12.2 Adult advanced life support algorithm

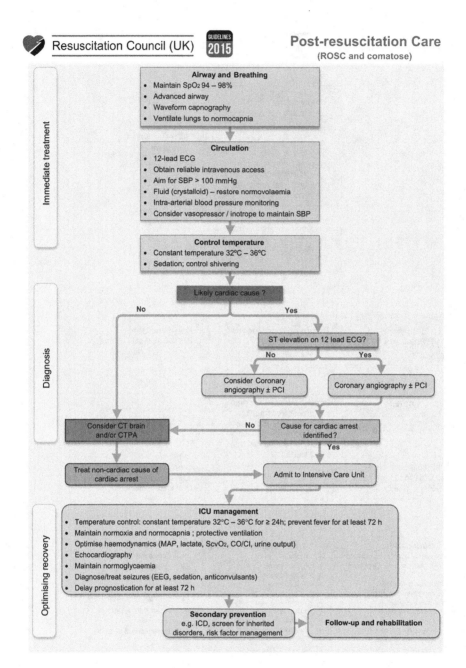

Figure 12.3 Return of spontaneous circulation care

Reproduced with kind permission from the Resuscitation Council (UK).

Drugs

Commonly used drugs in cardiac arrest are:

- adrenaline 1mg 1 in 10000;
- amiodarone 300mg.

Adrenaline

Shockable (VF/VT): Adrenaline in cardiac arrest should be given after the third shock once chest compressions have been resumed. Then every three to five minutes thereafter.

Non-Shockable (PEA/Asystole): Given as soon as circulatory access is obtained. Then repeated every three to five minutes thereafter. There should be no interruptions in chest compressions to secure IV/IO access or give drugs.

Amiodarone

Amiodarone is an anti-arrhythmic used to treat refractory VF or VT. The dose is 300mg bolus IV diluted in 5% dextrose to a volume of 20ml. It is given during chest compressions after three defibrillation attempts. A further dose of 150mg may be given if Ventricular Fibrillation (VF)/Ventricular Tachycardia (VT) persists after five defibrillation attempts (Resuscitation Council (UK), 2016).

Cardiac arrest rhythms

Ventricular fibrillation (VF)

Ventricular fibrillation (VF) is a bizarre irregular waveform (Figure 12.4), with uncoordinated electrical activity and no recognisable QRS complexes. VF can be coarse or fine. The treatment of VF is defibrillation.

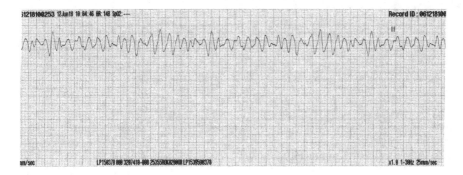

Figure 12.4 Ventricular fibrillation

Pulseless ventricular tachycardia (VT)

There are two types of ventricular tachycardia (VT): pulsed or pulseless. In a patient with a cardiac output (pulse) see the emergency tachycardia section below. Whereas for a patient that is pulseless the treatment is defibrillation.

There are two types:

- Monomorphic: A broad complex rhythm (Figure 12.5), rapid rate and has a constant QRS morphology.
- Polymorphic: Torsades de pointes (TdP) is rarely seen, but is associated with hypokalaemia and/or hypomagnesaemia.

Pulseless electrical activity (PEA)

PEA is a non-shockable rhythm, where there are clinical signs of a cardiac arrest (unconscious, apnoeic and no cardiac output), but the ECG looks normal and compatible with life (Figure 12.6).

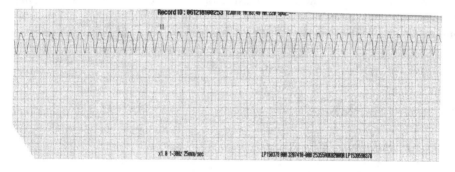

Figure 12.5 Ventricular tachycardia

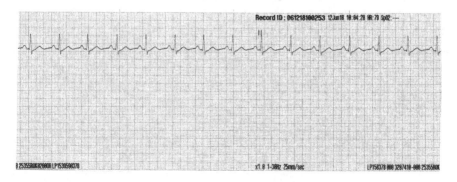

Figure 12.6 Pulseless electrical activity

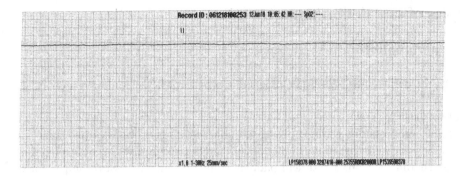

Figure 12.7 Asystole

Asystole

Asystole is rarely a flat line (Figure 12.7); there are sometimes P waves visible but never QRS complexes. It is important to check the leads are correctly attached and the monitor is working. In older monitors when a lead becomes detached you see a linear flat line, whereas with new monitors if a lead becomes detached a broken line appears to tell you. Asystole is a non-shockable rhythm.

Defibrillation

Traditionally external defibrillators used hand-held paddles; however, increasingly self-adhesive pads are being used in HIC, which means healthcare workers from HIC often have less experience of using hand-held paddles.

With hand-held paddles one should be placed to the right of the sternum and the other over the apex of the heart, lateral and inferior to the left nipple (MHRA, 2017) (Box 12.1). Sometimes the paddles are marked 'apex' and 'sternum'. When using paddles, it is important to maintain good electrical contact. Gel pads are highly conductive and placed between the paddle and the patient's chest. They should not touch each other during defibrillation. When using paddles you must press hard – approximately 8kg of pressure needs to be used. When using paddles on children, different sized paddles will need to be used. This may be an attachment which is placed onto adult paddles.

Self-adhesive pads are applied in the same position as outlined above. It is important to note there are currently no international standards on self-adhesive pad connections; therefore, you will need to check they fit the defibrillator connector.

The use of a precordial thump has a very low success rate for cardioversion of a shockable rhythm (Resuscitation Council (UK), 2016). This should only be considered if a defibrillator is not immediately available in a monitored VF/VT cardiac arrest.

Principles of safe defibrillation

Safety is paramount

- Ideally, the defibrillator should be plugged in when not in use and have a charged battery.
- Confirm cardiac arrest.
- Continue compressions while applying self-adhesive pads or monitoring leads.
- Ideally stop chest compressions for no longer than five seconds when confirming the cardiac rhythm. If using hand-held paddles, you can 'quickly' assess the patient's cardiac rhythm by applying the paddles to the patient's chest. This is termed 'quick look'. The defibrillator will need to be in 'paddles' mode (not lead II). 3 lead monitoring should then be applied during CPR.
- If a shockable rhythm is identified:
  - Continue effective CPR and ensure there is a coupling agent (e.g. gel pads or self-adhesive pads are applied to the patient's bare chest). Ensure the chest is dry and any medication patches on the chest have been removed.
  - Gloves routinely used in clinical settings do not provide protection from electrical current; therefore, safety during defibrillation is paramount.
  - Self-adhesive pads are likely to cause less risk of sparks and fire than hand-held paddles; however, the following precautions should be taken regardless of method used:
    - Remove any sources of oxygen, e.g. masks, at least 1m away from the patient's chest.
    - You can leave a self-inflating bag connected to an ETT or you can remove it and ensure it is at least 1m away.
    - If a patient is attached to a ventilator, you can leave them attached, as long as the FiO_2 has been increased to 1.0, a mandatory mode with adequate tidal volumes has been set. If you decide to remove the patient from the ventilator during defibrillation, ensure the tubing is at least 1m away; alternatively switch the ventilator off and use a self-inflating bag, as a disconnected ventilator will generate significant oxygen flows when disconnected.
  - The designated person:
    - selects an appropriate level on the defibrillator;
    - selects charge either on the defibrillator or via the paddles;
    - ensures nobody is touching the patient, the defibrillator operator shouts, 'stand clear' and performs a complete visual check of the bed area. Once safe the individual then delivers a shock. Nobody should be touching the patient; this includes holding IV fluids.
    - immediately following the shock, resumes CPR and returns the paddles to the defibrillator.

- Defibrillator users should:
  - know how to select and deliver a shock safely;
  - know how to discharge a shock that is no longer required;
  - be appropriately trained to recognise cardiac arrest rhythms and appropriate actions.

(MHRA, 2017; Resuscitation Council (UK), 2016)

References

Medicines and Healthcare Products Regulatory Agency (MHRA) (2017). Defibrillators. Available at: http://info.mhra.gov.uk/learning/Defibrillators/player.html.

Resuscitation Council (UK). (2016). Advanced life support. 7th Edition. London: Resuscitation Council (UK).

13 | Airway management

Most patients admitted to critical care require mechanical ventilation and have an endotracheal tube (ETT) or tracheostomy in place. Nurses need to be able to manage a variety of airway emergencies, ranging from attending a ward cardiac arrest and managing an airway, a patient arriving in critical care requiring emergency intubation to managing a tracheostomy in a long-term ventilation patient. In this chapter, the basic principles of airway management, including airway adjuncts, rapid sequence induction and tracheostomy care are covered.

Basic techniques

An airway obstruction can be partial or complete. Potential causes of airway obstruction are outlined in Box 13.1. In the event of severe obstruction follow the emergency sequence outlined in Figure 13.1. To remove secretions use a rigid suction catheter to remove fluids and/or turn the patient onto their side (lateral position) in order to allow fluids to drain out. When using a rigid suction catheter ensure the tip always remain visible.

Box 13.1   Causes of airway obstruction

- Central nervous system depression.
- Blood.
- Vomitus.
- Foreign body.
- Direct trauma to the face.
- Epiglottitis.
- Pharyngeal swelling, e.g. infection oedema.
- Laryngospasm.
- Bronchospasm.
- Bronchial secretions.
- Blocked tracheostomy or laryngectomy.

(Resuscitation Council (UK), 2016)

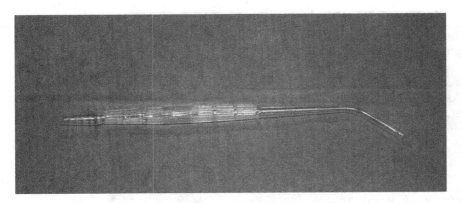

Picture 13.1 Rigid suction catheter

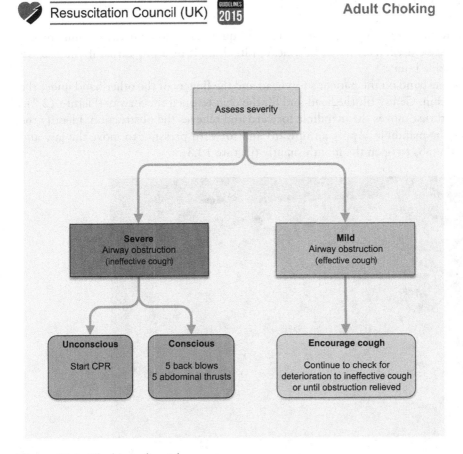

Figure 13.1 Choking algorithm

Reproduced with kind permission from the Resuscitation Council (UK).

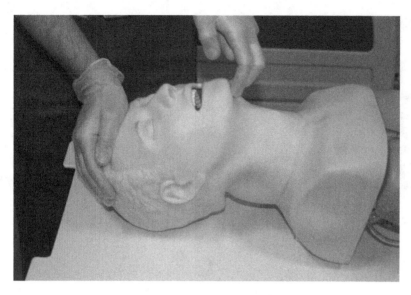

Picture 13.2 Head, tilt, chin lift

Prior to the arrival of specialist emergency equipment, basic airway opening procedures must be used. This could be a head, tilt, chin lift or a jaw thrust if you suspect cervical spine injury.

Place one hand on the patient's forehead and the fingers of the other hand under the patient's chin. Gently tilt the head and lift the chin to open the airway (Picture 13.2).

A jaw thrust moves the mandible forward and relieves the obstruction. Identify the angle of the mandible. Apply an upward and forward pressure to move the jaw and use the thumbs to open the mouth slightly (Picture 13.3).

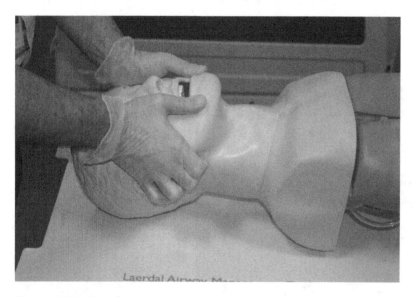

Picture 13.3 Jaw thrust

Following any airway procedure check the airway remains patent by looking, listening and feeling. If the airway is still obstructed, look and remove any solid foreign body in the mouth with forceps or suction. If there is no visible obstruction, follow the choking algorithm (Figure 13.1).

Airway adjuncts

Airway adjuncts assist in maintaining an open airway. Airway adjuncts include (Picture 13.4):

- nasopharyngeal airway (NPA);
- oropharyngeal airway (OPA)

Both NPA and OPA prevent soft palate obstruction and backward tongue displacement in an unconscious patient, but basic airway opening procedures including a head, tilt chin lift or jaw thrust may still be needed (Resuscitation Council (UK), 2016).

NP airways may be lifesaving in patients with clenched jaws (trismus), fitting, or maxillofacial trauma. However, they must be used with caution in patients with suspected fracture of the base of skull and insertion may cause epistaxis. To insert an NPA:

- Lubricate airway using a water soluble jelly.
- Insert the airway bevel end first, vertically along the floor of the nose with a slight twisting action. Try the right nostril first; if you are unable to pass the airway, stop and try the left (Picture 13.5).
- Once in place, check patency and ventilation (Picture 13.6).

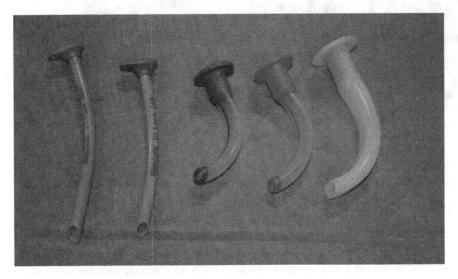

Picture 13.4 Airway adjuncts

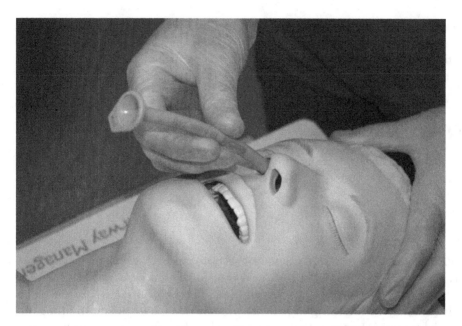

Picture 13.5 Insertion of an NPA

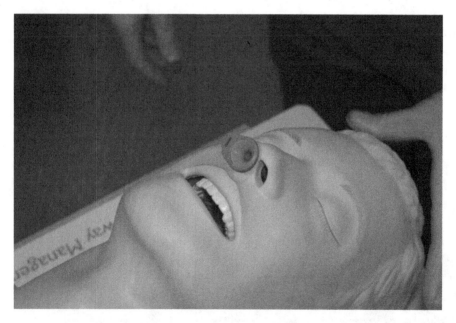

Picture 13.6 NPA in place

OPA is used in an unconscious patient only (GCS <8); attempting insertion in a semi-conscious patient may cause vomiting or laryngospasm. To insert an OPA:

- Estimate the size by selecting an airway with a length between the patient's incisors and the angle of jaw (Picture 13.7).
- Open the patient's mouth and ensure there is nothing visible.
- Introduce the airway past the teeth and gums 'upside down' (Picture 13.8).

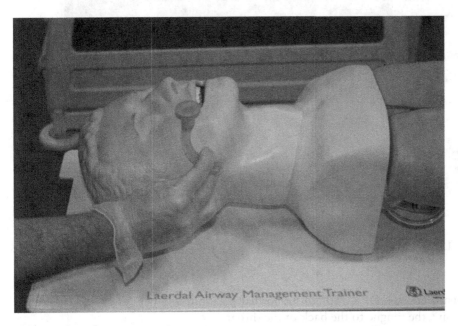

Picture 13.7 Estimating the size of an OPA

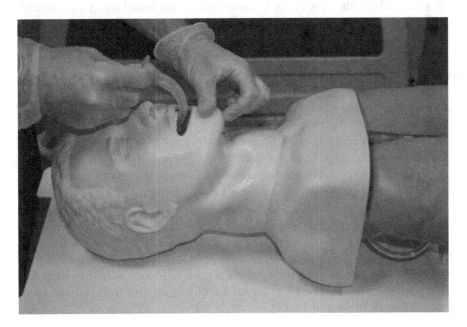

Picture 13.8 Insertion of an OPA

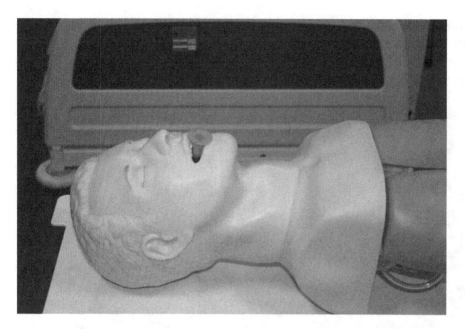

Picture 13.9 OPA in place

- Then rotate the OPA 180° to its normal position; this will lessen the chance of pushing the tongue to the back of the throat.
- If any reflect responses are seen, e.g. gagging, then remove the airway (Picture 13.9).
- After insertion, check the airway: look, listen and feel for breathing. You may still need to use a chin lift or jaw thrust to maintain a patent airway.

Advanced airway management

Advanced airway adjuncts include the laryngeal mask airway (LMA), I-Gel and the endo-tracheal tube.

The LMA and I-Gel are supraglottic airway devices. This means the airway adjunct sits above the larynx. They are often easier to insert than an ETT. Both airways do not guarantee protection of the airway and there is a risk of gastric aspiration. The patient must be deeply unconscious before attempting insertion of these airways. Insertion is deemed easy, and with a high success rate after a brief period of training they are often inserted by nurses, paramedics and medical staff in emergency situations, although they are routinely used in anaesthesia (Resuscitation Council (UK), 2016).

The LMA requires a cuff to be inflated, whereas the I-Gel has a 'jelly'-like material that does not require inflation. The I-Gel includes a bite block and an orogastric tube can be passed (Pictures 13.10 and 13.11).

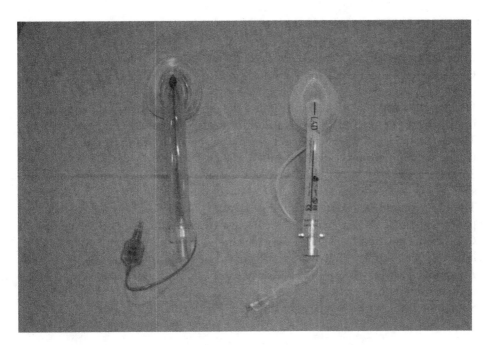

Picture 13.10 A laryngeal mask airway

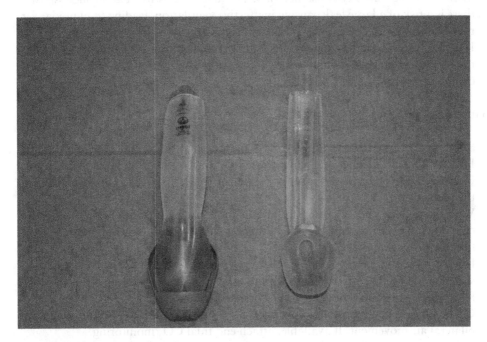

Picture 13.11 An I-Gel

To insert an LMA:

- Choose an appropriate size. Size 5 for adult males and size 4 for females.
- Check the cuff is deflated, apply lubricating gel to the outer face of the cuff area (the back).
- Holding the LMA like a pen, insert it into the mouth and advance the tip with the upper surface applied to the palate until it meets the posterior pharyngeal wall. Then press the mask backwards and downwards until resistance is felt.
- Connect the inflating syringe and inflate the cuff with air (40ml for a size 5 or 30ml for a size 4). Do not hold the LMA during inflation as the tube should lift slightly out of the mouth.
- The LMA should be inserted within 30 seconds; if there are any delays then the patient should be re-oxygenated with a bag, valve mask and insertion re-attempted.
- Confirm the position by listening over the chest during inflation and observing for bilateral air movement. If available, attach end tidal CO_2 monitoring.
- An audible leak may mean the LMA is not in position; a small leak is acceptable if chest rise is appropriate.
- Secure the LMA with a bandage or tape.

(Resuscitation Council (UK), 2016)

Limitations to the LMA include:

- In cases of high airway resistance or if the lungs are 'stiff', e.g. bronchospasm, there is a risk of a large leak causing ineffective ventilation, leading to hypoxia. Air may be forced into the patient's stomach increasing the risk of aspiration.
- If used in cardiac arrest, uninterrupted chest compressions can cause air leak from the LMA. If continuous compressions are not possible, return CPR ratio of 30 chest compressions to 2 ventilations.

To insert an I-Gel:

- Select an appropriately sized I-Gel – size 4 for most adults and size 3 for small adults.
- Lubricate the back, sides and front of the I-Gel cuff with a thin layer of lubricant.
- Holding the I-Gel, pass the tube, with the cuff outlet facing towards the chin of the patient.
- With the patient's head in the 'sniffing the morning air' position, gently press the chin down before inserting the I-Gel. Introduce the I-Gel into the mouth in a direction towards the hard palate.
- Do not force the airway during insertion. Glide the I-Gel downwards and backwards along the hard palate with a continuous but gentle push until resistance is felt. The device should now be in the correct position.
- Check for patency by listening over the chest during inflation and observing for bilateral air movement. If available, attach end tidal CO_2 monitoring.

(Resuscitation Council (UK), 2016)

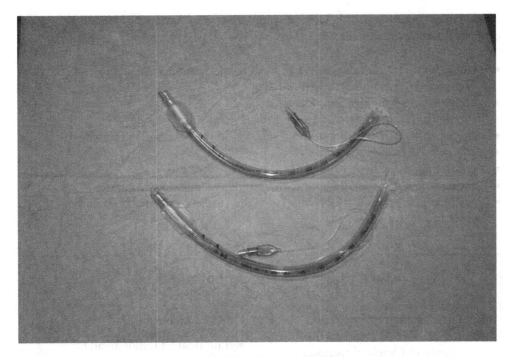

Picture 13.12 Adult ETT with cuff inflated and deflated

An ETT is inserted into the tracheal; the cuff creates an air-tight seal and is classed as the 'gold' standard in airway management. To insert an ETT this must be undertaken by a practitioner who is experienced in this procedure (Picture 13.12).

Rapid Sequence Induction (RSI) is used to insert an ETT, when there is risk of gastric aspiration. RSI involves:

- inducing loss of consciousness by the use of drugs;
- application of cricoid pressure;
- insertion of the ETT;
- confirmation of tube position.

The 'Six Ps' for RSI include:

- prepare;
- pre-oxygenation;
- pre-medication;
- paralysis;
- passage of endo-tracheal tube;
- post-intubation care.

Nurses may be required to help healthcare workers to intubate a patient. Box 13.2 outlines the equipment required. Prior to the procedure prepare by:

- working as a team to discuss the procedure and ensuring you all understand what is expected of each other;
- preparing/checking the equipment;
- stopping any enteral feed and aspirating the NG tube;
- ensuring the patient is monitored (ECG, blood pressure and pulse oximetry);
- checking IV access is patent;
- positioning the patient;
- checking and draw up any medications and labelling as appropriate;
- ensuring you have a working ventilator (pre-checks completed) and initial settings agreed.

Box 13.2   RSI equipment required

- Oxygen supply
- Effective suction (rigid suction catheter and tracheal suction catheters)
- Selection of OPAs and NPAs
- Lubricating gel
- Self-inflating bag (with reservoir)
- Catheter mount
- Magill forceps
- Two working laryngoscopes with selection of blades (2, 3, 4)
- Endotracheal tubes (sizes 7–9)
- Laryngeal mask airways
- Stylet, also termed introducer
- Bougie
- 10ml syringe to inflate the ETT cuff
- ETT ties
- Stethoscope

Other equipment:

- End tidal CO_2 monitoring
- Manometer to check cuff pressure
- Ventilator – switched on, ventilator tubing attached
- Drugs
- Patient monitoring
- Difficult airway equipment, this may include:

  o McCoy laryngoscope;
  o needle cricothyroidotomy set;
  o emergency surgical airway equipment.

The patient should be pre-oxygenated using a bag, valve, mask (BVM) or Water's Circuit +/– PEEP with 15l/min oxygen. Apply cricoid pressure; this should be applied from the moment the patient loses consciousness to the time the ETT has been passed, cuff inflated, and position verified. Cricoid pressure should only be removed when instructed to do so by the person inserting the tube.

Pre-medication sedation and paralysing agents are then administered. The ETT is then passed. The patient's condition should be monitored throughout for any changes. Post intubation:

- Ensure the patient's chest is moving bilaterally.
- Secure the tube using ties or tape.
- Auscultate the chest for air entry.
- Chest X-ray to confirm tube position.
- Attach the patient to the ventilator.
- Document the procedure including size of tube, length at teeth, grade of intubation.
- If available, measure cuff pressure and commence end-tidal carbon dioxide ($EtCO_2$) monitoring.
- Continue sedation +/– paralysing agents.
- Pass an oro- or naso-gastric tube.

Immediate potential complications following RSI are outlined in Box 13.3. Other complications include limited means of humidification, few nurses and anaesthetists resulting in ETT tube blockages (Towney & Ojara, 2008).

Box 13.3   Potential complications of intubation

- Right main bronchus intubation.
- Lacerated lips, tongue, pharynx or trachea.
- Vocal cord injury.
- Chipped teeth.
- Aspiration.
- Introduction of infection.
- ETT dislodgement.
- Obstruction.
- Pneumothorax.
- Equipment failure.
- Stomach full of air/vomiting.
- Hypoxia.
- Hypotension.
- Arrhythmias.

In resource limited environments, specialist tube securing devices, e.g. Anchor Fast or Thomas ETT tube holders, are unlikely to be unavailable. In consequence, nurses will need to secure ETT using ties. The following steps outline how to secure an ETT; this procedure may vary in units (Table 13.1).

Table 13.1 How to secure an ETT

Step 1: This is a two-person technique. Prior to releasing the ties, check the position of the tube. One nurse holds the ETT, while the second nurse releases the ties.

Step 2: Take the clean ties and have a short and long end.

Step 3: Wrap the ties around the ETT. Create a loop to pass the ties through (Picture 13.13).

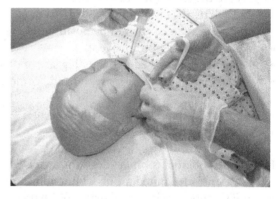

Picture 13.13 Securing ties to the ETT

Step 4: Pass the loose ends through the loop and pull tight. Tighten around the ETT, noting the position (Picture 13.14).

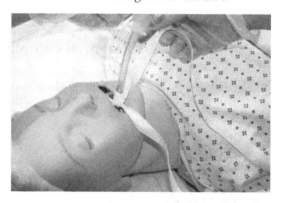

Picture 13.14 Securing ties to the ETT

Step 5: Pass the long tie around the neck and tie in a double knot. Check the ties are not too tight (Picture 13.15).

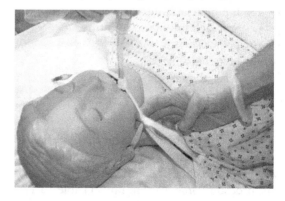

Picture 13.15 Securing ETT ties

Step 6: Confirm position of the ETT, re-assess patient and document care.

Humidification

The ETT passes the upper airway which warms, moistens and filers inspired air. In addition, oxygen is dry which dehydrates exposed membranes, making mucus and secretions more viscid (Woodrow, 2000). Humidification can be provided by either Heat Moisture Exchange (HME) and Heated Humidifiers (HH). A Cochrane Systematic Review (Gillies et al., 2017) reported 'no overall difference in the rates of airway blockage, pneumonia or death in adults who were ventilated through an HME compared to adults ventilated through a heated humidifier'. However, the quality of evidence was low, and further research is required. Within a resource limited environment it is advisable to use both an HME and HH; however, access to HMEs may be difficult as these are single-item use. In addition, evaporation of fluid from HH means they will need to be re-filled regularly and the increased environmental temperature may be a site for bacterial incubation and require high-level disinfection between patients (Restrepo & Walsh, 2012; Woodrow, 2000).

Extubation

Prior to extubation the patient should be assessed:

- conscious level (GCS >8);
- cough reflex;
- be on a spontaneous mode of ventilation with a low Positive End Expiratory Pressure (PEEP) and Pressure Support (PS);
- a rescue plan in case the procedure fails.

To remove an ETT (this is a two-person technique):

- Collect equipment.
- Obtain consent from the patient.
- Stop naso-gastric feed at least two hours prior to procedure.
- Wear PPE.
- Undo ETT ties, and hold ETT in place.
- Select appropriate sized suction catheter (see below). Attach suction catheter to suction tubing and switch on suction, checking the pressure is between 80 and 120mmHg.
- Disconnect the ETT from the ventilator and silence the ventilator alarms.
- Advance the suction catheter into the ETT until resistance is felt (this is the point the catheter tip has reached the carina), then remove 1–2cm.
- Apply continuous suction, while a second nurse deflates the cuff.
- Withdraw the ETT with the suction catheter in place and continuing to suction. This should take no longer than 10–15 seconds.
- Encourage the patient to cough, and suction any oral secretions with a rigid suction catheter.
- Commence oxygen therapy via a face mask.
- Reassure and assess the patient for any changes.
- Document the procedure.
- Dispose of any waste.

(Credland, 2016)

Tracheostomy

A tracheostomy tube (TT) is a surgical opening in the anterior wall of the trachea and the insertion of a tube. Reasons for insertions of TT include weaning from ventilation, tetanus, upper airway obstruction due to trauma of the mandible, laryngeal papillomas, Ludwig's angina, laryngotracheobronchitis, post-operative following thyroidectomy for a giant goitre, Guillain-Barré syndrome and severe head injury (Fasunla, 2010; Towney & Ojara, 2008). Although there is a paucity of evidence regarding when it is appropriate to insert a tracheostomy, the recognised benefits include:

- lower risk of laryngeal injury compared to prolonged intubation;
- improved comfort for the patient;
- assists with weaning from mechanical ventilation;
- improved tracheal secretion removal;
- enhanced patient communication;
- decreased sedation requirements.

Care of a tracheostomy tube

Tracheostomy tubes come in a variety of sizes and types. To reduce the risk of blockage some tracheostomy tubes have an inner tube which allows for the tube to be removed and cleaned (Leach, 2004).

Tracheostomy tubes need to be secured (Picture 13.16). To secure a tracheostomy tube either commercially available ties or ETT tapes can be used.

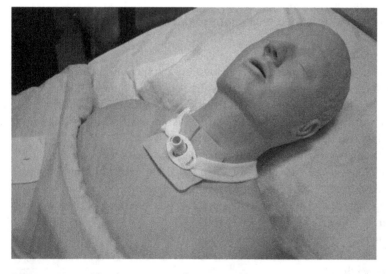

Picture 13.16 Tracheostomy tube secured

In resource limited environments TT may be secured using standard ETT tape; there are various methods to securing TT and may vary between units. The following procedure outlines how to secure a TT with ETT tapes (Table 13.2).

Table 13.2 How to secure a TT with ETT tapes

Step 1: Assemble the equipment.
- Two pieces of ETT tape
- Personal protective equipment
- Tracheostomy dressing if required
- Dressing pack
- Saline to clean site

Step 2: This is a two-person technique. Prior to releasing the ties, check the position of the tube. One nurse holds the TT, while the second nurse releases the ties.

Step 3: Pass the ties through the TT flange. Pass the ends through the loop and tighten (Picture 13.17).

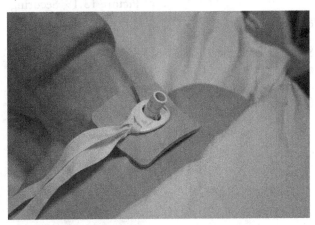

Picture 13.17 Securing ties to the TT

Step 4: Repeat for both sides of the TT (Picture 13.18).

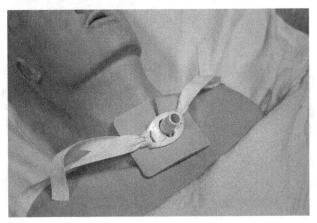

Picture 13.18 Securing ties to the TT

Table 13.2 Continued

Step 5: Take one of the long ties, pass around the patient's neck and tie off with the short tie on the other side (Picture 13.19).

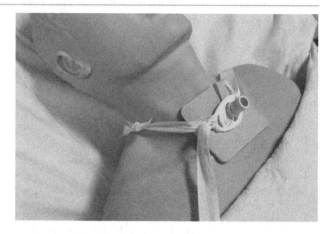

Picture 13.19 Securing TT ties

Step 6: Repeat.

Step 7: Check the TT ties are not too tight and re-assess the patient (Picture 13.20).

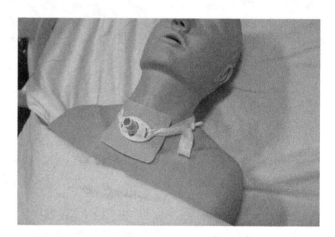

Picture 13.20 Securing TT ties

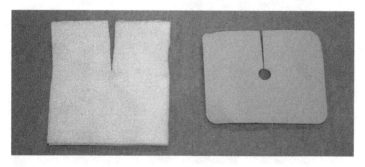

Picture 13.21 Examples of improvised and commercial 'keyhole' tracheostomy dressings

Tracheostomy sites should be dressed. Either an improvised or keyhole tracheostomy dressing (Picture 13.21) can be used. The site should be observed for signs of infection.

Blocked tracheostomy

A blocked TT is an airway emergency. Emergency equipment must always be at the patient's bedside, this includes:

- oxygen, BVM and oxygen masks;
- working suction and selection of suction catheters;
- sterile water;
- two spare tracheostomy tubes (one the same size as the one the patient currently has inserted and the other one size smaller);
- scissors;
- 10ml syringe;
- tracheal dilators;
- artery forceps;
- spare ties;
- suture cutter;
- lubricating gel;
- gloves, aprons and eye protection;
- access to emergency airway and cardiac arrest equipment.

In the event of a blocked tracheostomy, Figure 13.2 outlines the emergency treatment to be undertaken immediately.

Discharge planning

The decision to insert a tracheostomy in a resource limited environment is likely to increase the patient's stay, as ward areas may have few nurses to observe and respond to patients, have limited experience in nursing a patient with a tracheostomy and with limited equipment including suction machines (Towney & Ojara, 2008). In consequence, it may not be appropriate to discharge a patient to the ward with a TT in place.

Suctioning

Intubation impairs the cough reflex by bypassing the normal respiratory barriers. As a result, secretions accumulate in the lower respiratory tract, potentially reducing or obstructing the airway and allowing bacterial growth (Woodrow, 2000). The accumulation of secretions causes airway obstruction, hypoxia and acidosis; suctioning removes secretions, but can also introduce infection, cause trauma, hypoxia, atelectasis and bradycardias (Woodrow, 2000; Wang et al., 2017).

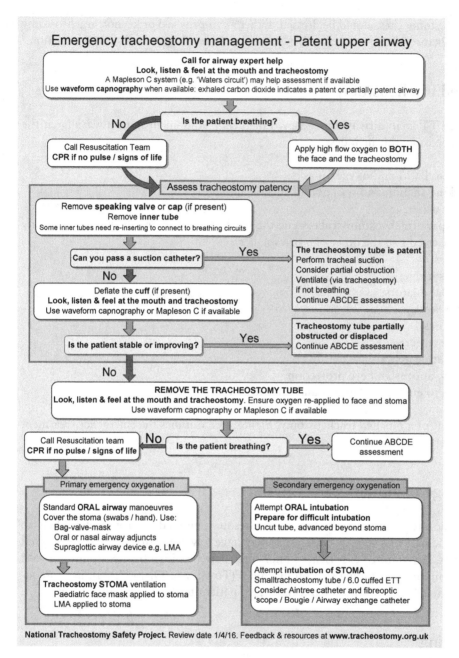

Figure 13.2 Emergency tracheostomy algorithm

Reproduced with kind permission from Wiley.

Selecting the appropriately sized suction catheter reduces hypoxia and atelectasis. To select the appropriate sized suction catheter use the following calculation.

Suction catheter size (French) = 2 × (size of ETT or TT mm) − 2

Suction using either an open or closed suction system may be used to clear tracheal secretions. Access to closed suction systems may not be possible due to the expense. When using open suction catheters there is an increased risk of introducing an infection as the ventilator circuit is broken. In addition, the patient may become hypoxic and take a longer time to recover post-suctioning due to the loss of oxygen and PEEP when disconnected from the ventilator.

Saline and suctioning

Maintaining a patent airway is a core role of a critical care nurse; this includes being able to suction an ETT or TT to remove secretions. A common but dated procedure involves the installation of saline prior to tracheal suctioning to loosen secretions. The proposed rational is to prevent/remove dried secretions which cause encrustation and potential blockage of ETT or TT. This practice is often based on a clinician's experience or as a routine, ritualistic procedure. The proposed rationale for using saline to 'loosen secretions' has no evidence base and has shown to reduce the PaO_2 by causing bronchospasm and a barrier for effective gas exchange (Woodrow, 2000). Wang et al. (2017) completed a meta-analysis of randomised control trials relating to the use of installation of normal saline. They concluded the use of saline does not provide any clinical benefits and can lead to complications including the reduction in oxygen saturations up to five minutes after suctioning. In consequence, the management of secretions involves regular suctioning as indicated, nebulisers and humidification.

References

Credland N. (2016). How to remove an endotracheal tube. Nursing Standard. 30. 36. 31–33.
Fasunla AJ. (2010). Challenges of tracheostomy in patients managed for severe tetanus in developing countries. International Journal of Preventive Medicine. 1. 3. 176–181.
Gillies D. Todd DA. Foster JP. Batuwitage BT. (2017). Heat and moisture exchangers versus heated humidifiers for mechanically ventilated adults and children. Cochrane Database of Systematic Reviews. 9. DOI: 10.1002/14651858.CD004711.pub3.
Restrepo RD. Walsh BK. (2012). Humidification during invasive and non-invasive mechanical ventilation. Respiratory Care. 57. 5. 782–788.
Resuscitation Council (UK). (2016). Immediate life support. 3rd Edition. London: Resuscitation Council (UK).
Towney RM. Ojara S. (2008). Practice of intensive care in rural Africa: an assessment of data from Northern Uganda. African Health Sciences. 8. 1. 61–64.
Wang CH. Tsai JC. Chen SF et al. (2017). Normal saline installation before suctioning: a meta-analysis of randomised controlled trials. Australian Critical Care. 30. 260–265.
Woodrow P. (2000). Chapter 5: Airway management. In: Woodrow P. Intensive Care Nursing: A framework for practice. Abingdon, Oxon; New York: Routledge.

14 Oxygen and mechanical ventilation

Oxygen and a patent airway are essential for life. Within a resource limited environment access to supplementary oxygen and mechanical ventilation can be the difference between life and death due to simple and preventable conditions. A lack of basic equipment including pulse oximetry, oxygen and skilled healthcare professionals have resulted in individuals and families having to decide on unsafe treatment or no treatment at all (Lifebox, 2017).

Access to supplementary oxygen may be only provided in areas where acutely ill patients are cohorted, e.g. emergency departments, acute bays on wards, theatres, recovery and critical care units and is only provided to those deemed most at risk. Oxygen may be provided from a wall supply, oxygen concentrators or oxygen cylinders. Regular access to oxygen has been identified as a challenge and the provision of oxygen cylinders is expensive and logistically difficult (Ojara & Towney, 2007). This means oxygen may be rationed; in this case pulse oximetry and patient assessment will need to be used to try to conserve supplies and prevent hypoxia. Each method of oxygen delivery system will have advantages and disadvantages (Table 14.1) and considerations when using oxygen concentrators and cylinders are outlined in Table 14.2.

Table 14.1 Advantages and disadvantages of using oxygen cylinders and concentrators in a resource limited environment

Characteristics	Cylinders	Concentrators
Capital cost	High when regulator and flowmeter costs included	High
Running cost	High particularly if leakage is significant	Low if power is inexpensive High if power is expensive
Ease of use	Training required	Considerable training required
Reliability	Good	Good on selected models
Physical robustness	Good	Fair
Regular maintenance	Needed	Needed

Table 14.1 Continued

Characteristics	Cylinders	Concentrators
Technical repairs	Needed (e.g. regulators to minimise leakage)	Needed (maintenance staff require specialist training)
Electricity	Not needed	Needed
Continuity of oxygen delivery	Liable to run out	Good if power is available
Portability	Poor for large cylinders	Good
Supply system	Transport needed Ordering needed	Transport not needed Ordering not needed

Source: Howie *et al.*, 2009

Table 14.2 Considerations when using oxygen concentrators and cylinders

Oxygen concentrator	The type of concentrator used will determine the maximum flow rates/oxygen concentrations. Factors which may affect the use of oxygen concentrators include: • Many require a continuous electricity supply. • Different countries use different voltage systems resulting in concentrators not working or alarming low pressure. • Elevated ambient temperature and humidity can result in concentrators not working.
Oxygen cylinder	Safety of cylinders when in use/stored, i.e. are they free standing or are they secured using an appropriate stand? Are empty cylinders kept separate from full cylinders? Are all cylinders kept in an area away from flammable liquids or other combustible materials? Who is responsible for changing cylinders and how is this done? Do you have emergency cylinders available? Are appropriate signs displayed prohibiting smoking/naked flames near cylinders? Poorly maintained cylinders and flow gauges result in leakage and increased oxygen consumption. When working with oxygen cylinders, you will need to work out the oxygen consumption so you can plan for the changes in the cylinder.

Sources: Peel *et al.*, 2013; Howie *et al.*, 2009

The challenges of oxygen administration are not only limited to the availability of oxygen. Healthcare professionals' understanding and perception of how oxygen is used can influence practice. Adipa *et al.* (2015) conducted a qualitative exploration of ward nurses' perspectives on using oxygen therapy in Ghana and identified the following challenges when initiating and using oxygen:

- Initiation of oxygen therapy may be at the direction of the doctor, which resulted in a delay in initiating this treatment.
- There may be no access to pulse oximetry or blood gas analyser to measure oxygen saturations and arterial blood gases. In consequence, assessment may be based on the patient's signs and symptoms and physiological observations. With few pulse oximeters they may need to be shared between patients, preventing continuous monitoring of the patient's condition.
- Nurses often receive minimal education on the use of oxygen and may administer the amount that they think is appropriate and use their discretion to initiate, increase and stop therapy. However, the nurses in this study did have insight into this knowledge deficit and requested in-service training to correct this.
- A lack of protocols to guide the delivery of oxygen therapy resulted in nurses waiting for patients to show signs of respiratory distress before initiating oxygen therapy and due to a lack of knowledge sometimes discontinued the therapy when the patient keeps removing it.
- Consumables such as oxygen masks and nasal prongs had to be purchased by families, who sometimes cannot afford this, so often they had to re-use them between patients.
- Oxygen therapy was provided by cylinders with limited nurses available; cylinders may run out and not be noticed. In addition, when waiting for cylinders to be replaced, nurses reported having to hand ventilate the patient for 10 to 20 minutes until an orderly changed the flow meter, as they are not trained to do this.

Identifying a patient who is hypoxic involves clinical assessment, pulse oximetry and arterial blood gases. In a resource limited environment, access to these interventions may be variable.

Clinical assessment

Assessment of a patient's respiratory system includes:

- ensuring the patient has a patent airway;
- looking for signs of respiratory distress (e.g. use of accessory muscles, sweating);
- assessing the respiratory rate, rhythm and depth. An increase is an indication of illness;
- observing for any signs of deformity to the chest, including abdominal distension that may splint the patient's diaphragm and prevent breathing;
- recording the amount of oxygen and type of oxygen delivery system used;
- assessing the patient's oxygen saturation (SpO_2);
- auscultating the chest to note any changes;
- checking the position of the trachea at the supra-sternal notch. A deviation may indicate a mediastinal shift due to a pneumothorax, pleural effusion or lung fibrosis.

(Smith & Bowden, 2017; Resuscitation Council (UK), 2016);
Towney & Ojara, 2008)

Hypoxia

The WHO recognises hypoxia is a significant risk for hospitalised patients. While the use of a pulse oximeter is universally accepted as essential when providing anaesthesia (WHO, 2009), in critical care the use can be variable and dependent on availability. Best practice requires every ventilated patient or patient at risk must have continuous pulse oximetry and monitoring.

The measurement of oxygen saturations of haemoglobin via a pulse oximeter is an essential part of patient assessment and monitoring, and deemed critical patient safety equipment (WHO, 2011; Lemanski, 2016; Towney & Ojara, 2008). The use of a pulse oximeter should be used with other vital signs to assess a patient's condition. If the patient has a low SpO_2 <95% a full assessment should be immediately conducted. Although developed for use in the operating theatre, the WHO hypoxia algorithm (Figure 14.1) provides a logical framework to follow and is useful when responding to a desaturating patient on a ventilator. Additional considerations when responding to a desaturating patient who is ventilated may include alarms which have alerted you to a problem.

Pulse oximeters provide two numerical values, the oxygen saturation of the haemoglobin in the blood and the pulse rate (WHO, 2011). In critical care, there may be limited monitoring, and a pulse oximeter may be the only equipment you have to look after a critically ill patient. Pulse oximeter readings do not provide information about respiratory rate, tidal volume, cardiac output or blood pressure. Therefore assessment, monitoring and recording of these additional observations are essential (WHO, 2009). When using a pulse oximeter (WHO, 2009):

- check it is plugged in/batteries charged;
- when you turn the oximeter on allow it to run through the internal calibration;
- select the appropriate probe. Probes are delicate and need to be used correctly and should be used where they are designed for, e.g. in a peripherally shut-down patient, using a finger probe on an ear should be avoided. Caution must also be exercised when using wraparound probes (normally children) as these may constrict the blood flow to the finger;
- remove any nail varnish before applying the probe;
- if possible, avoid using the arm with the blood pressure cuff on; when the cuff inflates it will interfere with the pulse oximeter signal;
- check you have a good trace;
- if in doubt, use your clinical judgement and assess your patient using the A–E approach;
- always make sure the alarms are on.

Alarms may include:

- low saturation (hypoxia), e.g. Spo2 <90%;
- no pulse detected;
- low pulse rate;
- high pulse rate.

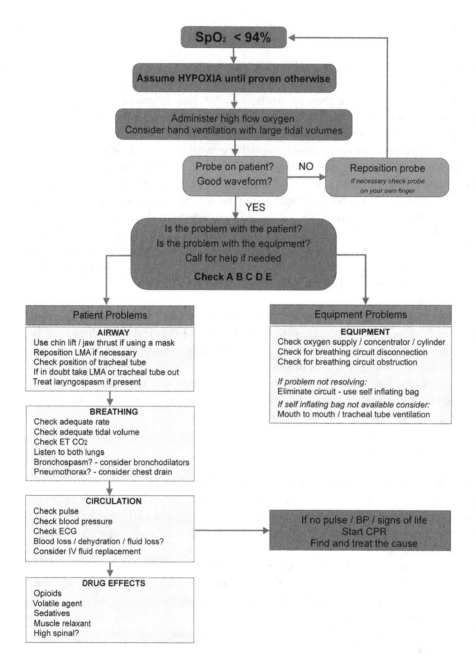

Figure 14.1 WHO hypoxia algorithm

Reproduced by kind permission from the World Health Organization.

When the monitor alarms it is important the nurse responds immediately and, depending on the alarm, assesses the patient and acts accordingly. Factors which can affect the correct functioning of a pulse oximeter include (WHO, 2011):

- light: bright lights, e.g. if used in an operating theatre, or sunlight can affect readings;
- shivering;
- pulse volume, e.g. due to hypovolemic shock, arrhythmias;
- vasoconstriction and poor perfusion to the peripheries;
- carbon monoxide poisoning may give you a falsely high saturation reading.

Arterial blood gases

While arterial blood gases (ABG) monitoring may be limited, staff may be unfamiliar with results due to the infrequent use of this test. Partial pressure of oxygen (PaO_2) and partial pressure of carbon dioxide ($PaCO_2$) may be measured in either kPa or mmHg. The equipment used will determine how the results are used. The following are normal ranges for arterial blood gases are as follows (Cowley *et al.*, 2013):

pH   7.35–7.45;

Hydrogen ion (H+) 35–45nmol/L

Partial pressure of oxygen (PaO_2) 10–13.3kPa 75–100mmHg;

Partial pressure of carbon dioxide (PaCO2) 4.8–6.1kPa 36–46mmHg;

Standard bicarbonate ($sHCO_3-$) 22–26mmol/L;

Base excess –2 to +2mmol/L;

Mechanical ventilation

In resource limited settings, ventilation may be provided for rescue interventions for young patients who have acute, curable diseases and conditions (Firth & Ttendo, 2012). The decision to intubate, ventilate a patient and admit a patient to critical care is a balance between potentially letting a patient die from an avoidable or preventable cause in a ward, or using an expensive, limited resource that may prove not to be clinically indicated later. Studies have shown most patients admitted to critical care require mechanical ventilation (Denney *et al.*, 2015; Tomlinson *et al.*, 2013. Ttendo *et al.*, 2016. Towney & Ojara, 2008). However, the availability of ventilators often exceeds demands (Dart *et al.*, 2016; Lillie *et al.*, 2015). In addition, many critical care units have insufficient beds meaning high dependency patients may be nursed on the ward or discharged earlier than expected, with minimal follow-up.

Providing mechanical ventilation is more than having access to ventilators; other considerations include:

- appropriately trained nurses who are competent to look after an endotracheal tube (including suctioning) and a ventilated patient;
- appropriate medical staff trained to adjust ventilator settings in response to patients' condition. In practice, nurses may be required to look after two or more ventilated patients at once;

- access to appropriate, working monitoring;
- provision of adequate sedation;
- access to technical staff who can care for and maintain ventilators;
- ventilators require electricity and compressed oxygen;
- protocols and care bundles, e.g. ventilator care bundle to reduce ventilator associated pneumonia (VAP).

(Krishnamoorthy *et al.*, 2014; Denney *et al.*, 2015)

Ventilator associated pneumonia

The incidence of hospital-acquired infection (HAI) in critical care units in low resource settings is difficult to ascertain; however, the WHO (2017) estimates HAIs are at least twice that of the United States, with ventilator associated pneumonia (VAP) incidence up to 19 times higher than in HICs. VAP is seen as potentially preventable (Rosenthal *et al.*, 2012). Care bundles provide standardisation in care for either a condition or an intervention (Denney *et al.*, 2015). The ventilator care bundle consists of (Institute for Health Improvement, 2012):

- raised head of the bed (minimises micro-aspiration);
- daily sedation hold and assessment of readiness to extubate;
- peptic ulcer prophylaxis;
- venous thrombo-embolism prophylaxis;
- oral care with chlorhexidine.

The ventilator care bundle is seen as simple and cost effective. Successful compliance and reduction in VAP has been identified in critical care units in low resource settings (Haque *et al.*, 2017; Rosenthal *et al.*, 2012; Molina, 2015). Smith *et al.* (2013) outline the realities: in a critical care unit in Ethiopia two nurses with no specific training in critical care looked after six patients, three of whom may be ventilated. Other challenges may include using beds which are fixed height; therefore it may not be possible to position patients 30° head up. A lack of 24-hour suction catheters means ventilation circuits are disconnected to use single-use suction catheters, resulting in loss of PEEP, hypoxia and increased risk of infection. A lack of single-use suction catheters requires them to be re-used, which leads to potentially introducing infections, poor hand hygiene due to a lack of water and a lack of access to drugs to provide gut protection and deep vein thrombosis (DVT) prophylaxis.

Implementation of the ventilator care bundle in resource limited settings requires appropriate resources and training prior to use (Haque *et al.*, 2017). Appropriate surveillance is needed before and after implementation to identify the incidence of VAP and compliance (Arabi *et al.*, 2008). Finally, other infection prevention strategies to prevent VAP, for example hand hygiene (Figure 14.2) must also be followed.

Weaning from ventilation

Weaning is defined as 'the gradual decrease of ventilator support and its replacement with the patient's own spontaneous ventilation' extubation (Intensive Care Society, 2007).

My 5 Moments for Hand Hygiene

Focus on caring for a patient with an endotracheal tube

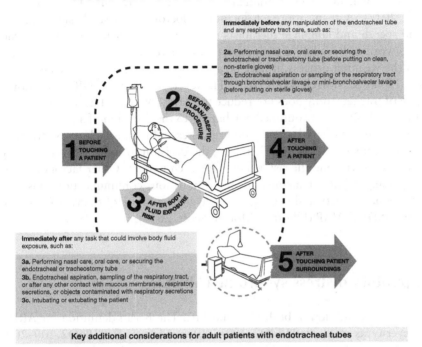

Immediately before any manipulation of the endotracheal tube and any respiratory tract care, such as:

2a. Performing nasal care, oral care, or securing the endotracheal or tracheostomy tube (before putting on clean, non-sterile gloves)
2b. Endotracheal aspiration or sampling of the respiratory tract through bronchoalveolar lavage or mini-bronchoalveolar lavage (before putting on sterile gloves)

2 BEFORE CLEAN/ASEPTIC PROCEDURE

1 BEFORE TOUCHING A PATIENT

4 AFTER TOUCHING A PATIENT

3 AFTER BODY FLUID EXPOSURE RISK

Immediately after any task that could involve body fluid exposure, such as:

3a. Performing nasal care, oral care, or securing the endotracheal or tracheostomy tube
3b. Endotracheal aspiration, sampling of the respiratory tract, or after any other contact with mucous membranes, respiratory secretions, or objects contaminated with respiratory secretions
3c. Intubating or extubating the patient

5 AFTER TOUCHING PATIENT SURROUNDINGS

Key additional considerations for adult patients with endotracheal tubes

- Avoid intubation and use non-invasive ventilation whenever appropriate.
- If possible, provide endotracheal tubes with subglottic secretion drainage ports for patients likely to require more than 48 hours of intubation.
- Elevate the head of the bed to 30°–45°.
- Manage ventilated patients without sedatives whenever possible.

- Assess readiness for extubation every day by performing spontaneous breathing trials with sedatives turned off (in patients without contraindications).
- Perform regular oral care aseptically using clean, non-sterile gloves.
- Facilitate early exercise and mobilization to maintain and improve physical condition.
- Change the ventilator circuit only if visibly soiled or malfunctioning.

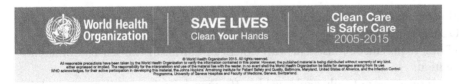

Figure 14.2 Caring for a patient with an endotracheal tube and preventing infection
Reproduced with kind permission from the World Health Organization.

Weaning can be simple (and rapid), difficult or prolonged, depending on the length of time and number of attempts to achieve.

A weaning plan should be in place for all patients and will be individual for each patient. Within resource limited environments the decision to wean may be difficult due to the complexity of the patient's condition, few staff and experience in using weaning protocols.

Prior to extubation a patient should be trialled on a spontaneous breathing trial; if they are unsuccessful, they should be trialled daily and after three attempts or longer than one week, a plan involving a gradual decrease in support should be followed (Adam et al., 2017). A team approach including doctors, nurses, physiotherapists, dieticians and speech and language therapists is required particularly in patients who are difficult to wean or have had a prolonged period of ventilation.

As part of the weaning process, it may be appropriate to consider a tracheostomy after >5 days (Elliott & Morrell-Scott, 2017). However, studies from HIC have shown early insertion of tracheostomy does not reduce mortality, VAP or duration of ventilation (Davidson et al., 2016). As outlined in Chapter 13 the insertion of a tracheostomy may increase the patient's length of stay on critical care due to a lack of experienced staff and suction units on the ward. Therefore, the decision to insert a tracheostomy should be based on reviewing the risk/benefits for each patient. Other factors to consider when weaning a patient include adequate nutrition, communication aids and interaction to reduce anxiety and isolation, oral hygiene and use of the ventilator care bundle to prevent DVT, VAP (Elliott & Morrell-Scott, 2017).

Acute respiratory distress syndrome (ARDS)

ARDS is a common condition in both HIC and LIC. The Berlin definition for ARDS categorises severity as mild (PaO2/FiO2 200–300), moderate (PaO2/FiO2 100–200) or severe (PaO2/FiO2 <100) on a PEEP >5. This definition was based on patients in a HIC setting; challenges when transferring these guidelines into resource limited environments include lack of mechanical ventilators (resulting in an inability to provide PEEP), arterial blood gases and chest radiographs (Riviello et al., 2016). The Kigali modified Berlin definition acknowledges the lack of these resources and uses the following criteria to assist with the diagnosis of ARDS:

- Within one week of a clinical insult or new or worsening respiratory deterioration.
- SpO2/FiO2 <315
- No PEEP requirement consistent with American European Consensus Conference Definition.
- Bilateral opacities not fully explained by effusions, lobar/lung collapse or nodules by chest X-ray or ultrasound.
- Respiratory failure not fully explained by cardiac failure or fluid overload.

The causes of ARDS are varied and may include topical infections, including malaria, and HIV (George et al., 2014. Taylor et al., 2012).

The management of ARDS includes:

- pre-oxygenation of patients prior to any intervention to prevent prolonged periods of desaturation. If available, use closed suction catheters;

- using lung-protective ventilation strategies (low volume, low pressure ventilation):

  o tidal volume 6ml/kg;
  o plateau airway pressure <30cmH$_2$O;
  o SpO$_2$ 88–93% or PaCO$_2$ 7.3–10.6kPa (55–80mmHg).

- avoiding disconnection of ventilator circuits; if available, use closed suction systems;
- using the prone position to improve oxygenation;
- using higher PEEP in patients with moderate to severe ARDS (PaCO$_2$/FiO$_2$ <200);
- conservative fluid management if no signs of shock.

In summary, access to oxygen, pulse oximetry and monitoring are taken for granted in HIC critical care units. Within low resource settings, these interventions are scarce resources saved for only the sickest of patients. In consequence, 'routine monitoring' may be not be available for every patient (Lifebox, 2017), resulting in variations in practice and potentially increasing the risk of harm and complications. Deciding to use and initiate treatments including mechanical ventilation needs to be balanced with the resources available and having appropriate staff available to respond and manage patients.

References

Adam S. Osbourne S. Welch J. (2017). Critical care nursing science and practice. 3rd Edition. Oxford: Oxford University Press.

Adipa FE. Aziato L. Zakariah AN. (2015). Qualitative exploration of nurses' perspectives on clinical oxygen administration in Ghana. International Journal of Africa Nursing Sciences. 2. 42–46.

Arabi Y. Al-Shirawi N. Memish Z. Anzueto A. (2008). Ventilator-associated pneumonia in adults in developing countries: a systematic review. International Journal of Infectious Diseases. 12. 5. 505–512.

Cowley NJ. Owen A. Bion JF. (2013). Interpreting arterial blood gas results. British Medical Journal. 346. F16.

Dart PJ. Kinnear J. Bould MD et al. (2016). An evaluation of inpatient morbidity and critical care provision in Zambia. Anaesthesia. 72. 2. 172–180.

Davidson C. Banham S. Elliott M et al. (2016). BTS/ICS guidelines for the ventilatory management of acute hypercapnic respiratory failure in adults. Thorax. 71. Suppl. 2. Ii1–135.

Denney JA. Capanni F. Herrera P et al. (2015). Establishment of a prospective cohort of mechanically ventilated patients in five intensive care units in Lima, Peru: protocol and organisational characteristics of participating centres. BMJ Open. 5. E005803.

Elliott S. Morrell-Scott N. (2017). Care of patients undergoing weaning from mechanical ventilation in critical care. Nursing Standard. 32. 13. 41–51.

Firth P. Ttendo S. (2012). Intensive care in low-income countries – a critical need. New England Journal of Medicine. 267. 21. 1974–1976. Doi: 10.1056/NEJMp1204957.

George T. Viswanathan S. Karnam ALF. Abraham G. (2014). Etiology and outcomes of ARDS in a rural-urban fringe hospital in South India. Critical Care Research and Practice. DOI: http://dx.doi.org/10.1155/2014/181593.

Haque A. Riaz Q. Ali SA. (2017). Implementation of ventilator bundle in paediatric intensive care unit of a developing country. Journal of College of Physicians and Surgeons of Pakistan. 27. 5. 316–318.

Howie SRC. Hill S. Ebonyi A. et al. (2009). Meeting oxygen needs in Africa: an options analysis from the Gambia. Bulletin of the World Health Organization. 87. 10. 763–771.

Institute for Health Improvement. (2012). How to guide: ventilator care bundle. Available at: www.ihi.org/resources/Pages/Tools/HowtoGuidePreventVAP.aspx.

Intensive Care Society. (2007). When and how to wean. Intensive Care Society Guidelines. London: ICS.

Krishnamoorthy V. Vavilala MS. Mock CN. (2014). The need for ventilators in the developing world: an opportunity to improve care and save lives. Journal of Global Health. 4. 1. 010303.

Lemanski C. (2016). Pulse oximetry for perioperative monitoring. Cochrane Nursing Care Review. Journal of Peri-Anaesthesia Nursing. 31. 1. 86–88.

Lifebox (2017). History of Lifebox. Available at: www.lifebox.org/history-of-lifebox/.

Lillie E. Holmes CJ. O'Donohoe EA et al. (2015). Avoidable perioperative mortality at the University Teaching Hospital, Lusaka, Zambia: a retrospective cohort study. Canadian Journal of Anesthesia. 62. 12. 1259–1267.

Molina F. (2015). Implementation of a bundle for prevention of ventilator-associated pneumonia in a developing country. Critical Care Medicine. 43. 12.

Peel D. Neighbour R. Eltringham RJ. (2013). Evaluation of oxygen concentrators for use in countries with limited resources. Anaesthesia. 68. 7. 706–712.

Resuscitation Council (UK). (2016). Immediate life support. 4th Edition. London: Resuscitation Council (UK).

Riviello ED. Kiviri W. Twagirumugabe T et al. (2016). Hospital incidence and outcomes of the acute respiratory distress syndrome using the Kigali modification of the Berlin definition. American Journal of Respiratory and Critical Care Medicine. 193. 1. 52–59.

Rosenthal VD. Alvarez-Moreno C, Villamil-Gomez W et al. (2012). Effectiveness of a multidimensional approach to reduce ventilator-associated pneumonia in paediatric intensive care units of 5 developing countries: international nosocomial infection control consortium findings. American Journal of Infection Control. 40. 497–501.

Smith D. Bowden T. (2017). Using the ABCDE approach to assess the deteriorating patient. Nursing Standard. 32. 14. 51–61.

Smith ZA. Ayele Y. McDonald P. (2013). Outcomes in critical care delivery at Jimma University Specialised Hospital, Ethiopia. Anaesthesia and Critical Care. 41. 3. 363–368.

Taylor WRJ. Hanson J. Turner GDH. White NJ. Dondorp AM. (2012). Respiratory manifestations of malaria. Chest. 142. 2. 492–505. DOI: https://doi.org/10.1378/chest.11-2655.

Tomlinson J. Haac B. Kadyaudzu C et al. (2013). The burden of surgical diseases on critical care services at a tertiary referral hospital in sub-Saharan Africa. Tropical Doctor. 43. 1. 27–29.

Towney RM. Ojara S. (2007). Intensive care in the developing world. Anaesthesia. 62. (suppl. 1). 32–37.

Towney RM. Ojara S. (2008). Practice of intensive care in rural Africa: an assessment of data from Northern Uganda. African Health Sciences. 8. 1. 61–64.

Ttendo SS. Was A. Preston MA et al. (2016). Retrospective descriptive study of an intensive care unit at a Ugandan Regional Referral Hospital. World Journal of Surgery. 40. 2847–2856.

World Health Organization. (2009). Implementation manual WHO surgical safety checklist 2009. Geneva: World Health Organization.

World Health Organization. (2011). Pulse oximetry training manual. Geneva: World Health Organization.

World Health Organization. (2017). The Burden of Health Care-Associated Infection Worldwide a Summary. Available at: www.who.int/gpsc/country_work/summary_20100430_en.pdf.

15 Cardiac monitoring and arrhythmias

Continuous cardiac monitoring allows for cardiac rate and rhythm to be monitored. Monitoring is used to detect a change in clinical condition, to assist assessment and responses to therapy in real time. Monitoring aids assessment but does not replace staff and the need for a comprehensive assessment. Cardiac monitors will have alarms which can be set to identify any significant changes in condition. They must be checked and appropriate parameters set for each patient (Leach, 2004).

A normal adult heart rate is between 60 and 100 beats per minute. Electrocardiogram (ECG) monitoring provides a tracing of the cardiac conduction system. Lead II provides the best view and should be used as the default setting for monitoring. As the atria depolarises a P wave is seen on the monitor, followed by ventricular contraction (QRS wave), then repolarisation (T wave) (Swift, 2013a). This is termed sinus rhythm (Figure 15.1). Bradycardia is defined as a heart rate <60 beats per minute. Tachycardia >100 beats per minute.

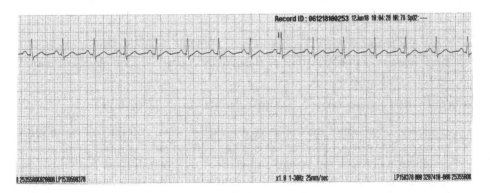

Figure 15.1 Sinus rhythm

Interpreting a cardiac rhythm

To interpret a cardiac rhythm, you will need to print a rhythm strip. The following steps can be followed to interpret cardiac rhythms:

Step 1: Is there any electrical activity?

- Check the patient has a pulse. If no pulse:
- Check a lead has not become disconnected.
- If no pulse, immediately begin CPR (Chapter 12).

Step 2: What is the ventricular (QRS) rate?

To calculate the rate:

- ECG paper is calibrated in mm, with bolder lines every 5mm.
- Standard ECG paper speed is $25mm^{-3}$. One second = 5 large squares or 25 small squares.
- To work out the rate count the number of cardiac cycles (R to R wave) that occur in 6 seconds (30 large squares) and multiply by 10. This provides an estimated heart rate, even when the heart rate is irregular. For shorter rhythm strips, count the number of cardiac cycles in 3 seconds (15 large squares) and multiply by 20.

Step 3: Is the QRS rhythm regular or irregular?

- Measure each R to R wave and compare it to others to detect irregularity. This is done by using a piece of paper and marking R-R waves then moving the paper along to another section and seeing if the R-R waves line up.

Step 4: Is the QRS complex duration normal or prolonged?

- The upper limit for QRS duration is 0.12 seconds (three small squares).

Step 5: Is atrial activity present?

- Look for P waves. Atrial activity may be difficult or impossible to identify as the P wave may not be visible, or the activity is partly or completely obscured by QRS or T waves.

Step 6: Is atrial activity related to ventricular activity and if so how?

- Look for a consistent interval between each P wave and the following QRS complex. The normal PR interval is 0.12–0.20 seconds. This will demonstrate conduction between the atrium and ventricle is intact. If there is no relationship between the P wave and QRS complexes, atrial and ventricular depolarisation is occurring independently. This is referred to as atrioventricular dissociation.

(Resuscitation Council (UK), 2016)

Bradycardia

Bradycardia is defined as a QRS rate <60/min (Resuscitation Council (UK), 2016). Causes of bradycardia which may require treatment include:

- first degree atrioventricular (AV) block (heart block) (Figure 15.2);
- second degree AV block;
  - o Mobilitz type I AV (also termed Wenckebach AV block) (Figure 15.3);
  - o Mobilitz type II AV block (Figure 15.4);
- Third degree IV block (Figure 15.5).

First degree atrioventricular block

First degree atrioventricular block occurs when there is a delay conducting through the atrioventricular junction. This results in a PR interval of >0.20s (Figure 15.2). This rhythm rarely causes any symptoms and can be identified during routine investigations, for example prior to surgery. Unless symptomatic patients rarely require treatment.

Second degree atrioventricular block

Second degree atrioventricular block results in a progressive prolongation of the PR interval, until a P waves occurs without a resulting QRS complex. There are two types:

- Mobilitz Type I (Figure 15.3) results in a progressively longer PR interval until the atrial impulse is blocked and no QRS complex follows.
- Mobilitz Type II (Figure 15.4) constant PR interval, with some P waves not followed by QRS complexes. There is an increased risk of developing complete heart block and asystole. This can be further divided into 2:1 block whereby alternate P waves are followed by a QRS complex. A 3:1 block is rare.

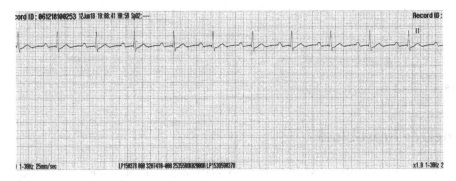

Figure 15.2 First degree atrioventricular block

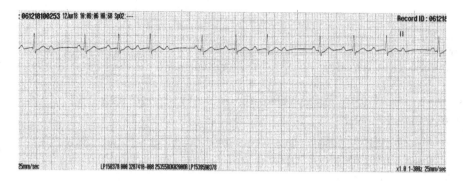

Figure 15.3 Second degree atrioventricular block

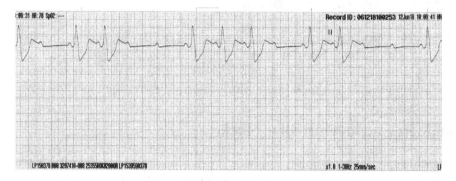

Figure 15.4 Second degree heart block 2:1

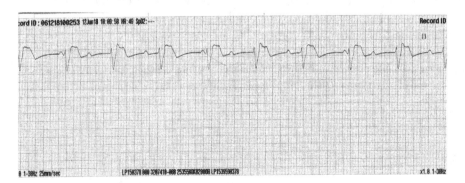

Figure 15.5 Third degree heart block

Third degree heart block

Third degree heart block occurs when there is no relationship between the P waves and QRS complexes. These patients are at high risk of developing asystole and are rarely asymptomatic.

Cases of atrioventricular blocks

Potential temporary causes of atrioventricular blocks include:

- myocardial infarction usually associated with inferior wall MI;
- digoxin toxicity;
- acute myocarditis;
- calcium channel blockers;
- beta-adrenoceptor blocking drugs (beta-blockers);
- cardiac surgery.

Permanent causes include:

- congenital abnormalities;
- MI usually associated with anteroseptal MI;
- cardiomyopathy;
- cardiac surgery.

(Resuscitation Council (UK), 2016; Swift, 2013a)

Assessment

Patients with severe bradycardia (30–40bpm) may be symptomatic due to poor cardiac output and coronary perfusion, decreased myocardial function and perfusion (Swift, 2013a). Patients may experience a wide range of signs and symptoms and treatment will be guided by the patient's overall condition and the existence of other co-morbidities (Resuscitation Council (UK), 2016). Adverse signs are critical signs and symptoms which will assist in determining if treatment is required include:

- shock. Hypotension, confusion, oliguria, delayed capillary refill;
- syncope caused by reduced blood flow to the brain causing a brief loss of consciousness;
- myocardial ischaemia. Chest pain with/without 12 lead ECG changes;
- heart failure. Pulmonary oedema with or without raised jugular vein pressure, peripheral oedema and/or liver enlargement.

(Swift, 2013a; Resuscitation Council
(UK), 2016)

Patients should be assessed using the A–E approach. Electrolytes should be checked to maintain serum potassium level >4.5mmol/L and magnesium levels >1.2mmol/L. Treatment involves both pharmacological and cardiac pacing.

Atropine 500mcg can be administered intravenously every five minutes to a maximum dose of 3mg. If the cause of the bradycardia is due to a beta-blocker overdose, glucagon can be given. Glycopyrronium bromide and adrenaline (epinephrine) may be used in the operating theatre or critical care settings.

Atropine is contra-indicated in patients who have myocardial ischemia or MI and those who have undergone cardiac transplant. For bradycardia in post-cardiac transplant patients, it may be appropriate to use theophylline as an alternative, as the patient may not have a vagal nerve (Swift, 2013a).

Cardiac pacing involves the use of percussion pacing, transcutaneous or transvenous. In an emergency, percussion pacing may be used until a cardiac pacing unit is available. Percussion pacing is performed by providing serial rhythmical blows with a closed fist over the left lower edge of the sternum at a rate of 60–90bpm.

Transcutaneous pacing can be either fixed or demand. Demand mode involves the pacing unit detecting an intrinsic QRS complex, whereas fixed mode pacing involves the delivery of a set number of electrical impulses regardless of an intrinsic QRS. Transcutaneous pacing is painful, therefore sedation is often provided with specialist airway support available in case of any airway compromise. When establishing transcutaneous pacing a pacing spike will be seen on the ECG trace followed by a QRS complex; a carotid pulse should be checked to confirm mechanical capture. The pacing current should be increased until the desired effect has been achieved. Capture may not occur in 'non-viable myocardium' and conditions including hyperkalaemia (Swift, 2013a). Transcutaneous pacing is used until transvenous pacing has been established. If no capture is achieved, then the patient is in cardiac arrest with pulseless electrical activity. CPR should be immediately commenced as outlined in Chapter 12. A summary of key interventions to be undertaken in an emergency situation is outlined in Figure 15.6.

Tachycardias

During diastole (relaxation phase of the cardiac cycle) myocardial oxygen perfusion occurs (Swift, 2013b). When an individual develops a tachycardia, the diastolic phase is reduced, resulting in the heart pumping less efficiently and blood flow to the heart reduced (Swift, 2013b). Types of life-threatening tachycardias include:

- broad complex tachycardia:
  - regular broad-complex tachycardia: ventricular tachycardia (VT) (with pulse);
  - irregular broad-complex tachycardia: atrial fibrillation;
- narrow complex tachycardia:
  - atrial flutter;
  - supraventricular tachycardia (SVT);

Monomorphic ventricular tachycardia

Monomorphic ventricular tachycardia (VT) (Figure 15.7) originates in the ventricles below the Bundle of His and results in a severe reduction in cardiac output (Swift, 2013b). The QRS morphology can be monomorphic and less commonly polymorphic.

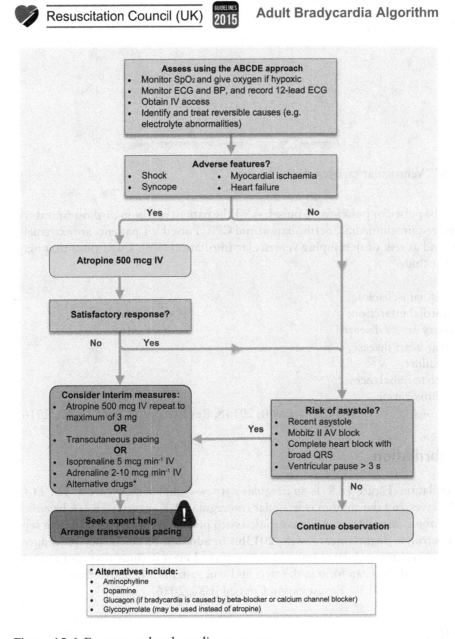

Figure 15.6 Emergency bradycardia treatment

Reproduced with kind permission from the Resuscitation Council (UK).

Monomorphic VT has a rapid ventricular (QRS) rate and P waves are absent. Polymorphic VT (Torsades de Pointes) may be caused by hypokalaemia and/or hypomagnesaemia, cerebrovascular accident and certain anti-arrhythmic drugs (Swift, 2013b).

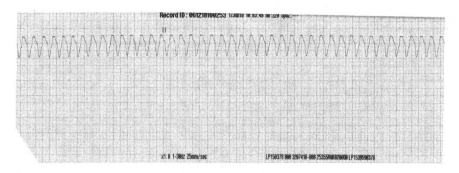

Figure 15.7 Ventricular tachycardia

VT can be pulsed or pulseless. In pulseless VT the patient will be in cardio-respiratory arrest and require immediate defibrillation and CPR. Pulsed VT patients are extremely unstable and at risk of developing ventricular fibrillation (VF). Conditions that may cause VT include:

- myocardial ischaemia;
- myocardial infarction;
- coronary artery disease;
- valvular heart disease;
- heart failure;
- electrolyte imbalances;
- drug intoxication.

(Swift, 2013b; Resuscitation Council (UK), 2016)

Atrial fibrillation

Atrial fibrillation (Figure 15.8) is an irregular narrow-complex tachycardia. The ECG has no P waves and the rhythm is irregular (no regular R-R waves). AF can be either acute or chronic onset. Acute AF is associated with precipitating factors including sepsis and electrolyte disturbances (Swift, 2013b). In addition to emergency procedures outlined below, anticoagulants must be administered even if sinus rhythm has been restored as blood clots can form in the atria and sent systemically due to reduced atrial contraction (Swift, 2013b; Resuscitation Council (UK), 2016).

Atrial flutter

Atrial flutter (Figure 15.9) is caused by conditions that enlarge the atrial tissue and elevate atrial pressure, for example patients with severe mitral valve disease, hyperthyroidism, pericardial disease and chronic obstructive pulmonary disease (Swift, 2013b). The ECG has no flat baseline between P waves and the rhythm looks like a 'saw-tooth pattern' (Swift, 2013b). The QRS is usually narrow; however, a broad QRS complex may be seen if there is aberrant ventricular conduction (Swift, 2013b).

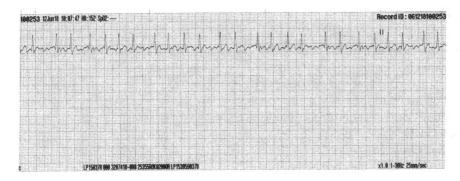

Figure 15.8 Atrial fibrillation

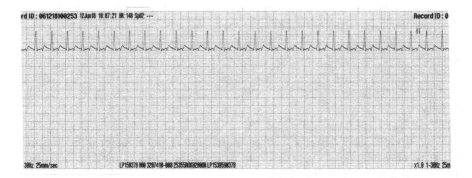

Figure 15.9 Atrial flutter

Supraventricular tachycardia

Supraventricular tachycardia (Figure 15.10) originates above the atrioventricular node. Care must be taken not to mistake this rhythm for a sinus tachycardia due to other sources, for example sepsis, hypovolaemic shock, e.g. post-operative haemorrhage.

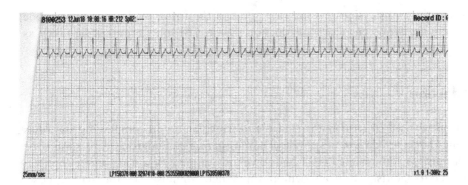

Figure 15.10 Supraventricular tachycardia

Treatment

Patients with a tachyarrhythmia must be assessed using the A–E approach. Interventions should include:

- high flow oxygen;
- continuous cardiac monitoring established;
- 12 lead ECG;
- IV access obtained;
- cardiac electrolytes checked and optimised;
- urgent medical assistance.

Patients should be assessed to identify if they are stable or unstable. The reduction in cardiac output results in reduced vital organ perfusion and the patient may present with life-threatening adverse signs including:

- shock;
- syncope;
- myocardial ischaemia;
- heart failure.

A patient with adverse signs is likely to be unstable and require urgent intervention. Emergency treatment includes the use of vagal manoeuvres, drugs (amiodarone, adenosine) and DC cardioversion (Figure 15.11).

Vagal manoeuvres

Vagal manoeuvres include asking patients to perform the Valsalva manoeuvre, for example blowing into a 20ml syringe.

Carotid sinus massage

Stimulating the carotid sinus by massage inhibits the firing of the sino-atrial node and slowing the atrio-ventricular conduction (Swift, 2013b). Care must be taken as patients may have undiagnosed carotid atherosclerosis.

Amiodarone

Amiodarone is used to treat both regular and irregular broad-complex tachycardias (excluding Torsades de Pointes). When administering amiodarone care should be taken. It must be administered via a central venous catheter or a wide bore peripheral cannula due to the risk of thromboembolism. When administering the loading dose, care must be taken as amiodarone can cause hypotension.

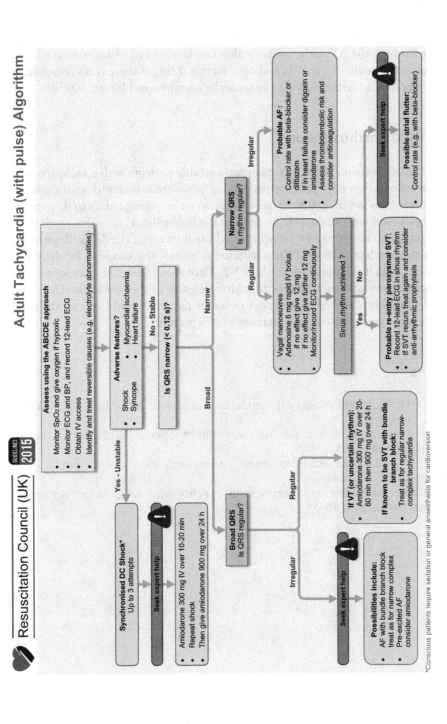

Figure 15.11 Emergency tachycardia treatment

Reproduced with the kind permission of the Resuscitation Council (UK).

Adenosine

Adenosine slows the conduction time through the atrioventricular node. By interrupting the pathway through the AV node, sinus rhythm can be restored. Adenosine is administered in boluses, initially 6 mg followed by a further 12mg if there is no response. If there is no response, a further dose of 12mg can be administered (Swift, 2013b).

Synchronised cardioversion

Synchronised cardioversion is the treatment for unstable patients with a tachyarrhythmia. Cardioversion allows the primary pacemaker (sino-atrial node) to regain control of cardiac conduction (Swift, 2013b). Cardioversion can be attempted up to three times and the energies used vary and are dependent on the defibrillator.

When planning to undertake DC synchronised cardioversion, the defibrillator must be able to deliver a 'sync' shock. When selected it allows the shock to be delivered on the R wave, which minimises the risk of VF. Care should be taken, as some defibrillators immediately switch off the setting after delivery of the shock; therefore, the defibrillator should be checked each time. Conscious patients should be anaesthetised or sedated before synchronised cardioversion as it is painful.

References

Leach R. (2004). Acute and critical care medicine at a glance. 2nd Edition. New York: Wiley Blackwell.

Resuscitation Council (UK). (2016). Advanced Life Support. 7th Edition. London: Resuscitation Council (UK).

Swift J. (2013a). Assessment and treatment of patients with acute unstable bradycardia. Nursing Standard. 27. 2. 48–56.

Swift J. (2013b). Assessment and treatment of patients with acute tachyarrhythmias. Nursing Standard. 28. 5. 50–59.

16 | Acute kidney injury .

Acute kidney injury (AKI), formerly termed acute renal failure, is a global concern, but is potentially preventable and treatable (Anand *et al.*, 2015). Evidence has shown knowledge of AKI amongst healthcare professionals tends to be poor in both HIC and LIC (Adejumo *et al.*, 2017; Evans *et al.*, 2015; Stevens *et al.*, 2001; Muniraju *et al.*, 2012). In resource limited settings, further challenges include accessing most hospitals as they tend to be based in urban areas, coupled with a limited hospital infrastructure and having to find funds to pay for hospital admission, making it difficult to access treatments early (Olowu *et al.*, 2016). If detected early enough, AKI can be reversed (Olowu *et al.*, 2016). Causes of AKI are divided into three main types (Griffiths & Kanagasundaram, 2011):

- Pre-renal uraemia. Caused by reduced renal perfusion, e.g. poor cardiac output due to haemorrhage.
- Intrinsic AKI uraemia. Caused by a lack of oxygen to the tubular death resulting in acute tubular necrosis by ischaemia, hypotension nephrotoxins (drugs) and systemic vascular disease.
- Post renal uraemia. Caused by obstruction, e.g. tumour, thrombi, urinary tract obstruction or enlarged prostate gland.

Specific causes of AKI in low resource settings include (Li *et al.*, 2013; Lameire *et al.*, 2013; Bagasha *et al.*, 2014; White *et al.*, 2008):

- diarrhoeal diseases with dehydration due to poor sanitation and water hygiene, e.g. gastroenteritis, cholera, typhus outbreaks;
- infectious diseases, e.g. dengue, malaria, tetanus, HIV, schistosomiasis, TB, hepatitis B and C;
- treatments from HIV and TB;
- sickle cell disease;
- animal venoms, e.g. snakes, bees, spiders, caterpillars;
- septic abortion;
- pre-eclampsia;

- use of dyes, natural and local medicines and remedies;
- poverty;
- overuse of nephrotoxic drugs;
- poorly controlled or undiagnosed diabetes mellitus and hypertension;
- many patients are young.

AKI can be classified in three stages:

- Stage 1:
    - Serum creatinine 1.5 to 1.9 times baseline or >0.3mg/dL (>26.5micromol/L) increase.
    - Urine output <0.5ml/kg/hr for 6–12 hours.

- Stage 2:
    - 2.0 to 2.9 times baseline.
    - Urine output: <0.5ml/kg/hr for >12hours.

- Stage 3:
    - 3.0 times baseline or increase in serum creatinine to >4.0mg/dL (>353.6micromol/L) or initiation of renal replacement therapy (RRT) or in patients under 18, decrease in eGFR <35mL/min per 1.73m^2.
    - Urine output <0.3ml/kg/hr for >24hours or anuria >12hours.

Management of AKI includes the following:

- Early identification of those at risk of developing AKI in 'real time' to ensure diagnosed immediately and clinical management adjusted.
- Good fluid resuscitation and early use of anti-malarial and antibiotics for sepsis.
- Haemodynamic optimisation.
- Recognition a patient can have a normal urine output or serum creatinine and have an AKI.
- Avoid overuse or not reviewing nephrotoxic drugs.
- Use of continuous renal replacement therapy (CRRT) to remove waste products, restoration of acid base balance, correction of electrolyte imbalance, stabilisation of cardiovascular system and maintenance of fluid balance (Richardson & Whatmore, 2013).

(Pickkers et al., 2017; Perico & Remuzzi, 2016;
Olowu et al., 2016; Anand et al., 2015; Bagasha et al., 2014)

Continuous renal replacement therapy (CRRT)

In resource limited environments, there is limited published evidence on the use of continuous renal replacement therapy (CRRT) in the critical care setting. Perico and

Table 16.1 Types of CRRT

Type	Process	Indications
Slow continuous ultrafiltration (SCUF)	Ultrafiltration	Fluid overload without uraemia or significant electrolyte imbalance.
Continuous veno-venous haemofiltration (CVVH)	Ultrafiltration Convection	Uraemia or severe acid-base or electrolyte imbalance, with or without fluid overload.
Continuous veno-venous haemodialysis (CVVHD)	Ultrafiltration Diffusion	Removal of fluid and small to medium sized molecules. Severe uraemia, acid-base and electrolyte imbalance.
Continuous veno-venous haemodiafiltration (CVVHDF)	Ultrafiltration Diffusion Convection	Effective metabolic control if CVVH is not being achieved.

Source: Richardson & Whatmore, 2013

Remuzzi (2016) identified acute haemodialysis is not only unaffordable for patients but also healthcare systems due to the cost of machines, consumables, unreliability of electricity and water supply and few trained personnel. The limited availability of critical care facilities and CRRT means patients simply die (Perico & Remuzzi, 2016). However, Stanifer and Sharma (2017) propose for patients with AKI that require CRRT it is an appropriate intervention in critical care given most people affected are younger, economically active, whereas the provision of dialysis is for chronic renal failure and patients tend to be older and chronically ill. In consequence, Stanifer and Sharma (2017) argue the provision of life-sustaining technologies such as CRRT is appropriate in the resource limited environment. The decision to initiate CRRT poses complex ethical, clinical and resource challenges, including a need for a continuous electrical supply, sufficient extracorporeal circuits, filtrate fluid to deliver treatments, access to regular blood tests (e.g. arterial blood gases, coagulation, electrolytes) and staff to manage CRRT (Jha *et al.*, 2017). Types of CRRT include (Richardson & Whatmore, 2013) (Table 16.1):

- slow continuous ultrafiltration (SCUF);
- continuous veno-venous haemofiltration (CVVH);
- continuous veno-venous haemodialysis (CVVHD);
- continuous veno-venous haemodiafiltration (CVVHDF).

The type of CRRT used will determine the mechanism used. This can be either a combination or only one method (Table 16.1) (Richardson & Whatmore, 2013):

- Ultrafiltration: movement of fluid through a semi-permeable membrane along a pressure gradient. The blood side causes a positive pressure and a negative pressure on the fluid side; this results in fluid being removed from the patient.
- Convection: one-way movement of solutes through a semi-permeable membrane. Hydrostatic pressure in the blood is higher than the pressure in the ultrafiltrate, causing plasma water with solutes to cross the membrane (termed 'solute drag'). The faster the flow rate the higher the clearance.
- Diffusion: movement of particles from higher concentration to regions of lower concentration. Solutes move from high concentration (blood side) across the membrane to a low concentration in the dialysate. Removes small to medium molecules but not large molecules.

To maintain the CRRT circuit good vascular access is required. Specialist wide-bore access CVCs are required to maintain high blood flow, anticoagulation may be required to try and prevent clots in the extracorporeal circuit. Indications clots may be forming result in increasing circuit pressures. The type of anticoagulant depends on the patient's condition, for example patients with coagulopathy, sepsis or hepatic failure may not require anti-coagulation (Dirkes & Hodge, 2007). Types of anticoagulation include:

- heparin. Most common type of anticoagulant used in CRRT;
- prostacyclin. Used as an alternative to heparin in patients with increased risk of bleeding. Prostacyclin should not be used in patients with low platelet counts and hypotension as it is a powerful vaso-dilator;
- regional citrate. Citrate binds to calcium in blood and prevents clotting. Hypocalcaemia is caused, and intravenous calcium replacements is required. Citrate is used if the patient is actively bleeding, at high risk of bleeding or heparin-induced thrombocytopenia. It is contra-indicated in patients with severe liver failure;
- thrombin inhibitors: Alternative anticoagulants for patients with heparin-induced thrombocytopenia. Patients are at high risk of bleeding and there are no reversal agents.

Complications of CRRT include haemodynamic instability, haemorrhage, hypothermia, electrolyte and acid-base imbalance, inappropriate drug dosing, infection and circuit failure (Richardson & Whatmore, 2013). The nursing care of patients on CRRT include observation for signs of any complications. 'Filter observations' should be recorded hourly and any trends noted. Types of continuous CRRT monitoring include (Richardson & Whatmore, 2013):

- blood pump speed (mL/min). Speed blood is removed from the patient;
- access pressure (mmHg). Pressure generated to remove blood from the patient;
- return pressure (mmHg). Pressure generated to return blood to the patient;
- transmembrane pressure (TMP) (mmHg). Pressure gradient exerted across the semi-permeable membrane. TMP needs to be adequate to enable ultrafiltration;
- pre-filter pressure (mmHg). Positive pressure generated in the circuit immediately before the blood enters the haemofilter.

Although CRRT machines have alarms, these may be mistaken for other types of alarms, which may result in a delay in responding if solely relying on the filter alarms to detect problems. In consequence, patients on CRRT require one to one nursing care. Alarms may include:

- low access pressure;
  - potential causes: CVC 'sucking' against vessel wall; CVC partially clotted or fully clotted; lumen kinked or clamped;
  - action: Ensure both lumens and tubing are straight and unclamped.

- High return pressure;
  - potential causes: CVC lumen is clotted or occluded; lumen or lines are kinked; circuit clotted;
  - action: ensure lumens and tubing are straight and unclamped.

- Low return pressure;
  - potential causes: low blood pump speed; return tubing disconnected;
  - action: ensure tubing is securely connected.

- High TMP;
  - potential causes:
    - rapid rise: filtrate tubing or bags occluded by clamp or kinking;
    - slow rise: filter clotting slowly;
    - high TMP at start of treatment: ratio of pressure between the blood flow and replacement fluid is too high.
  - action: ensure all tubing is unclamped and straight.

- High pre-filter;
  - potential causes: tubing kinked; 'return chamber' clotting; filter clotting;
  - action: ensure tubing is straight and not kinked. Consider more pre-dilution on next CRRT cycle.

- Air detection;
  - potential causes: air in the tubing returning to the patient; blood level is too low in 'return chamber', return tubing is not in the air detector clamp correctly;
  - action: when setting up circuit ensure air detector is securely fitted. When priming circuit ensure all air is cleared.

- Blood leak;
  - potential causes: filter membrane ruptured causing a leak of blood into the ultrafiltrate; blood leak detection chamber not correctly housed; sensor in housing in unclean;
  - action: when setting up circuit, ensure blood leak detection chamber is housed in correct position and machine sensor cleaned.

- Fluid balance;
    - ○ potential causes: fluid bags moving or swinging below machine; fluid bags not connected properly; fluid tubing kinked or clamped;
    - ○ action: ensure tubing is straight and free from obstruction and fluid bags are unclamped.

CRRT on deployed military operations

The challenges and demands of providing CRRT in resource limited environments are not only an issue for low-income settings but also deployed military medical facilities. Both the UK and US military do not have CRRT immediately available, and plan for the rapid evacuation of patients who require CRRT. Specialist teams are on standby to deploy with the equipment and provide in-theatre CRRT to stabilise patients prior to the transfer, as CRRT cannot be provided in-flight (Nesbitt et al., 2011). Military CRRT teams deploy infrequently, and there are few documented cases (Nesbitt et al., 2011). The US research into the use of CRRT in the Iraq conflict reported AKI secondary to traumatic injuries is a rare complication, albeit one with poor outcome (Perkins et al., 2008). Perkins et al. (2008) reported the challenge of providing CRRT to local nationals when there are no renal services or critical care units with a CRRT capability; they identified this as an ethical dilemma. The need for CRRT on deployed operations should be risk assessed and considered during the planning of operations. As equipment and technology improves the increased opportunity to provide life-sustaining interventions in the deployed setting will potentially increase the gulf between military, NGO and civilian healthcare facilities all within the same area of responsibility. As outlined in Chapter 4, the professional and ethical dilemmas in providing care to local nationals will be a challenge military critical care nurses will face on operations.

References

Adejumo OA. Akinbodewa AA. Alli OE. Pirisola OB. Abolarin OS. (2017). Knowledge of acute kidney injury among nurses in two government hospitals in Ondo City, Southwest Nigeria. Saudi Journal of Kidney Diseases and Transplantation. 28. 5. 1092–1098.

Anand S. Cruz DN. Finkelstein FO. (2015). Understanding acute kidney injury in low resource settings: a step forward. BMC Nephrology. 16. 5.

Bagasha P. Nakwagala F. Kwizera A et al. (2014). Cross-sectional study of acute kidney injury among adult patients admitted with sepsis in low-income country: clinical pattern and short term outcomes. BMC Nephrology. 16. 4.

Dirkes S. Hodge K. (2007). Continuous renal replacement therapy in the adult intensive care unit: history and current trends. Critical Care Nurse. 27. 61–80.

Evans R. Rudd P. Hemmila U. Dobbie H. Dreyer G. (2015). Deficiencies in education and experience in the management of acute kidney injury among Malawian healthcare workers. Malawi Medical Journal. 27. 101–103.

Griffiths L. Kanagasundaram NS. (2011). Assessment and initial management of acute kidney injury. Medicine. DOI: https://doi.org/10.1016/j.mpmed.2011.04.010.

Jha V. Martin BE. Bargman JM *et al*. (2017). Ethical issues in dialysis therapy. The Lancet. 389. 1851–1856.

Lameire NH. Bagga A. DeMaeseneer JD *et al*. (2013). Global kidney disease: acute kidney injury: an increasing global concern. The Lancet. 382. 170–179.

Li PKT. Burdmann EA. Mehta RL. (2013). Acute kidney injury: global health alert. Advances in Chronic Kidney Disease. 20. 3. 114–117.

Muniraju TM. Lillicrap MH. Horrocks JL *et al*. (2012). Diagnosis and management of acute kidney injury: deficiencies in the knowledge base of non-specialist, trainee medical staff. Clinical Medicine (London). 12. 216–221.

Nesbitt I. Almond MK. Freshwater DA. (2011). Renal Replacement in the Deployed Setting. Journal of the Royal Army Medical Corps. 157. 2. 179–181.

Olowu WA. Safo C. Ashuntantang G *et al*. (2016). Outcomes of acute kidney injury in children and adults in sub-Saharan Africa: a systematic review. The Lancet. 4. E242–250.

Perico N. Remuzzi G. (2016). Acute kidney injury in low-income and middle-income countries: no longer a death sentence. The Lancet. 4. E216–217.

Perkins S. Simon J. Jayakuma A *et al*. (2008). Renal replacement therapy in support of Operation Iraqi Freedom: a tri-service perspective. Military Medicine. 173. 11. 1115–1121.

Pickkers P. Ostermann M. Joannidis M *et al*. (2017). The intensive care medicine agenda on acute kidney injury. Intensive Care Medicine. 43. 1198–1209.

Richardson A. Whatmore J. (2013). Chapter 9: Continuous renal replacement therapies: assessment, monitoring and care. In: Mallett J. Albarran JW. Richardson A (eds). Critical care manual of clinical procedures and competencies. 1st Edition. Chichester, West Sussex: John Wiley & Sons Ltd.

Stanifer JW. Sharma A. (2017). Life-sustaining technologies in resource-limited settings. The Lancet. 390. 1024.

Stevens PE. Tamimi NA. Al-Hasani MK *et al*. (2001). Non-specialist management of acute renal failure. QJM: Monthly Journal of the Association of Physicians. 894. 533–540.

White SL. Chadban SJ. Jan S. Chapman JR. Cass A. (2008). How can we achieve global equity in provision of renal replacement therapy? Bulletin of the World Health Organization. 86. 3. 229–237.

17 | Sepsis

Sepsis is a time-critical medical emergency and a global problem. Within resource limited settings sepsis has been identified as likely to contribute to the high burden of infectious disease (Jacob *et al.*, 2009; WHO, 2015). However, there remains a significant paucity of evidence, appropriate consensus guidelines and recommendations specifically for this setting. With few national organisations to represent countries at international meetings, this means many international definitions and standards are based on HIC environments (Singer *et al.*, 2016). While international consensus definitions are useful for standardisation, limited access to continuing professional development and resources makes the implementation of these evidence-based interventions difficult. A survey of anaesthetic providers in sub-Saharan African hospitals explored the implementation and delivery of international sepsis standards and revealed just 1.2% of hospitals could implement these standards (Baelani *et al.*, 2011).

Factors which make it difficult to use evidence from HIC includes the fact that life expectancy in LICs and LMICs is often less. Younger patients may be able to compensate and/or present in later stages of diseases, there may be underlying pathologies including HIV, TB and malnutrition, which make people (particularly children) more susceptible due to the associated poor immunological response. Potential causes of sepsis, including bacterial, fungal, viral, protozoal (malaria) or tropical disease, add complexity to the presentation and management of sepsis (Kwizera *et al.*, 2016).

Like many critical care conditions, care often commences before admission to critical care. Key interventions in sepsis care involve early recognition of patients with sepsis, assessment and screening for the cause of sepsis, early administration of oxygen and antibiotics and treatment of the underlying cause. Potential barriers to initiating treatment outside of the critical care unit are outlined in Box 17.1.

Box 17.1 Potential barriers to sepsis care (Singhi *et al.*, 2009)

- Limited availability of critical care services; this includes technology for monitoring and equipment to deliver care.
- Inadequate number of trained staff.

- Limited availability of medications.
- Inadequate transport facilities to move critically ill patients to hospitals with critical care facilities, especially paediatrics.
- Delay in seeking and accessing care.
- Other diseases, e.g. malaria, dengue.
- Higher incidence of malnutrition.
- The issue of antimicrobial resistance.
- Prohibitive cost of care, which families may be required to pay for specialist tests or drugs.

In extreme cases, sepsis may be linked to an outbreak, for example cholera or H1N1 influenza; this results in a balance between a high caseload of patients and a low supply of resources and personnel (Jacob *et al.*, 2013). With few countries having national surveillance programmes (WHO, 2017a), the identification and monitoring of disease progression may be difficult. The recent Ebola outbreak in West Africa highlighted the importance of surveillance monitoring to identify potential outbreaks early. From a hospital perspective, infectious disease outbreaks should be included in major incident plans.

Recognition

Jacob *et al.* (2009) highlighted the material and human resources which impacted on sepsis care in Uganda. With low nurse to patient ratios, limited amounts of IV fluids available in ward areas and access to supplementary oxygen and monitoring resulted in delays in imitating care.

The revised international definitions of sepsis recommended the use of the Sequential (Sepsis – Related) Organ Failure Assessment (SOFA). In practice, with limited access to microbiology services, it may not be possible to use the SOFA screening tool in a resource limited environment due to limited microbiology services. However, the quick-SOFA (q-SOFA) (Box 17.2) was developed to quickly identify high-risk patients with suspected infection outside of the intensive care and prompt further action (Seymour *et al.*, 2016; Vincent *et al.*, 2016). With limited monitoring, early warning scoring tools and many unwell patients on wards, the use of the q-SOFA may provide benefits as a screening tool. The q-SOFA has been used and effective in a hospital in Gabon. Huson *et al.* (2016) conducted 329 complete data sets of adult patients and found the q-SOFA was good predictive value for in-hospital mortality and could identify high-risk patients with bacterial infection or malaria, when diagnostic tests are not available.

Box 17.2   q-SOFA

Systolic blood pressure <100mmHg

Respiratory rate >22/min

Altered mental state (Glasgow Coma Scale <15)

(q-SOFA 2017)

Antibiotics and antimicrobial resistance

Rapid administration of antibiotics in sepsis is linked to reduced mortality; however, the rise in antimicrobial resistance (AMR) is a global concern and there are conflicting messages between these two areas (Reinhart *et al.*, 2017). The WHO (2017b) identifies AMR is already occurring with malaria, TB, HIV, influenza, E. coli, gonorrhoea, Klebsiella pneumoniae treatments. The WHO (2017b) recognises AMR potentially puts the successes of the Millennium Development Goals and Sustainable Development Goals (SDG) reaching their full potential at risk. Not including AMR in the SDGs has been criticised as a missed opportunity, particularly as TB, malaria and HIV reduction has been identified and resistance to medicines is already seen (Fitchett & Atun, 2016). AMR is multi-factorial and specific challenges within low-income settings include overuse, inappropriate use of antibiotics or taken with no professional oversight, coupled with restricted access to antibiotics and microbiology services to process samples and monitor antibiotic levels (WHO, 2017b; Thwaites *et al.*, 2016). Early administration of antibiotics in sepsis has been showed to decrease mortality, but it should also include rapid de-escalation once the causative organism has been identified (Reinhart, 2016).

Education

Like many conditions specialist input from a variety of healthcare professionals is required to prevent sepsis and promote early recognition. When a patient presents with sepsis and organ dysfunction, it may be the critical care nurse who has the most knowledge. Their role may be to assess, initiate treatment and co-ordinate patient care; however, care often begins before the patient arrives at the hospital. The following steps outline logical time-critical steps to be taken for a patient with suspected sepsis.

1. Education and training of staff and nations focusing on prevention, recognition and treatment.

    a. The term 'sepsis' should be used as a standard term amongst healthcare workers and when speaking to patients and families.

2. Prevention, e.g. HIV prevention, malaria, cholera, Ebola, hand washing, flu, access to clean water, education, to prevent the spread of infection or to recognise signs and symptoms of sepsis early.

3. Recognition

    a. Assess patient:

        i. Do you think it is sepsis? Treat it as sepsis until proved otherwise.
        ii. Take a structured history.
        iii. Assess patient using Airway, Breathing, Circulation, Disability (neurological), Exposure approach.
        iv. Use q-SOFA.

      v. Early recognition of organ hypoperfusion; do not rely on hypotension to diagnose septic shock, as often this is a preterminal sign and associated with high mortality.

     vi. Early recognition of septic shock and escalation in care.

    vii. Consider potential sources of sepsis including local infections and disease epidemiology. Use radiological, ultrasound, laboratory results as available.

  b. Identify causative microbiology pathogen:

      i. Blood cultures and any other swabs/specimens as appropriate.

     ii. Use rapid testing or microscopy to screen for malaria.

    iii. Consider testing for other viruses, e.g. Ebola, dengue, influenza.

    iv. Consider other causes of immunosuppression, e.g. HIV, TB and malnutrition.

4. Initial treatment – within hour:

  a. Oxygen.

  b. IV access and blood cultures.

  c. If available measure lactate level.

  d. Intravenous antibiotics within one hour of recognition.

  e. Nurse in an observation area (e.g. acute bay on a ward).

  f. Increase the frequency of observations.

  g. Urinary catheter/fluid balance charting.

  h. IV fluid resuscitation.

5. Urgent senior review and plan:

  a. Regular reviews and escalate if concerned.

  b. Consider critical care.

6. Ongoing care:

  a. Continue one-hourly observations.

  b. Start fluid balance chart.

  c. Continue oxygen and titrate SpO_2 >94%.

  d. Review laboratory, radiological and ultrasound results. Does this change your treatment plan?

  e. Assess all interventions – are they working?

  f. Establish a source of infection and treat, e.g. drain surgical infection.

  g. Daily medical review by the critical care team.

  h. Daily review of antibiotics in response to condition and microbiology. Aim to change antibiotics or de-escalate as appropriate.

  i. Continue team approach.

  j. Daily medical review and plan including appropriate parameters.

  k. Continuous monitoring and manage situation.

  l. If poor response, re-consider if this is sepsis:

      i. pneumothorax;

     ii. pleural effusion;

    iii. heart failure;

    iv.   poisoning;

    v.   TB;

    vi.   PCP associated with HIV.

  m. Nutrition (consider NG feeding).

  n. Microbiology and antimicrobial review. Aim to change antibiotics or de-escalate as appropriate.

> (Reinhart *et al.*, 2017. Kwizera *et al.*, 2016.
> Thwaites *et al.*, 2016. Jacob *et al.*, 2013)

In summary, the recent historic World Health Assembly resolution to improve the prevention, diagnosis and clinical management of sepsis (WHO, 2017c) will provide priorities to improve education and resources for healthcare professionals. For sepsis care to be effective, clinicians from all settings need to be involved in the development and promotion of guidelines (Kissoon, 2014). Sepsis requires action on many levels, from a variety of healthcare organisations including public health, primary health-care and hospital services to ensure a seamless transition and escalation in sepsis care. Variations in disease aetiology, high antimicrobial resistance and restricted antibiotics, resources and trained workforce will continue to pose significant challenges in sepsis care in resource limited environments. There is an urgent need to develop research and consensus guidelines into the treatment of sepsis in resource limited environments.

References

Baelani I. Jockberger S. Laimer T *et al.* (2011). Availability of critical care resources to treat patients with severe sepsis or septic shock in Africa: a self-reported, continent-wide survey of anaesthesia providers. Critical Care. R10. DOI: https://doi.org/10.1186/cc9410.

Fitchett JR. Atun R. (2016). Antimicrobial resistance: opportunity for Europe to establish global leadership. Lancet Infectious Diseases. 16. 388–389.

Huson MAM. Kalkman R. Grobusch MP. Van der Poll T. (2016). Predictive value of the qSOFA score in patients with suspected infection in a resource limited setting in Gabon. Travel Medicine and Infectious Disease. 15. 76–77.

Jacob ST. Lim M. Banura P. *et al.* (2013). Integrating sepsis management recommendations into clinical care guidelines for district general hospitals in resource-limited settings: the necessity to augment new guidelines with future research. BMC Medicine. 11. 107.

Jacob ST. Moore CC. Banura P *et al.* (2009). Severe sepsis in two Ugandan hospitals: a prospective observational study of management and outcomes in predominantly HIV-1 infected population. PLOS one. 4. 11. E7782.

Kissoon N. (2014). Sepsis guideline implementation: benefits, pitfalls and possible solutions. Critical Care. 18. 207. Available at: http://ccforum.com/content/18/2/207.

Kwizera A. Festic E. Dünser MW. (2016). What's new in sepsis recognition in resource-limited settings? Intensive Care Med. DOI: 10.1007/s00134-016-4222x.

q-SOFA. (2017). What is qSOFA? Available at: http://qsofa.org/what.php.

Reinhart K. Daniels R. Kissoon N *et al.* (2017). Recognizing Sepsis as a Global Health Priority – A WHO Resolution. New England Journal of Medicine. DOI: 10.1056/NEJMp1707170.

Seymour SW. Liu VX. Iwashyna TJ *et al.* (2016). Assessment of clinical criteria for sepsis: for the Third International Consensus definition for sepsis and septic shock (sepsis-3). Journal of the American Medical Association. 315. 8. 762–774.

Singer M. Coopersmith CCM. Hotchkiss RRS *et al.* (2016). The third international consensus definitions for sepsis and septic shock (Sepsis-3). Journal of the American Medical Association. 315. 8. 801–810.

Singhi SC. Khilnani P. Lodha R *et al.* (2009) Guidelines for treatment of septic shock in resource limited environments. Journal of Paediatric Infectious Diseases. 4. 173–192.

Thwaites CL. Lundeg G. Dondrop AM. (2016). Recommendations for infection management in patients with sepsis and septic shock in resource-limited settings. Intensive Care Med. DOI: 10.1007/s00134-016-4415-3.

Vincent JL. Martin GS. Levy MM. (2016). qSOFA does not replace SIRS in the definition of sepsis. Critical Care. 20. 210. DOI: https://doi.org/10.1186/s13054-016-1389-z.

World Health Organization. (2015). The 10 leading causes of death by country income group 2012. Available at: www.who.int/mediacentre/factsheets/fs310/en/index1.html.

World Health Organization. (2017a). The burden of health care-associated infection worldwide: a summary. Available at: www.who.int/gpsc/country_work/summary_2010 0430_en.pdf.

World Health Organization. (2017b). Antimicrobial resistance. Available at: www.who.int/mediacentre/factsheets/fs194/en/.

World Health Organization. (2017c). 70th World Health Assembly improving the prevention, diagnosis and clinical management of sepsis. Available at: http://apps.who.int/gb/ebwha/pdf_files/WHA70/A70_R7-en.pdf.

18 Vascular access

Critically ill patients often require vascular access to administer drugs and fluids. Types of devices include peripheral cannulas, central venous catheters (CVCs), intra-osseous lines and venous cut-downs. Choosing the type of vascular access will be determined by the situation, e.g. cardiac arrest, resources available, medication and fluids to administer and the skills of the person inserting the line.

Peripheral cannulas

In resource limited critical care units peripheral cannulas are likely to be the commonest type of vascular access used. Challenges with peripheral cannulas include limited skin antiseptics, dressings which do not allow inspection of the insertion site, and cannulas may stay in longer than expected. Also, drugs which may cause extravasation and necrosis may be administered via this route due to a lack of CVCs or operators skilled to insert this type of line. For example, vasopressors may need to be given carefully through a peripheral IV line placed in the ante-cubital fossa due to a lack of central access (WHO, 2013).

Allegranzi et al. (2011) conducted a systematic review of the burden of endemic healthcare associated infections in low resource settings and found the incidence of infection acquired in critical care was 47.9 per 1000 bed days, compared to the 13.6 per 1000 bed days in the USA. Vascular access devices were identified as one of the highest sources of infection in this environment. Principles of caring for a peripheral IV cannula are outlined in Figure 18.1. To minimise the risk of complication, peripheral cannula care includes:

- carefully observing for signs of extravasation and necrosis;
- observing for signs of infection and phlebitis every time the cannula is used;
- removing cannulas that are no longer required;
- following the principles of infection control prevention when siting and handling cannulas including hand hygiene, wearing of clean gloves;

- re-siting cannulas that have been in place for longer than 24–48 hours;
- documenting when the line was inserted and any concerns or complications.

Tools including the Visual Infusion Phlebitis Scoring Tool (VIPS) (Table 18.1) can assist nurses to monitor insertion sites and identify potential complications early.

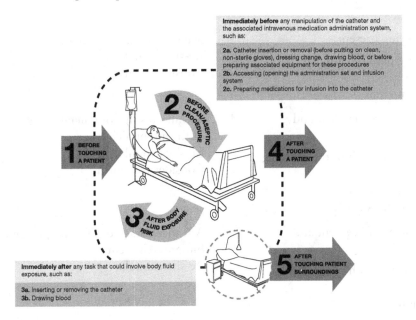

My 5 Moments for Hand Hygiene
Focus on caring for a patient with a peripheral venous catheter

Immediately before any manipulation of the catheter and the associated intravenous medication administration system, such as:

2a. Catheter insertion or removal (before putting on clean, non-sterile gloves), dressing change, drawing blood, or before preparing associated equipment for these procedures
2b. Accessing (opening) the administration set and infusion system
2c. Preparing medications for infusion into the catheter

1 BEFORE TOUCHING A PATIENT

2 BEFORE CLEAN/ASEPTIC PROCEDURE

3 AFTER BODY FLUID EXPOSURE RISK

4 AFTER TOUCHING A PATIENT

5 AFTER TOUCHING PATIENT SURROUNDINGS

Immediately after any task that could involve body fluid exposure, such as:

3a. Inserting or removing the catheter
3b. Drawing blood

Key additional considerations for peripheral intravenous catheters

1. Indication: Ensure that a peripheral venous catheter is indicated. Remove the catheter when no longer necessary/clinically indicated.
2. Insertion/maintenance/removal
2.1 Prepare clean skin with an antiseptic (70% alcohol, tincture of iodine, an iodophor, or alcohol-based 2% chlorhexidine gluconate) before catheter insertion.
2.2 Wear clean, non-sterile gloves and apply an aseptic procedure (with non-touch technique) for catheter insertion, removal, and blood sampling.

2.3 Replace any dry gauze-type dressings every 2 days.
2.4 Consider scheduled catheter change every 96 hours.
2.5 Change tubing used to administer blood, blood products, chemotherapy, and fat emulsions within 24 hours of infusion start. Consider changing all other tubing every 96 hours.
3. Monitoring: Record time and date of catheter insertion, removal and dressing change, and condition (visual appearance) of catheter site every day.

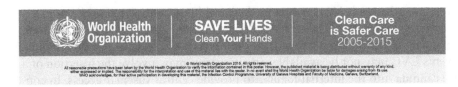

World Health Organization | **SAVE LIVES** Clean **Your** Hands | **Clean Care is Safer Care** 2005-2015

Figure 18.1 Principles of caring for a peripheral IV cannula

Table 18.1 Visual Infusion Phlebitis Scoring Tool

IV site appears healthy	0	No signs of phlebitis. Observe cannula.
One of the following evident: • slight pain near IV site; • slight redness near IV site.	1	Possible first signs of phlebitis. Observe cannula.
Two of the following evident: • pain near IV site; • erythema; • swelling.	2	Early stage of phlebitis. Re-site cannula.
All the following present: • pain along path of cannula; • erythema; • induration.	3	Medium stage of phlebitis. Re-site cannula. Consider treatment.
All the following are evident and extensive: • pain along the path of the cannula; • erythema; • induration; • palpable venous cord.	4	Advanced stage of phlebitis or start of thrombophlebitis. Re-site cannula. Consider treatment.
All the following are evident and extensive: • pain along the path of the cannula; • erythema; • induration; • palpable venous cord; • pyrexia.	5	Advanced stage of thrombophlebitis. Initiate treatment. Re-site cannula.

Source: VIPS, 2018. Reproduced with kind permission from IV Team

Central venous catheters

Central venous catheters (CVC), also termed central lines, central venous line or central venous access, (Picture 18.1) are special lines inserted either into the subclavian, internal jugular or femoral veins to provide intravenous access. In resource limited environments CVC may not be available; an alternative may involve the insertion of a wide bore cannula into the internal jugular to provide central vascular access. In consequence, nurses may have varying experiences of using CVCs in practice.

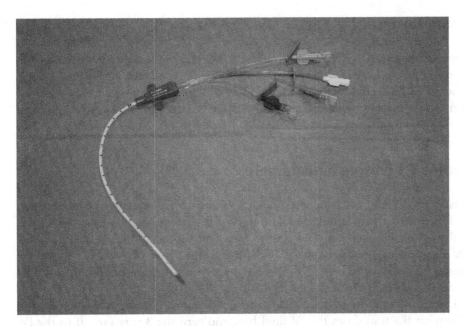

Picture 18.1 Central venous catheter. NB the different coloured ports indicate different sized lumen

In critical care, CVCs are inserted for the following reasons:

- Rapid fluid resuscitation, e.g. trauma, burns, major surgery.
- To measure central venous pressure (CVP).
- To administer drugs that cannot be administered via peripheral lines, e.g. vasopressors, amiodarone, potassium.
- To administer multiple continuous infusions.
- To take blood, e.g. central venous oxygen saturation measurements.

Potential CVC complications include:

- pneumothorax;
- catheter related blood stream infection (CRBSI);
- haemorrhage;
- haematoma;
- air embolism;
- misplacement, e.g. into the carotid artery;
- cardiac arrythmias;
- cardiac tamponade;
- thrombosis;
- catheter occlusion.

CVP monitoring

CVP monitoring can be either via a transducer attached to a monitor or the use of a manometer (Cole, 2007). Regardless of the method used, the distal port of the CVC should be dedicated for measuring CVP. Transducers are measured in millimetres of mercury (mmHg), whereas, manometers are measured in centimetres of water (cmH$_2$O). Normal ranges are 5–10cmH$_2$O or 2–6mmHg.

Measuring CVP using a manometer

To measure a CVP with a manometer, first check the CVC is patent. The manometer will be attached to a drip stand; therefore to zero the manometer, use the spirit level attached to the manometer to line up the 'zero' on the manometer with the phlebostatic axis (fourth intercostal space, mid-axillary line). You may need to move the manometer up or down to zero. To maintain consistency in results the same position and landmarks on the patient should be used.

Turn the 3-way tap off to the patient, and slowly fill the manometer column with fluid. Turn off the flow from the IV fluid bag, and turn the 3-way tap off to the IV fluids and open to the manometer and patient. The fluid should then fall to the level of pressure in the central vessels. The fluid will move every time the patient breaths; you should record the lower number. Finally, turn off the 3-way tap to the manometer and document the reading.

Measuring CVP using a transducer

To measure CVP using a transducer set requires a monitor with a transducer cable attached to a special transducer giving set. A pressure bag inflated to 300mmHg with 0.9% sodium chloride maintains line patency and provides pressure to measure the CVP. The position of the transducer is the fourth intercostal mid-axillary line and can be taped or attached to a transducer table on a drip stand.

When the transducer set is run though, attached and zeroed a continuous trace will appear on the monitor and provide real-time CVP measurements.

CVC infection

CVCs are high-risk for infection, particularly femoral lines, and there is a higher incidence of central line associated blood stream infections (CLABSI) (Allegranzi et al., 2011). Arrieta et al. (2015) found the development of CLABSI occurred due to health-care workers not following evidence-based or standardised healthcare practices. In addition, Parajuli et al. (2017) reported the need of development and implementation of infection prevention control practices and protocols, surveillance and antimicrobial stewardship was required to reduce the incidence of CLABSI. Principles of preventing CLABSI are outlined in Figure 18.2.

My 5 Moments for Hand Hygiene

Focus on caring for a patient with a central venous catheter

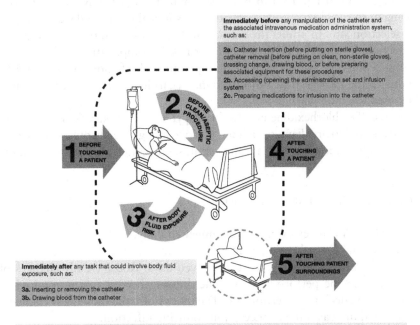

Immediately before any manipulation of the catheter and the associated intravenous medication administration system, such as:

2a. Catheter insertion (before putting on sterile gloves), catheter removal (before putting on clean, non-sterile gloves), dressing change, drawing blood, or before preparing associated equipment for these procedures
2b. Accessing (opening) the administration set and infusion system
2c. Preparing medications for infusion into the catheter

1 BEFORE TOUCHING A PATIENT

2 BEFORE CLEAN/ASEPTIC PROCEDURE

3 AFTER BODY FLUID EXPOSURE RISK

4 AFTER TOUCHING A PATIENT

5 AFTER TOUCHING PATIENT SURROUNDINGS

Immediately after any task that could involve body fluid exposure, such as:

3a. Inserting or removing the catheter
3b. Drawing blood from the catheter

Key additional considerations for central intravenous catheters

1. Indication: Ensure that a central intravenous catheter is indicated. Remove the catheter when no longer needed/clinically indicated.
2. Insertion/maintenance/removal
2.1 Avoid inserting catheters into the femoral vein.
2.2 Prepare clean skin with an antiseptic (alcohol-based 2% chlorhexidine-gluconate preferred) before insertion.
2.3 Use full sterile barrier precautions during insertion (cap, surgical mask, sterile gloves, sterile gown, large sterile drape).
2.4 Replace gauze-type dressings every 2 days and transparent dressings every 7 days; replace dressings whenever visibly soiled.

2.5 Change tubing used to administer blood, blood products, chemotherapy, and fat emulsions within 24 hours of infusion start. Consider changing all other tubing every 96 hours.
2.6 Use aseptic procedure (with non-touch technique) for all catheter manipulations.
2.7 "Scrub the hub" with alcohol-based chlorhexidine-gluconate for at least 15 seconds.
3. Monitoring: Record time and date of catheter insertion, removal and dressing change, and condition (visual appearance) of the catheter skin site every day.

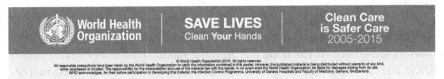

World Health Organization | **SAVE LIVES** Clean **Your** Hands | **Clean Care is Safer Care** 2005-2015

Figure 18.2 Principles of caring for a patient with a central venous catheter

Reproduced by kind permission from the World Health Organization.

In resource limited environments evidence has shown compliance with insertion and maintenance CVC care bundles reduced the incidence of CLABSI (Arietta *et al.*, 2011). The principles of the CVC insertion care bundle include the following (Scottish Intensive Care Society Audit Group, 2012):

- Use of an insertion checklist and documentation. This provides a record and prompts the operator and assistant to follow best practice. The checklist can also be used for audit purposes to ensure compliance.
- Hand hygiene and maximal barrier precautions. Strict aseptic techniques on insertion including surgical hand scrub prior to donning surgical gowns and gloves. The wearing of sterile gloves, gowns, theatre hat, surgical masks and sterile drapes.
- Catheter selection site. In adults the subclavian line has shown to have a reduced risk of infection; however, this carries a higher risk of complication (e.g. pneumothorax) and requires a greater skill of the operator. The femoral site should be avoided due to the increased risk of infection. Regardless of location, ultrasound should be used to guide placement.
- Skin antisepsis. 2% chlorhexidine in 70% isopropyl alcohol should be used to clean the skin and allowed to dry. Fanning, wiping or blow drying should not be undertaken.
- The site should be addressed with a transparent, semi-permeable dressing to allow inspection of the site.

CVC maintenance bundle include the following:

- The need for the CVC is reviewed and documented daily.
- Check to ensure the CVC dressing is intact.
- Ensure the CVC dressing is changed every seven days. Routine/daily changes of dressing should not be performed unless the dressing becomes compromised or you are unable to check the insertion site. The more times the dressing is changed/line manipulated increases the chances of introducing infection.
- 2% chlorhexidine gluconate in 70% isopropyl alcohol should be used for cleaning the insertion site during dressing changes.
- 'Scrub the hub' for 15 seconds prior to accessing any of the access hubs, e.g. to administer drugs.
- Ensure hand hygiene is performed before accessing the line.

Intra-osseous

The insertion of an IO cannula involves the insertion of a special needle through the skin, periosteum, the cortex of the bone and into the medullary cavity (Resuscitation Council (UK), 2011). While the intra-osseous (IO) route is routinely used in pre-hospital and paediatric emergencies, the use in adult hospital emergencies remains less frequent. Advantages of IO access include the following:

- Easy and quick to insert. IO insertion is faster than establishing IV access, and takes less than one minute (Day, 2011), with speeds of <20 seconds reported (Ong et al., 2009). However, the decision to use the IO route may be delayed, for example policies and training courses may recommend the IO route should be considered. Practitioners should choose the route they deem most appropriate at the time (Garside et al., 2015).
- Less training is required than for other forms of vascular access and it has fewer associated complications (Garside et al., 2015).

- Fluids, medications and blood products can be delivered with an IO. Flow rates of up to 125ml/min can be achieved (Day, 2011).
- Rapid administration of medications, with plasma concentrations reaching the equivalent to central venous catheters (Resuscitation Council (UK), 2011).
- Allows for bone marrow aspiration which can be used for analysis. If using bone marrow for tests, do not use point of care testing machines, e.g. blood glucose, arterial gas analysers, as the sample can damage the machines; therefore, all bloods will need to be sent to the laboratory and marked via the route taken.

While the IO route is predominately used in the pre-hospital/emergency setting, patients may be admitted to critical care units with an IO in place; therefore, nurses need to understand what they are used for and how to remove them (Garside *et al.*, 2015).

There are several types of IO insertion devices including 'screw' type devices, drills or gas pressurised guns. If no IO cannula is available, bone marrow aspiration or spinal (lumbar puncture) needles can be used (Resuscitation Council (UK), 2011) (Pictures 18.2 to 18.4). Locations for an IO in an adult is proximal humerus, proximal or distal tibia. In children proximal or distal tibia.

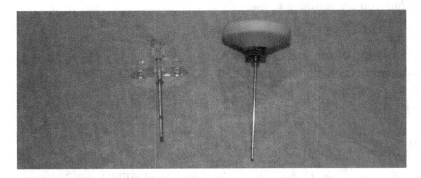

Picture 18.2 IO needle with trocar

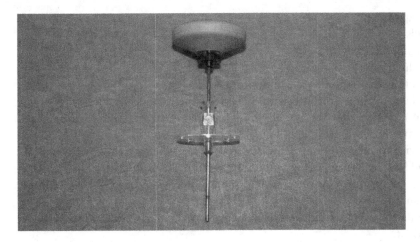

Picture 18.3 IO needle with trocar

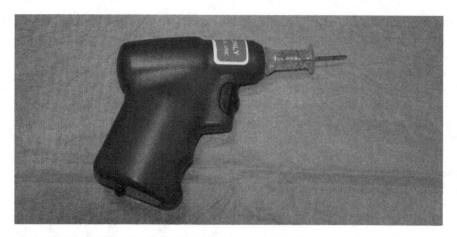

Picture 18.4 IO drill

Contra-indications include:

- fracture in bone you are planning to use;
- osteogenesis imperfecta;
- coagulation disorders, e.g. haemophilia;
- previous orthopaedic surgery near insertion site;
- IO previously within last 24 hours in the bone you are planning to use;
- infection at site;
- inability to locate landmarks.

IO insertion

The procedure for inserting an IO depends on the device used (WHO, 2013; Resuscitation Council (UK), 2011).

- Assemble equipment.
- Wash hands and wear PPE.
- Attach needle to IO device.
- Locate landmarks.
- Clean the site with alcohol-based solution.
- If appropriate, infiltrate the site with local anaesthetic and allow to work. Ong *et al.* (2009) identify that the actual effects of using local anaesthetic prior to IO insertion have not been evaluated.
- Use the device to insert IO needle as directed by manufacturer instructions. Stop when a sudden 'give or pop' is felt and the desired depth is obtained.
- Release the driver and remove the stylet. Immediately dispose of the stylet in an approved sharps box.
- Secure the IO to prevent accidental dislodgement particularly if you need to transfer the patient.

- Flush the line with 10ml of normal saline (no flush = no flow) then repeated flushes as required. The insertion of an IO is relatively painless; however, the administration of drugs is painful in the conscious patient (Garside *et al.*, 2015). Some operators administer a local anaesthetic; however, caution should be taken as administration of local anaesthetic into the circulating volume is dangerous.
- Connect the primed giving set to the line. Unless a syringe pump is available, gravity giving sets will not allow administration of fluids. Therefore, a 50ml syringe connected via a 3-way tap allows for fluids/drugs to be 'pushed'.
- Monitor the site for complications.
- Document the procedure.
- IO should be removed within 24 hours. When removing the line be careful not to rock or bend needles. Once removed immediately dispose of the needle in a sharps bin. Apply pressure at the site if needed and cover via a dry dressing.

Potential complications include (Resuscitation Council (UK), 2011):

- extravasation;
- embolism;
- infection, e.g. osteomyelitis or cellulitis;
- compartment syndrome;
- skin necrosis;
- fracture.
- In hospitalised patients, if the line is not documented or handed over, there is a risk the line may get covered by sheets and blankets and stay in longer than expected, which could then lead to other complications.

In critical care, the IO route may be used in the emergency resuscitation and stabilisation of a patient, for example on admission, a collapsed patient on the ward or in the emergency department. Once the patient has been sufficiently volume resuscitated, peripheral or central venous catheters may be easier to insert, or skilled help will have arrived, and the IO needle can be removed to prevent potential complications as outlined above.

Venous cut-down

Venous cut-downs have been largely replaced by the use of IO; therefore, this technique is not frequently performed and tends to be the last attempt when all other routes have failed. The great saphenous vein is the commonest vein used in both adults and children and performed at the ankle. The procedure involves the following:

- Assemble equipment.
- Wash hands and apply PPE.
- Immobilise the patient's lower limb.
- Clean the skin using appropriate skin antisepsis and identify the saphenous vein.
- Infiltration with local anaesthetic.

- The vein is identified following incision of the skin and blunt dissection of the subcutaneous tissue with haemostat forceps.
- 1–2cm of the vein is identified. Ligatures are passed around the proximal and distal part of the vein. The distal end is tied off.
- A small hole is made into the upper part of the exposed vein and a cannula is inserted into the vein.
- The cannula is then secured in place.
- The line is flushed with normal saline. If it does not work, the cannula may not be in the vein.
- The wound should be sutured around the cannula and the site covered with a sterile dressing.

References

Allegranzi B. Nejad SB. Combescure C. (2011). Burden of endemic health-care associated infection in developing countries: systematic review and meta-analysis. The Lancet. 377. 228–241.

Arrieta J. Delgado P. Orrego C et al. (2015). Reducing the incidence of CLABSI in Latin American ICUs: A multi-country quality improvement collaborative. Preliminary results from the second phase. BMJ Quality & Safety. 24. 728–729.

Cole E. (2007). Measuring central venous pressure. Nursing Standard. 22. 7. 40–42.

Day MW. (2011). Intraosseous devices for intravascular access in adult trauma patients. Critical Care Nurse. 31. 2. 76–90.

Garside J. Prescott S. Shaw S. (2015). Intraosseous vascular access in critically ill adults: a review of the literature. Nursing in Critical Care. 21. 3. 167–177.

Ong MEH. Chan YH. Oh JJ. Ngo S-Y. (2009). An observational, prospective study comparing tibial and humeral intraosseous access using the EZ-IO. The American Journal of Emergency Medicine; 27: 8–15. DOI: 10.1016/j.ajem.2008.01.025.

Parajuli NP. Acharya SP. Dahal S. et al. (2017) Epidemiology of device-associated infections in an intensive care unit of a teaching hospital in Nepal: a prospective surveillance study from a developing country. American Journal of Infection Control. Doi: 10.1016/j.ajic.2017.02.040.

Resuscitation Council (UK). (2011). Paediatric immediate life support. 2nd Edition. London: Resuscitation Council (UK).

Scottish Intensive Care Society Audit Group. (2012). Central line insertion bundle. Version 2. NHS National Service Scotland. Edinburgh: ISD Scotland Publications.

Visual Infusion Phlebitis Score. (2018). VIP Score introduction. Available at: www.vipscore.net/introduction/.

World Health Organization. (2013). Pocket book of hospital care for children: guidelines for the management of common childhood illnesses. 2nd Edition. Geneva: World Health Organization.

19 | Pain management and sedation

While communicable, non-communicable diseases, child and maternal health have attracted significant international focus within the UN SDGs, there remains no reference to pain management, yet acute pain can be accompanied with all these conditions (Vijayan, 2011; Bond, 2010). The effects of not managing pain in a critically ill patient include delayed healing and recovery, poor sleep, increased stress response (increased catabolism, hyperglycaemia, immunosuppression), discomfort, suffering, higher risk of morbidity, prolonged critical care and hospital stay and risk of developing chronic pain (Throp & James, 2010; Vijayan, 2011).

A lack of access to appropriate drugs and resources is a daily challenge when trying to provide analgesia; in addition, limited access to education and ongoing professional development opportunities result in poor pain management strategies. Nursing and medical schools may not include pain management as part of the education programmes; coupled with limited access to professional development opportunities, prescription patterns may not have changed even though newer drugs may be available within the department (Vijayan, 2011). A survey of the International Association for the Study of Pain (IASP) (2010) members in low resource settings revealed 91% of members reported limited education was the main barrier to pain management (Bond, 2010). In practice, healthcare professionals may rely on following what others do, learning from books or by didactic training, with little practical experience (Johnson *et al.*, 2015).

The perception amongst healthcare professionals can influence pain management strategies; for example, Chan *et al.* (2008) reported while surgeons recognised effective pain management improved recovery, they also found 70% of surgeons felt patients should expect pain post-operatively. Johnson *et al.* (2015) found Rwandan anaesthetists had little time to follow up patients post-operatively and relied on nurses to assess and direct pain management, who often requested a pain review only if the patient complained.

A lack of training and experience can also affect healthcare professionals' use of opioids; for example, concerns of overuse of strong opioids exist for fear of causing addiction, or patients being too sensitive to them, leading to healthcare professionals not wanting to use opioids (opiophobia) or withholding strong medications, and opting for sedation and restraint (Soyannwo, 2010; Boni, 2010). Vijayan *et al.* (1994)

found 40% of patients who reported moderate to severe pain cited analgesia was either not given or inadequate. This study lead to the development of an acute pain service in all university and major hospitals in Malaysia and the concept of pain being the '5th vital sign' (Vijayan, 2011).

Additional challenges with managing pain in resource limited environments include opioids not being freely available and having restrictive laws to prevent abuse. Families and patients can have negative attitudes towards opioids; with limited information given to patients pre-operatively regarding post-operative pain management options, this can lead to patients afraid to ask or report pain and accept the care they receive (Vijayan, 2011; Johnson *et al.*, 2015).

Most patients in critical care will experience pain (Throp & James, 2010). The sources of pain can vary, from the primary pathology (e.g. burns, wounds, fractures), complications of the original problem, pain from critical care interventions (e.g. insertion of central or peripheral lines), painful joints and pain during position changes (Throp & James, 2010). Exacerbating factors also may include:

- fear, helplessness and loss of control due to the situation that made them require admission or the unfamiliar critical care environment itself;
- loss of memory due to drugs that have been given, so loss of time. Drugs and/or condition may not allow them to communicate or understand the situation;
- anxiety and uncertainty about the present and future for the individual and family;
- background noises, e.g. alarms, phones ringing;
- ongoing activity 24 hours a day, e.g. admissions, patients deteriorating, lights not being turned down;
- inability to sleep;
- frustration, e.g. not being able to do things for themselves or feeling they are not getting better;
- other sensations: thirst, hunger, hot, cold, cramps, nausea, itching;
- boredom.

Effective pain management in critical care allows ETT tolerance, mechanical ventilation, suctioning and other distressing procedures to be undertaken, co-operation with care, reduce stress response and cause less disturbing memories (Throp & James, 2010). Patients should not be restrained as this will cause injury and increase the patients' distress. In addition, to the multi-modal pharmacological approaches outlined above, non-pharmacological approaches should be followed (Box 19.1).

Box 19.1   Non-pharmacological and pharmacological approaches to pain management within critical care

Non-pharmacological approaches:

- Talk to the patient and use their name.
- Encourage visitors to talk to the patient.

- Tell recovering patients they are doing well; tell those who are less well about some positive aspects.
- Include the patient; ask them if they are in pain or explain what you are doing so they feel involved in the care.
- Reduce additional sources of discomfort.
- Splint and stabilise fractures.
- Use distraction therapies, e.g. music.
- Try to maintain day and night routines.
- Provide good nursing care, e.g. position changes, mouth care to prevent thirst, ensure patients are not too hot, cold or hungry.
- Therapeutic touch.
- Appropriate use of alarm settings.

Pharmacological approaches:

- Ask the patient if they are in pain at regular intervals.
- Pre-empt pain, e.g. prior to dressing changes, position changes.
- Ensure 'as required' analgesia is prescribed for breakthrough pain.
- Daily assessment of pain during the ward round.

(Throp & James, 2010)

Assessing pain in a critically ill patient can be challenging, due to sedation or an endotracheal tube preventing communication, resulting in pain often being under-assessed and undertreated (Throp & James, 2010; Vijayan, 2011). If the patient is conscious and can communicate, it may be possible to use the Numerical Rating Scale (NRS) (0–3 or 0–10 scale) to assess pain and interventions. In unconscious patients, subjective observation of pain-related behaviours (movement, facial expression and posturing) and physiological measurements (heart rate, blood pressure and respiratory rate) may be used to assess pain (Throp & James, 2010). There are specially developed scoring tools for use in unconscious patients, for example the Behavioural Pain Score (BPS) or the Critical Care Pain Observation Tool (CCPOT). While validated, they tend to be linked to sedation scores, with pain scores becoming less sensitive as the patient becomes more sedated, suggesting sedation may be used to inappropriately control pain (Whitehouse et al., 2014). Although subjective and less than ideal, pain assessments are important as they allow standardised, consistent information to be gathered by healthcare professionals to assess the interventions provided.

Critically ill patients often require continuous infusions of both short-acting analgesia and sedations if ventilated. Examples include:

- analgesics: morphine or fentanyl;
- sedations: midazolam or propofol.

With few syringe pumps, sometimes boluses of analgesia are administered; this is risky as it may lead to potential complications, and it leads to peaks and troughs resulting in poor pain management. If this method is used, the drugs should be prescribed regularly to avoid troughs (Throp & James, 2010). The enteral route is unpredictable, and the absorption of opioids is poor, therefore analgesics in critical care should be given intravenously.

Analgesics including alfentanil and remifentanil are more expensive and unlikely to be used in a resource limited environment. Pethidine/meperidine may be used as boluses for procedural pain relief but should not be used as an infusion. Ketamine can be used for short procedures and when other analgesics are not available (Throp & James, 2010; Hodges *et al.*, 2007).

A combination of non-opioid and opioid analgesics may achieve better quality pain management, and may include:

- paracetamol/acetaminophen (intravenous (IV) if available, or via nasogastric tube regularly);
- nonsteroidal anti-inflammatory drugs (NSAID), e.g. diclofenac, ibuprofen or keto-profen (via nasogastric tube, or IV) given regularly unless contra-indicated;
- opioids (preferably as a continuous IV infusion);
- nerve blocks (single-shot nerve blocks or epidural analgesia).

(Throp & James, 2010)

Nerve blocks

Nerve blocks may be a bolus or continuous infusion and will be determined by the situation, resources and availability of ultrasound (Johnson *et al.*, 2015). Sites include intercostal, paravertebral, epidural analgesia, transversus abdominis plate (TAP), femoral nerve and interscalene/brachial plexus nerves (Throp & James, 2010). The commonest method is likely to be a spinal block (Johnson *et al.*, 2015). If using a continuous infusion, the catheter and infusion device must be clearly labelled, and a filter should be used to reduce the risk of infection (Throp & James, 2010).

Patient controlled analgesia (PCA)

The use of patient controlled analgesia (PCA) is increasing (Jain & Chatterjee, 2010; Hoda *et al.*, 2007; Anwari *et al.*, 2005; Barros & Lemonica, 2003). To deliver a PCA specialist syringe pumps are required, which may not be available. Alternative methods include the use of elastomeric pumps (Picture 19.1). An elastomeric pump has a balloon reservoir which holds the drug. Used successfully for over 20 years, they have been used to deliver analgesics, chemotherapy, antibiotics, anaesthetics, post-operative pain control and chronic pain management (Theodorides, 2017).

Depending on the type of pump used, pumps can either deliver a set rate of an analgesic, e.g. for a continuous peripheral nerve block, or via a device to give a bolus of a drug (Theodorides, 2017). Factors which affect flow include: atmospheric pressure, e.g. aircraft at altitude, back pressure from IV access, e.g. bent elbows, either over- or underfilled pumps at the start, temperature, viscosity of fluids used and storage of drugs, e.g. if the drug was kept in a fridge prior to adding to the pump. Studies have shown although the flow rates vary, they have been deemed minimal and acceptable

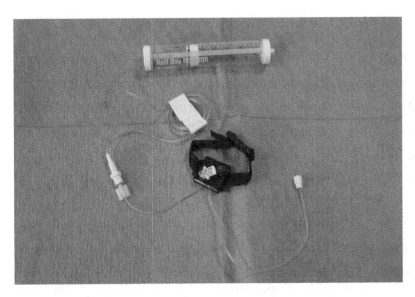

Picture 19.1 Example of a PCA elastomeric infusion device

(Theodorides, 2017). If using an elastomeric PCA, it is important to observe the patient for any signs of over- or under-dosing.

Sedation

If using continuous infusions of sedation, a sedation scoring tool should be used; examples include Ramsay Sedation Scale (RSS) (Box 19.2), Richmond Agitation Sedation Score (RASS) (Table 19.1) and the Riker Sedation Agitation Score (SAS). There is no one best sedation score and it will depend on the type of unit. Evidence has shown using a sedation score is better than not using a scoring tool (Whitehouse *et al.*, 2014). The optimum sedation level depends on the type of patient, but the ideal for most patients will be a balance of preventing anxiety and being not too deeply sedated that they are un-rousable.

Box 19.2   Ramsay Sedation Scoring Tool

1. Patient is anxious and agitated or restless, or both.
2. Patient is co-operative, oriented and tranquil.
3. Patient responds to commands only.
4. Patient exhibits brisk response to light glabellar tap or loud auditory stimulus.
5. Patient exhibits a sluggish response to light glabellar tap or loud auditory stimulus.
6. Patient exhibits no response.

(Anaesthesia UK, 2018)

Table 19.1 Richmond Agitation Sedation Score

+4	Combative	Overtly combative, violent, immediate danger to staff
+3	Very agitated	Pulls or removes tube(s) or catheter(s); aggressive
+2	Agitated	Frequent non-purposeful movement, fights ventilator
+1	Restless	Anxious but movements not aggressive, vigorous
0	Alert and calm	
−1	Drowsy	Not fully alert, but has sustained awakening (eye-opening/eye contact) to voice (>10 seconds)
−2	Light sedation	Briefly awakens with eye contact to voice (<10 seconds)
−3	Moderate sedation	Movement or eye-opening to voice (but no eye contact)
−4	Deep sedation	No response to voice, but movement or eye-opening to physical stimulation
−5	Unarousable	No response to voice or physical stimulation

Source: ICU Delirium, 2018

Summary

In resource limited settings, limited specialist pain practitioners means nurses at the bedside often deal with acute pain. A misconception amongst healthcare workers is that a non-complaining, non-combative patient is deemed pain free. Pain is termed the '5th vital sign' and asking patients if they are in pain regardless of the perception will help provide effective pain relief and prevent complications. However, to do this healthcare professionals must have the confidence to deal with pain and this can only be achieved through effective education programmes, experience in practice and role-modelling. Unrelieved pain causes significant suffering for patients. Nurses spend the most time with the patients and can prevent or intervene early when a patient is in pain; this is the cornerstone of good nursing care. Interventions may include both non-pharmacological and pharmacological approaches.

References

Anaesthesia UK. (2018). Ramsay sedation scale. Available at: www.frca.co.uk/article.aspx?articleid=100192.

Anwari JS. Ahmed F. Mustafa T. (2005). An audit of acute pain service in Central, Saudi Arabia. Saudi Medical Journal. 26. 298–305.

Barros GA. Lemonica L. (2003). Patient controlled analgesia in a university hospital. Revista Brasileira Anestesiologia. 53. 69–82.

Bond M. (2010). Foreword. In: Kopf A. Patel NB (eds). Guide to pain management in low-resource settings. Washington, DC: International Association for the Study of Pain. Available at: www.iasp-pain.org/files/Content/ContentFolders/Publications2/FreeBooks/Guide_to_Pain_Management_in_Low-Resource_Settings.pdf.

Boni F. (2010). Chapter 14: Pain management after major surgery. In: Kopf A. Patel NB (eds). Guide to pain management in low-resource settings. Washington, DC: International Association for the Study of Pain. Available at: www.iasp-pain.org/files/Content/ContentFolders/Publications2/FreeBooks/Guide_to_Pain_Management_in_Low-Resource_Settings.pdf.

Chan SKC. Chui PT. Lee A et al. (2008). Surgeons' attitudes and perception of an acute pain service. Hong Kong Medical Journal. 14. 5. 342–347.

Hoda MQ. Hamid M. Khan FA. (2007). Audit of an acute pain service in a tertiary care hospital in a developing country. Journal of the Pakistan Medical Association. 57. 560–562.

Hodges SC. Mijumbi C. Okello M et al. (2007). Anaesthesia services in developing countries: defining the problems. Anaesthesia. 62. 1. 4–11.

ICU Delirium. (2018). Richmond Agitation-Sedation Scale (RASS). Available at: www.icudelirium.org/docs/RASS.pdf.

International Association for the Study of Pain. (2010). Guide to pain management in-low resource settings. Available at: www.iasp-pain.org/files/Content/ContentFolders/Publications2/FreeBooks/Guide_to_Pain_Management_in_Low-Resource_Settings.pdf.

Jain PN. Chatterjee A. (2010). Development of acute pain service in an Indian cancer hospital. Journal of Pain and Palliative Care Pharmacotherapy. 24. 129–135.

Johnson AP. Mahaffey R. Egan P. Twagirumugabe T. Parlow JL. (2015). Perspectives, perceptions and experiences in postoperative pain management in developing countries: a focus group study conducted in Rwanda. Pain Research and Management. 20. 5. 255–260.

Soyannwo OA. (2010). Chapter 2: Obstacles to pain management in low-resource settings. In: Kopf A. Patel NB (eds). Guide to pain management in low-resource settings. Washington, DC: International Association for the Study of Pain. Available at: www.iasp-pain.org/files/Content/ContentFolders/Publications2/FreeBooks/Guide_to_Pain_Management_in_Low-Resource_Settings.pdf.

Theodorides AA. (2017). The role of elastomeric pumps in post-operative analgesia in orthopaedics and factors affecting their flow rate. Journal of Perioperative Practice. 27. 12. 276–282.

Throp JM. James S. (2010). Chapter 37: Pain management in the intensive care unit. In: Kopf A. Patel NB (eds). Guide to pain management in low-resource settings. Washington, DC: International Association for the Study of Pain. Available at: www.iasp-pain.org/files/Content/ContentFolders/Publications2/FreeBooks/Guide_to_Pain_Management_in_Low-Resource_Settings.pdf.

Vijayan R. (2011). Managing acute pain in the developing world. Pain Clinical Updates. XIX. 3. 1–7. Available at: www.iasp-pain.org/files/Content/ContentFolders/Publications2/PainClinicalUpdates/Archives/PCU_19-3_web_revised_1390260400113_4.pdf.

Vijayan R. Tay KH. Tan LB et al. (1994). Survey of postoperative pain in University Hospital, Kuala Lumpur. Singapore Medical Journal. 35. 502–504.

Whitehouse T. Snelson C. Grounds M. (2014). Intensive Care Society Review of best practice for analgesics and sedation in critical care. London: Intensive Care Society.

20 | Nutrition, rehabilitation and discharge from critical care

Nutrition

Nutrition is essential for recovery from critical illness, but is often neglected in the clinical setting (Azim & Ahmed, 2016). The evidence supporting early enteral feeding in the critically ill patient has been well documented. Over- or under-feeding patients are associated with complications; nutritional requirements depend on multiple factors including the patient's baseline nutritional status, severity of illness, the progression of illness, use of mechanical ventilation, sedation and analgesics (Azim & Ahmed, 2016). In low resource settings, additional challenges may include patients who are malnourished prior to admission; in consequence, balancing the correct nutritional requirement is highly specialised (Giannou et al., 2013). Critically ill patients are also at risk of developing malnutrition resulting in loss of body mass, poor wound healing, impaired immune function, poor diaphragmatic strength, and increased risk of hospital-acquired infection and organ dysfunction (Azim & Ahmed, 2016; Kim & Choi-Kwon, 2011). Studies have shown patients' nutritional status changes and can deteriorate during their hospital stay, even though enteral nutrition was provided (Kim & Choi-Kwon, 2011).

Overfeeding can also lead to hepatic dysfunction, hyperglycaemia and increased risk of infection. Causes of over-feeding can come from poor nutritional monitoring/lack of dietician input, not including non-nutritional energy sources, e.g. propofol infusions, and not changing the energy requirements to meet the changing physiology (Azim & Ahmed, 2016).

Patients with severe malnutrition require specialist dietician input. Specialist guidelines developed by the WHO provide practical guidelines, which consider limited resources when treating severely malnourished children (Ashworth et al., 2003).

Nutritional assessment on admission is a useful tool to provide a baseline. There are various methods for measuring nutritional status including weight and body mass index (BMI), nutritional screening tools, e.g. Malnutrition Universal Screening Tool (MUST), Nutritional Risk Scores (NRS) or the Nutritional Risk in the Critically Ill (NUTRIC) scores. To calculate nutritional requirements, predictive equations for calculating energy requirements are used, with the Harris-Benedict equation being the most commonly used method (Azim & Ahmed, 2016; Kim & Choi-Kwon, 2011).

In critically ill patients, the enteral route of nutrition is the preferred method with the aim of establishing feed within 24 to 48 hours of critical care admission (Azim & Ahmed, 2016). All patients should be enterally feed unless contra-indicated and high-risk conditions that require a greater need for nutritional support include:

–   severe trauma;
–   sepsis;
–   fasting for more than seven days post-surgery;
–   post-operative weight loss greater than 15%;
–   serum albumin level <30g/gl;
–   severe burns;
–   upper gastro-intestinal injuries;
–   pancreatic injury;
–   high-output bowel fistula;
–   chronically discharging sinus or chronic wound;
–   severe maxillo-facial injuries;
–   tracheostomy that makes swallowing difficult.

(Giannou *et al.*, 2013)

Conventional standard feeds are unlikely to be available and alternative sources of enteral feed may be used. These include milk and egg feeds, watery porridge or soups; however, the nutritional content may be difficult to establish (Azim & Ahmed, 2016; Carter & Snell, 2016). With limited resources and staff to feed patients, family members may be used to mix and deliver enteral feeds to patients; this allows patients to receive regular bolus feeds and observation for any complications (Mahoney *et al.*, 2017; Maude *et al.*, 2011).

Enteral feeding may be continuous feeding via gravity or volumetric pumps or by bolus feeding (Kim *et al.*, 2012). Strategies to prevent complications of enteral feeds may include (Giannou *et al.*, 2013; Rutledge & Nesbitt, 2013):

–   warm feeding solution;
–   metoclopramide, to decrease nausea and increase peristalsis and absorption;
–   acid suppression;
–   Imodium and dilution of the feeding solution for diarrhoea;
–   awareness of the possibility of constipation in the immobile patient;
–   attention that the NG tubes may become blocked by crushed tablets;
–   keep the patient's head >30° up during feeding and keep up for 30 minutes afterwards to prevent aspiration;
–   the size of the tube and type of fluid being administered as tubes may become blocked. Flushes of boiled, bottled or sterile water should be used to prevent blockages;
–   start continuous enteral feeds at a rate of 25–50ml/hr then gradually increase until the target regimen has been reached.

During enteral feeding, the stomach contents should be aspirated to confirm the feed has been absorbed and reduce the risk of vomiting (Table 20.1).

Table 20.1 Flow chart for NG aspiration of stomach contents when
establishing enteral feeding and ongoing care

Step 1: Insert NG tube and confirm position

Step 2: Commence feed at 25–50ml/hr

Step 3: Aspirate NG tube after six hours of feeding

Step 4:	Aspirate <300ml	Aspirate 300–400ml	Aspirate 400–500ml	Aspirate >500ml	Vomiting
	Replace aspirate	Replace 300ml	Replace 300ml	Replace 300ml	Stop feed
	Increase feed as tolerated/ indicated until target rate reached	Discard balance Continue at same rate	Discard balance Reduce rate to 15–20ml/hr	Discard balance Reduce rate to 10–20ml/hr	Aspirate and discard stomach contents Restart feed after one hour at half the original rate

Source: Rutledge & Nesbitt, 2013

Naso-gastric tubes

Enteral feeding and administration of medications may be provided via naso-gastric (NG) tubes, e.g. Ryles tubes, fine-bore feeding tubes or Foley, Foley catheters inserted to provide gastrostomy and jejunostomy feeding (Giannou *et al.*, 2013). Potential risks of NG tube insertion include (Rutledge & Nesbitt, 2013):

- insertion into the lungs;
- insertion into the brain in cases of fractured base of skull;
- coiling in the throat. In an intubated patient, the NG tube can wrap around ('lasso') the ETT. Refrigerating the tube helps to reduce the risk of coiling;
- perforation of the oesophagus;
- retropharyngeal abscess;
- damage to the epithelium;
- confirmation of NG position may be difficult due to a lack of pH test strips and the risk of aspiration is high.

Confirmation of position involves the following:

- Train staff involved in NG tube care to check the position of the tube prior to use.
- Record the length of the tube at the nostril and check the position prior to use.
- pH testing of NG aspirate. A pH of between 1 and 5.5 is deemed within the safe range (Picture 20.1).
- X-ray should be used as a second-line test when no NG aspirate can be obtained or the pH test is out of range.

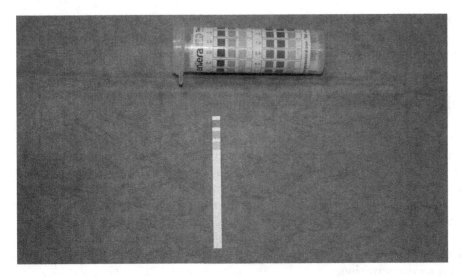

Picture 20.1 pH test strips for confirming NG tube position

- The position of the tube should be documented, including how the position was confirmed. Any tube not inserted correctly must be removed immediately.
- NG tubes must not be used (e.g. flushed or feeding commenced) until the position has been confirmed.

(Rutledge & Nesbitt, 2013)

Methods which must not be used include:

- the 'whoosh' test (listening for air while injecting air through the NG tube);
- Blue litmus paper to confirm acidity or alkalinity;
- absence of respiratory distress;
- bubbling at the end of the tube;
- appearance of feed in the NG tube.

(Rutledge & Nesbitt, 2013; NHS Improvement, 2016)

Total parental nutrition

When the oral and/or enteral route is unable to meet the nutritional needs of the patient, the Total Parental Nutrition (TPN) route may be an option (Rutledge & Nesbitt, 2013). In resource limited environments access to TPN may be limited. Complications of TPN include (Rutledge & Nesbitt, 2013):

- central venous catheter related sepsis;
- hypo- or hyperglycaemia;
- liver dysfunction;
- electrolyte and mineral disturbances;
- volume overload.

In critical care, TPN tends to be administered via a dedicated line on a central venous catheter and administered the same way as other intravenous infusions. Regular electrolyte monitoring and specialist dietician input will be required.

Rehabilitation following critical illness

The WHO recognises as part of the provision of acute care, rehabilitation services are an essential part of service provision, but often services are fragmented, with a greater focus on emergency care (Hirshon *et al.*, 2013). Physiotherapists, also termed physical therapists, provide an important component of care for the critically ill patient. There are no universal standards relating to the number of physiotherapists, occupational therapists, speech and language therapists and specialist doctors to support rehabilitation care. However, the number of trained physiotherapists in the low income settings is estimated to be fewer than 10 per 1 million (WHO, 2017), which is a significant shortfall in service provision.

The role of physiotherapist differs throughout the world, and little has been published on the role of physiotherapists in resource limited environments. Physiotherapists may focus more on treating respiratory conditions; this may be due to few staff to develop and deliver complex rehabilitation plans (Tadyanemhandu & Manie, 2015; Kumar *et al.*, 2007; WHO, 2017). With few healthcare professionals, often there is an overlap of roles and nurses may be required to co-ordinate or deliver treatment plans set by physiotherapists. Specific challenges may include, overcrowding on wards, resulting in few bedside chairs for patients. A lack of specialist equipment including wheelchairs and prosthesis mean patients remain in bed.

A lack of manual handling equipment and training mean patients need to be lifted when repositioning in bed or moving from bed to chair; this increases the risk to injury to both patients and healthcare professionals.

Limited manual handling equipment and staff mean unconscious patients may not be repositioned frequently, resulting in patients developing pressure sores. While patients may survive critical illness, the development of a chronic pressure sore can lead to depression and stress as the individual recognises they are no longer independent or able to work and be financially stable (Nthumba, 2016). The assessment and management of pressure sores are outlined in Chapter 36. When re-positioning patients, check limbs are not trapped and that they are well supported with pillows and blankets.

Venous thromboembolism (VTE)

Venous thromboembolism is a term used to describe both deep vein thrombosis (DVT) and pulmonary embolism (PE) (Davies & Pilcher, 2014). Predisposing factors for VTE include (Davies & Pilcher, 2014):

- venous stasis;
- vein wall injury;
- hypercoagulopathy of the blood.

Patients in critical care are at risk of developing a DVT due to a variety of factors including immobility (bed-rest), surgery, trauma, burns, malignancy, pregnancy, thrombophilia, obesity, smoking, central venous catheter and heart failure (Davies & Pilcher, 2014). Ascertaining the true extent of DVT incidence and prophylaxis may be unclear. Good practice includes finding out if:

- there is access to DVT prophylaxis and if local colleagues routinely prescribe anti-coagulate drugs;
- anti-embolism stockings are available and/or used;
- the unit has any guidelines or audits.

DVT prophylaxis includes use of anti-coagulant drugs, anti-embolism stockings, intermittent compression devices (if available); non-pharmacological methods include good pain management allowing for early patient mobilisation, physiotherapy and leg exercises (Giannou *et al.*, 2013; Davies & Pilcher, 2014).

Discharge for critical care

The decision to discharge a patient from critical care in a resource limited environment depends on several factors including the pressure for beds and the quality of care to be found on the ward (WHO, 2003). Often there is no 'high dependency area', and patients go from intensive nursing care to ward-based care with low nursing numbers (Carter & Snell, 2016). The discharge criteria may follow the WHO (2003) standards:

- conscious;
- good airway, extubated and stable for several hours after extubation;
- breathing comfortably;
- stable blood pressure and urine output;
- haemoglobin >6g/dl or blood transfusion in progress (the patient should not be transferred with a transfusion in progress);
- minimal naso-gastric drainage and bowel sounds, abdomen not distended;
- afebrile;
- not confused.

Preparing a patient for discharge involves liaising with the patient and family, the medical team and admitting ward. All patients should be assessed prior to discharge using the A–E approach and any concerns addressed before transfer.

Medical/nursing handover

Once accepted by the ward medical team, a detailed handover from critical care doctors and nurses to the receiving team should be undertaken. The medical notes should be updated and include discharge summary and plan.

Preparing the patient and family

Explain the discharge plan to the patient and their family. Provide information including the ward name, telephone number, location, visiting time and any additional relevant information. When appropriate gradually start to reduce the frequency of monitoring and equipment attached to the patient, to prepare them for the ward where less monitoring will be available.

Patient assessment

Table 20.2 Patient assessment

Preliminary information	Discharge criteria met? Ward bed identified? Accepted handover by medical team? Patient/family informed? Background information: • date of admission to hospital; • number of days on critical care; • reason for admission/diagnosis; • summary of procedure/stay on critical care; • past medical history; • allergies; • name band checked and correct.
Airway	Patent? Any airway adjuncts? Date extubated? If tracheostomy tube in place: • date inserted; • size and type; • inner tube last checked/changed?
Breathing	Self-ventilating? Oxygen therapy? Respiratory rate and oxygen saturations Productive cough Chest physiotherapy input/plan? Chest drain in place/date removed? Date of last chest X-ray?
Circulation	Pulse Blood pressure Any cardiac medication? Most recent blood results Intravenous fluids in progress?

Table 20.2 Continued

	Urinary catheter: • size; • date inserted/removed? • output? Signs of infection: • barrier nursing required; • source of infection? • antibiotics/microbiology results. Intravenous access: • type/size/location; • date inserted; • any signs of infection? • is IV access still required?
Disability/ neurological	Neurological assessment (Glasgow Coma Scale and pupil size and reaction) Blood glucose level Pain assessment Prescribed analgesia (regular or as required) – is it effective? Sleep pattern Mood
Exposure	Core temperature Pressure areas assessment Any wounds: • location; • type, e.g. surgical, pressure sore; • wound care plan completed including dressing regimen; • when was dressing last completed? Nutrition status (oral fluids/diet/enteral feeding) NG tube size/measurement at nostril/date inserted Enteral feeding regimen agreed by dietician Any complications, e.g. nausea/vomiting, constipation/loose stool Bowels last opened? Any aperients required? Mobility assessment: • physiotherapist input; • assistance required to re-position in bed, transfer from bed to chair, stand, and walk; • any aids available, e.g. crutches, wheelchair?
Other considerations	Do you have all the notes and X-rays? Check patient has a name band Has the doctor completed a discharge summary or letter? Have enough intravenous fluids been prescribed for next 12–24 hours? Ward observation and fluid chart commenced

Time of discharge and follow-up

The time of discharge is an important consideration. Hospital staffing tends to be at its lowest at night and at weekends; in consequence, admission or transfer to a ward during these times is associated with increased mortality. Studies have shown in-hospital cardiac arrests occur 'out of hours' and are likely to be 'un-witnessed events' (Resuscitation Council (UK), 2016). When planning a discharge from critical care, 'out of hours' should be avoided due to the limited staff available to adequately assess and respond to any deterioration.

Depending on staff availability, discharged patients should be followed up to find out what happened to them. If the patient dies, try to find out where the death took place and learn from it (WHO, 2003). However, finding this information can be difficult. Smith *et al.* (2013) conducted a retrospective observational study in one hospital in Ethiopia to assess outcomes following admission to a critical care unit. Smith *et al.* (2013) found overall critical care mortality was 50.4%; they concluded poor record-keeping prevented accurate follow-up of discharged patients and survival from hospital is unknown. All critical care units should have an admission and discharge book. This will allow follow-up of patients post-discharge. Nurses should be encouraged to take responsibility to record the discharge information and feedback given to teams on the outcome.

References

Ashworth A. Khanum S. Jackson A. Schofield C. (2003). Guidelines for the inpatient treatment of severely malnourished children. Available at: http://apps.who.int/iris/bitstream/10665/42724/1/9241546093.pdf.

Azim A. Ahmed A. (2016). Nutrition in neurocritical care. Neurology India. 64. 1. 105.

Carter C. Snell D. (2016). Nursing the critically ill surgical patient in Zambia. British Journal of Nursing. 25. 20. 1123–1128.

Davies AR. Pilcher DV. (2014). Chapter 34: Pulmonary embolism. In: Bersten AD. Soni N (eds). Oh's intensive care manual. 7th Edition. Oxford: Butterworth Heinemann Elsevier.

Giannou C. Baldan M. Molde A. (2013). War surgery: working with limited resources in armed conflict and other situations of violence. Volume 2. Available at: https://shop.icrc.org/la-chirurgie-de-guerre-travailler-avec-des-ressources-limitees-dans-les-conflits-armes-et-autres-situations-de-violence-volume-416.html.

Hirshon JM. Risko N. Calvello EJB *et al.* (2013). Health systems and services: the role of acute care. World Health Organization Bulletin. 91. 386–388. DOI: http://dx.doi.org/10.2471/BLT.12.112664.

Kim H. Choi-Kwon S. (2011). Changes in nutritional status in ICU patients receiving enteral tube feeding: a prospective descriptive study. Intensive and Critical Care Nursing. 27. 194–201.

Kim H. Stotts NA. Froelicher ES *et al.* (2012). Adequacy of early enteral nutrition in adult patients in the intensive care unit. Journal of Clinical Nursing. 21. 2860–2869.

Kumar JA. Maiya AG. Pereira D. (2007). Role of physiotherapists in intensive care units in India: a multicenter trial. Indian Journal of Critical Care Medicine. 11. 4. 198–203.

Mahoney PF. Jayanathan J. Wood P *et al.* (eds). (2017). Anaesthesia handbook. Geneva: International Committee of the Red Cross.

Maude RJ. Hoque G. Hasan MU *et al*. (2011). Timing of enteral feeding in cerebral malaria in resource-poor settings: a randomized trial. PLOS one. 6. 11. E27273.

NHS Improvement. (2016). Resource set initial placement checks for nasogastric and orogastric tubes. July. Publication code: IG20/16. Available at: https://improvement.nhs.uk/documents/193/Resource_set_-_Initial_placement_checks_for_NG_tubes_1.pdf.

Nthumba PN. (2016). Chapter 17: Pressure ulcers. In: Carter LL. Nthumba PM (eds). Principles of reconstructive surgery. Available at: www.paacs.net/wp-content/uploads/2012/09/PAACS-Reconstructive-Surgery-Text-v.-2-072516.pdf.

Resuscitation Council (UK). (2016). Advanced life support. 7th Edition. London: Resuscitation Council (UK).

Rutledge K. Nesbitt I. (2013). Chapter 8: Assessment and support of hydration and nutrition status and care. In: Mallett J. Albarran JW. Richardson A (eds). Critical care manual of clinical procedures and competencies. Chichester, West Sussex: Wiley Blackwell.

Smith ZA. Ayele Y. McDonald P. (2013). Outcomes in critical care delivery at Jimma University Specialised Hospital, Ethiopia. Anaesthesia and Critical Care. 41. 3. 363–368.

Tadyanemhandu C. Manie S. (2015). Profile of patients and physiotherapy patterns in intensive care units in public hospitals in Zimbabwe: a descriptive cross-sectional study. BMC Anaesthesiology. 15. 136. DOI: https://doi.org/10.1186/s12871-015-0120-y.

World Health Organization. (2003). Chapter 14.7: Post-Operative management. In: Surgical Care at the District Hospital. Geneva: World Health Organization.

World Health Organization. (2017). The need to scale up rehabilitation. Available at: www.who.int/disabilities/care/NeedToScaleUpRehab.pdf?ua=1.

21 | Critical care transfer

In a resource limited environment, a critically ill patient may need to be transferred for a variety of reasons including transfer from the ward to a critical care unit, from a critical care unit to another part of the hospital or transferred to another hospital for specialist care, e.g. neurosurgery. There is little evidence surrounding the transfer of critically ill patients in resource limited settings, but it is recognised inter-hospital transfers are likely to be high given the geographical spread of hospitals and few specialist services (Verma *et al.*, 2013).

The decision to transfer must be based on a risk/balance benefit, as there are many complications which may adversely affect the patient (Kulshrestha & Singh, 2016; Intensive Care Society, 2011). The regionalisation of specialist centres, for example paediatrics, level 1 trauma centres and neurosurgery, is accepted as best practice. However, Goh *et al.* (2003) hypothesised the regionalisation of services would have an impact on overall morbidity and mortality due to transfers being undertaken by non-specialist teams. They argued given the high critical care workload in some specialities, for example paediatrics, healthcare professionals in rural and regional hospitals would receive the frequency of patients to attain and retain their proficiency, if appropriate education and resourcing were to be made available. While specialist services are essential, Goh *et al.*'s study demonstrated the need for specialist services and resources in all hospitals, as transfers are likely to be undertaken by non-specialist teams, increasing the risk of potential complications.

For inter-hospital transfers the move is likely to be by road, over a long distance and may involve periods of off-road driving. The availability of skilled transfer nurses and doctors and specialist equipment may be varied. Many critical care units vary from basic units with limited resources and staff to tertiary referral centres. There may be only one nurse to transfer the critically ill patient, and while the nurse and escort team are away the hospital critical care and anaesthetic services may be significantly reduced, until they return.

Undertaking inter-hospital transfers

In the absence of an anaesthetist, it is likely the nurse is the most qualified person to undertake the transfer. Dedicated ambulances may be available; however, the skills of the crew may be varied. All transfers involve changes in momentum, acceleration and deceleration forces, which can affect patients. Potential respiratory effects associated with transfer (Baker & Whiteley, 2013) include the following:

- Gravitational forces affect the distribution of blood within the lungs, which could lead to blood being forced away from the well-perfused areas of the lungs to other areas, resulting in a ventilation – perfusion mismatch, leading to increased hypoxia.
- Exacerbation of bronchospasm in patients with asthma and chronic obstructive airways disease.

Cardiovascular effects may include (Baker & Whiteley, 2013):

- fluid shifts;
- hypotension;
- myocardial ischaemia;
- arrythmias.

Critically ill patients may have an impaired ability to maintain their temperature. When exposed to environmental changes, patients may become hypothermic. This leads to depression of cardiovascular and respiratory function, reduced consciousness and metabolic derangements and coagulopathy. Patients' temperature should be regularly checked and hypo- and hyperthermia should be prevented (Baker & Whiteley, 2013).

Other potential complications associated with transfers, include:

- the effect of noise and vibration on the patient;
- challenges with communication due to noise;
- effect of acceleration and deceleration forces (e.g. braking) on physiology and the increased the risk of gastric aspiration;
- risk of injury due to equipment not being secured;
- light may be limited, particularly when travelling at night, which may result in you not being able to observe your patient;
- being unable to access the patient due to their position in the vehicle, e.g. IV access may be under blankets.

When planning a transfer the following considerations should be undertaken regardless of the type of transfer (Intensive Care Society, 2011):

- Who will be doing the transfer? What is their experience? Talk through your plans and any complications that you think may happen and how you will deal with them.
- Check emergency transfer equipment, including sufficient oxygen and drugs for the journey. Some units have dedicated transfer equipment and checklists to help you prepare.
  - What equipment do you have available?
  - Have you checked it?

- Establish the patient on transfer monitor and ventilator.

  – Monitor to include: ECG, blood pressure, oxygen saturation, end tidal carbon dioxide, temperature.

- Transfer the patient onto the ambulance trolley, ensuring they are not lying on any lines, bungs, etc.
- Cover the patient with blankets and keep them warm.
- All lines and infusions running are adequately secured and labelled.
- Do not rest pumps or oxygen cylinders on the patient as this may cause pressure damage or they may move during transfer.
- Airway.

  – Consider C-spine immobilisation prior to transfer.
  – Patients with a Glasgow Coma Scale of less than 8 should be intubated prior to transfer.
  – Check the endotracheal tube is secured and patent.
  – If required, the cervical spine needs to be protected.
  – Tracheal tube position confirmed on chest X-ray.
  – Adequate sedation, analgesia and muscle relaxation needs to be given, while avoiding hypotension and reduced cerebral perfusion pressure (CPP).

- Breathing.

  – Adequate spontaneous respiration or ventilation established on transport ventilator. Ventilation should target PaO_2 levels of greater than 13kPa and $PaCO_2$ levels of 4.5–5.0kPa.
  – If available end tidal CO_2 monitoring should be used.
  – Adequate gas exchanged confirmed by arterial blood gas.
  – If the patient has a pneumothorax, this must be drained prior to transfer. Drains should never be clamped, and care should be taken to check the position and that they are not raised above the level of the patient.

- Circulation.

  – Heart rate and blood pressure optimised. Hypovolaemic patients should be fluid resuscitated prior to transfer. If the patient remains hypotensive, other sources of bleeding/fluid loss should be investigated prior to starting vasopressors.
  – Assess tissue and organ perfusion is adequate.
  – Potassium <6mmol/l.
  – Ionised calcium >1mmol/l.
  – Acid-base balance acceptable.
  – Haemoglobin adequate.
  – Minimum of two routes of venous access.
  – Arterial line and central venous access if appropriate.

    o Check the patient has peripheral IV access in case the central venous catheter becomes dislodged or you are unable to access it when in the ambulance.
    o If the patient has an arterial line in place, still take a non-invasive blood pressure (NBP) cuff, in case the arterial line becomes dislodged.

    o   NBP can be unreliable due to motion and can be a significant drain on battery supply monitors; therefore, if available, an arterial line may be indicated.

- – Intra-thoracic and intra-abdominal bleeding controlled.
- – Intra-abdominal injuries adequately investigated and appropriately managed.
- – Urinary catheter inserted and draining adequate amounts?

- Disability (neurological).

  - – Care must be taken with brain injured patients as a poorly conducted transfer can lead to secondary brain injury and poor outcome. Causes of secondary brain injury include: raised intra cranial pressure (ICP), hypotension, hypoxia, hypercarbia, cardiovascular instability and hyperpyrexia.
  - – Seizures controlled and metabolic causes excluded.
  - – Raised intracranial pressure appropriately managed.
  - – Analgesia provided.
  - – Sedated and paralysed as appropriate.
  - – Blood glucose >4mmol/l.

- Exposure/environmental.

  - – Long bone/pelvic fractures stabilised and splinted to provide neurovascular protection and analgesia.
  - – Temperature maintained.
  - – Oro-/naso-gastric tube on free drainage.

Other considerations:

- Prior to departure, assess the patient to confirm they remain stable.
- Telephone the department/hospital to let them know you are on your way, the patient's current condition and estimated time of arrival.
- Do you have named medical and nursing personnel at the receiving hospital?
- Do you have the address?
- Patient notes, X-rays, etc.
- Does the patient's family know about the transfer?
- How will you get back to your hospital?
- Do you need warm clothing, snacks, etc?

During the transfer:

- For the majority of cases high-speed travel is not required. When in the ambulance you should remain seated and wear a seatbelt. In the event of a deterioration, do not attempt to undertake any intervention in a moving vehicle – ask the driver to stop.
- Check the patient's trolley is secured.
- If available, plug electrical devices into the ambulance power supply.
- Use the ambulance oxygen supply for the ventilator.
- Check all equipment safely mounted or stowed.

Droogh *et al.* (2015) identified that common complications during transfer may include:

- respiratory: inadequate ventilation, oxygen desaturation;
- cardiovascular: hypo-/hypertension, brady-/tachycardia, arrythmias;
- technical: power failure, gas supply failure, missing or damaged equipment.

Handover

Throughout the transfer clear records should be maintained including the patient's condition and any intervention undertaken. Monitoring should include:

- pupillary size and reaction to light;
- continuous ECG;
- continuous pulse oximetry;
- non-/invasive blood pressure;
- urine output by urinary catheter;
- continuous capnography trace;
- central venous pressure monitoring where indicated;
- temperature (preferably core and peripheral);
- this should be documented on an observation chart or specialist transfer paperwork.

On arrival, a formal handover should be given by the transfer team to the receiving medical and nursing team who will then assume responsibility for the patient's care (see 'Medical/nursing handover' on pp. 177–179). A summary of the transfer should be documented in the patient's notes.

References

Baker A. Whiteley SM. (2013). Chapter 15: Transfer of the critically ill patient. In: Mallett J. Albarran J. Richardson A (eds). Critical care manual of clinical procedures and competences. Chichester, West Sussex: Wiley-Blackwell.

Droogh JM. Smit M. Absalom AR. Ligtenberg JJM. Zijlstra JC. (2015). Transferring the critically ill patient: are we there yet? Critical Care. 19. 62. DOI: https://doi.org/10.1186/s13054-015-0749-4.

Goh AYT. Abdel-Latif Mel-A. Lum LCS. Abu-Bakar MN. (2003). Outcome of children with different accessibility to tertiary paediatric intensive care in a developing country – a prospective cohort study. Intensive Care Medicine. 29. 97–102.

Intensive Care Society (2011). Guidelines for the transport of the critically ill adult. 3rd Edition. London: Intensive Care Society.

Kulshrestha A. Singh J. (2016). Inter-hospital and intra-hospital patient transfer: recent concepts. Indian Journal of Anaesthesia. 60. 451–457.

Verma V. Singh GK. Carvello EJ et al. (2013). Inter-hospital transfer of trauma patients in a developing country: a prospective descriptive study. Indian Journal of Community Health. 15. 309–315.

22 Human immunodeficiency virus (HIV)/ acquired immune deficiency syndrome (AIDS)

Human immunodeficiency virus (HIV) is a complex retrovirus that uses a ribonucleic acid (RNA) to replicate itself. There are two types of HIV: HIV-1 and HIV-2. HIV-1 is the commonest form of the virus and HIV-2 is predominately found in West Africa and thought to first have infected humans in the 1940s (Coughlan & Nevin, 2014). HIV is transmitted by three routes:

- sexual transmission;
- transmission by body fluids including unscreened blood and blood products;
- transmitted vertically from mother to child.

Significant improvements have been made in the prevention, diagnosis and treatment of HIV worldwide. In 2017, the UN estimated 36.9 million people were living with HIV, and 21.7 million people were accessing anti-retroviral treatment (ART) (UN, 2019). The WHO (2017) estimated 54% of adults and 43% of children receive lifelong ART. HIV is a chronic, life-threatening disease with no cure. Newly diagnosed HIV sufferers who commence treatment can remain well with a life expectancy comparable to those without HIV and it can be considered and managed as a long-term condition (Crock, 2017). People with HIV may not develop AIDS and without treatment AIDS is usually fatal. The UN SDG has an ambitious aim of ending the AIDS epidemic by 2030 (UN, 2017).

Fear of transmission and stigma that leads to discrimination remains. In consequence, there are many people who do not receive ART early and are associated with poor outcome. Acute deterioration may require admission to critical care and it is only during this time that a diagnosis is made.

CD4 cell count is used to stage HIV infections to assess the disease progression and immune status of a patient (Taegtmeyer et al., 2014). The normal CD4 count is 800 to 1500 × 106/L. A count of <200 × 106/L indicates severe immunosuppression and makes the patient at risk for opportunistic infection. The clinical stages are outlined in Box 22.1. HIV patients develop many critical illnesses due to one of the following reasons (Timsit, 2005; Ganesan & Masur, 2013; Dart *et al.*, 2017):

- Those with a known HIV diagnosis or due to complication of their disease, e.g. an opportunistic infection (Table 22.1).
- Those admitted for a non-HIV-related condition such as complications of elective surgery, trauma-related admissions, pancreatitis, and gastrointestinal bleeding.
- Those unaware of their HIV status and diagnosed during their admission.
- Those on ART and living longer and non-HIV-related conditions may require critical care treatment.

Box 22.1   Clinical staging (Taegtmeyer, *et al.*)

Clinical Stage 1:

- Primary HIV infection: asymptomatic or seroconversion syndrome.
- Asymptomatic or persistent generalised lymphadenopathy (PGL).

Clinical Stage 2:

- Weight loss <10% of presumed body weight.
- Recurrent respiratory tract infections.
- Herpes zoster.
- Oral ulcers.
- Seborrhoeic dermatitis.
- Fungal nail infections.
- Angular cheilitis.

Clinical Stage 3:

- Weight loss >10% presumed body weight.
- Unexpected diarrhoea for >1 month.
- Unexpected fever for >1 month.
- Oral candida.
- Oral hairy leukoplakia.
- Pulmonary tuberculosis.
- Severe bacterial infections (meningitis, empyema, pneumonia, bone and joint sepsis).
- Vulvo-vaginal candidiasis for >1 month.

Clinical Stage 4:

- HIV wasting syndrome.
- Pneumocystis pneumonia.
- Cryptosporidiosis or cystoisosporiasis and diarrhoea for >1 month.
- Chronic herpes simplex infection for >1 month.
- Oesophageal candidiasis.
- Extrapulmonary tuberculosis.
- Kaposi's sarcoma.
- Cerebral toxoplasmosis.
- HIV encephalopathy.
- CMV infection.
- Cryptococcal infection.
- Atypical mycobacterial infection.
- Lymphoma.

Patients may present with pyrexia of unknown origin. Fever with or without localisation is a common presentation among individuals with HIV. If fever lasts longer than a few days, it is likely to be TB. HIV infection increases the risk of TB and should always be suspected in HIV-infected individuals with the following symptoms and signs:

- fever;
- cough;
- weight loss;
- malaise;
- night sweats;
- chest pain;
- abdominal pain;
- lymphadenopathy.

(Hoffman & Chaisson, 2009)

Common causes of febrile illness among HIV-infected individuals include:

- TB;
- bacteraemia (Salmonella, Pneumococcal);
- malaria;
- Cryptococcus neopformans;
- lymphoma;
- Mycobacterium avium complex (MAC);
- Penicillium marneffei (particularly found in Asia);
- visceral leishmania (found in Bangladesh, India, Brazil, Nepal, Sudan and Ethiopia).

(Hoffman & Chaisson, 2009)

Table 22.1 Opportunistic infections

Type	Infection	Clinical features	Treatment
Fungal	Pneumocystis jiroveci pneumonia (PJP)	AIDS defining illness usually seen in people presenting late in the course of HIV infection or poor complication to HRT or PJP prophylaxis. Clinical features include: – fever; – cough – non-productive; – shortness of breath; – tachypnoea; – tachycardia. Chest X-ray may show peri-hilar interstitial infiltrates or diffuse alveolar shadowing or may be normal (seen in approximately 10% of cases).	Co-trimoxazole (IV/oral) Atovaquone (oral) Pentamidine isethionate (IV/nebulised)
	Cryptococcus neoformans	Cryptococcal meningoencephalitis (CM) is the most frequent and severe form with mortality reported between 20% and 70%; untreated it is fatal. Causes meningitis: – fever; – headache; – Reduced level of consciousness/mental changes.	Amphotericine B (IV/oral) Flucytosine (IV) Fluconazole (IV/oral)

Table 22.1 Continued

Type	Infection	Clinical features	Treatment
	Candida albicans	Oral and vaginal thrush Oral infections can extend to the oesophagus. Features include: – sore mouth; – loss of taste and appetite; – difficulty in swallowing.	Fluconazole (IV/oral) Nystatin (suspension or pastilles) Amphotericine B (IV)
Bacterial	Tuberculosis	Reactivation of old infection or exposure to bacterium. Not only confined to the lungs but can include bone marrow, liver and gastro-intestinal tract. Clinical features: – fever; – chills; – cough; – shortness of breath; – weight loss.	Combination anti-tuberculosis drugs: Isoniazid (oral Rifampicin (oral) Ethambutol (oral) Pyrazinamide (oral)
	Mycobacterium avium complex	Disseminated, multi-organ disease. Clinical features: – fever; – night sweats; – weight loss; – fatigue; – diarrhoea; – abdominal pain.	Clarithromycin (oral) Ethambutol (oral) Rifabutin (oral)
Viral	Cytomegalovirus (CMV)	Common presentation is CMV retinitis if untreated will lead to blindness.	Ganciclovir (IV) Valganciclovir (oral) Foscarnet sodium (IV)

Table 22.1 Continued

Type	Infection	Clinical features	Treatment
Parasitic	Taxoplasma gondii	Central nervous system presentation is the commonest form. Common when CD4 count falls below 50×10^9/L in previously infected individuals. Common features include encephalitis progressing to seizures and coma if untreated. Clinical features: – headache; – confusion; – motor weakness. Cerebral abscess and encephalitis is common, but retinochoroidits is rare in adults.	Pyrimethamine and sulfadiazine and leucovorin Co-trimoxazole (oral) Atovaquone (oral)
	Cryptosporidium	Clinical features: – non-bloody, watery diarrhoea; – fever; – sometimes malabsorption.	Patients who have not commenced on HARRT should do so.
Opportunistic	Karposi Sarcoma	AIDS defining illness. Since introduction of HARRT it is less common and the progression is slower. Can range from localised cutaneous lesion to widespread multi-organ condition. Four types: – classical or sporadic form; – endemic African form; – iatrogenic immunosuppression form; – endemic or HIV-related form.	Antineoplastic drugs may be used to slow the progression in rapidly advancing conditions. Pain relief.

Sources: Coughlan & Nevin, 2014; Post, 2018; Chitman, 2018; Chang & Clezy, 2018; Chang & Kelly, 2018

Often other conditions including malaria, hepatitis B and C and TB co-exist, adding complexity to treatment. Opportunistic infections may result in the requirement for critical care and include:

- respiratory failure requiring mechanical ventilation, e.g. PJP. This may be complicated by pneumothoraces;
- complications of ART including dyslipidemias, insulin resistance, diabetes;
- central nervous system dysfunction. Meningitis or toxoplasma encephalitis causing sepsis, reduced consciousness, fitting coma and an inability to maintain a patent airway;
- sepsis;
- gastro-intestinal bleeding;
- end stage liver failure, secondary to viral hepatitis;
- renal disease secondary to HIV-associated nephropathy, hepatitis B or C coinfection, diabetes, or hypertension.

(Post, 2018; Coughlan & Nevin, 2014; Chiang et al., 2011; Huang, 2006; Pathak et al., 2012)

Decision to admit to critical care

The decision to admit and initiate critical care treatments with patients with HIV or AIDS, with a potentially reversible and treatable condition, poses ethical decisions for healthcare workers when trying to balance limited resources (Kar et al., 2015). Admission guidelines may help guide decision-making; however, patients may not be identified as HIV positive on admission to critical care (Chiang et al., 2011). Patients may be admitted without their HIV status known or a confirmed diagnosis. Given HIV-infected patients may have multiple processes and continue to deteriorate despite appropriate therapy for the known condition or disease, this may promote the healthcare team to consider HIV testing (Hoffmann & Chaisson, 2009). Routine HIV screening may be appropriate if the HIV status is unknown, to enable appropriate care to be provided. However, the routine testing of patients without consent, e.g. unconscious, should not be performed unless agreed as part of hospital protocol and deemed in the patient's best interest (Bisanzo et al., 2016; Thornhill et al., 2014). If performed and the result is positive it is important to provide appropriate counselling, confidentiality and discussion regarding options for partners' testing. The pre- and post-testing discussion should be undertaken by someone trained in this area.

Given the variety of reasons for admission, the nursing management will be determined by the reason for admission and may or may not be related to their HIV/AIDS diagnosis, for example a trauma patient involved in a road traffic collision versus a patient with an acute respiratory deterioration due to PJP. The nurse's role is to recognise the potential consequences of a HIV diagnosis, e.g. immunosuppression, delayed wound healing and optimising patient care; this includes nutrition and maintaining confidentiality. In addition, often HIV and other infections including TB and malaria co-exist and add complexity to treatment strategies.

Any patient admitted to critical care with a new diagnosis or chronic disease is complex and will require input from other specialties including HIV specialists. It is often recommended if the patient is already on ART this should continue during an acute HIV admission. Adequate drug delivery and absorption of ART may be a challenge; with limited access to syrups or IV sources, crushing of tablets may be appropriate. However, pharmacist input will be required. In addition, ART can affect certain drugs used in critical care, for example protease inhibitors significantly potentiate the effects of midazolam (Padiglione & McGloughlin, 2014).

The timing of when to start ART is controversial and is often delayed until the patient has recovered. The potential early improvements in immune function need to be balanced against the potential side effects from introducing new drugs and increasing the risk of complications from immune reconstruction. Evidence currently suggests early use of ART therapy is associated with improved survival in most opportunistic infections; however, specialist HIV expert input is required (Padiglione & McGloughlin, 2014).

References

Bisanzo M. Gema F. Wangoda R. (2016). Chapter 127: Malaria. In: Wallis LA. Reynolds TA (eds). African Federation of Emergency Medicine: Handbook of Acute and Emergency Care. Oxford: Oxford University Press.

Chang CC. Clezy K. (2018). Toxoplasmosis. Available at: http://hivmanagement.ashm.org.au/index.php/clinical-manifestations-of-hiv/key-opportunistic-infections/toxoplasmosis#.

Chang CC. Kelly M. (2018). Cryptococcosis. Available at: http://hivmanagement.ashm.org.au/index.php/clinical-manifestations-of-hiv/key-opportunistic-infections/cryptococcosis#.

Chiang HH. Hung CC. Lee CM et al. (2011). Admissions to intensive care unit of HIV-infected patients in the era of highly active antiretroviral therapy: etiology and prognostic factors. Critical Care. 15. R202. DOI: https://doi.org/10.1186/cc10419.

Chitman M. (2018). Kaposi's sarcoma. Available at: http://hivmanagement.ashm.org.au/index.php/clinical-manifestations-of-hiv/key-opportunistic-infections/kaposi-s-sarcoma#.

Coughlan M. Nevin M. (2014). Chapter 18: Nursing care of conditions related to the immune system. In: Brady AM. McCabe C. McCann M (eds). Fundamentals of medical-surgical nursing: a systems approach. Chichester, West Sussex: Wiley Blackwell.

Crock EA. (2017). HIV and AIDS: an overview of the current issues, treatment and prevention. Nursing Standard. 32. 15. 51–62.

Dart J. Kinnear J. Bould D et al. (2017). An evaluation of inpatient morbidity and critical care provision in Zambia. Anaesthesia. 72. 172–180.

Ganesan A. Masur H. (2013). Critical care of persons infected with human immunodeficiency virus. Clinics in Chest Medicine. 34. 2. 307–323.

Hoffmann CJ. Chaisson RE. (2009). Section 3: Systems orientated disease. Chapter 20: HIV/AIDS & opportunistic illnesses. In: Cook GC. Zumla AI (eds). Manson's tropical diseases. 22nd Edition. Edinburgh: Saunders Elsevier.

Huang L. Quarten A. Jones D. Havlir DV. (2006). Intensive care of patients with HIV infection. The Lancet. 355. 173–181.

Kar SK. Chakraborty B. Ghosh S. Sarkar M. Ray R. (2015). HIV in intensive care unit: concerns and constraints of intensivists. Translational Biomedicine. 6. 4. DOI: 10.21767/2172-0479.100028.

Padiglione AA. McGloughlin S. (2014). Chapter 68: HIV & acquired immunodeficiency syndrome. In: Besten AD. Soni N (eds). OH's intensive care manual. 7th Edition. Oxford: Butterworth Heinemann Elsevier.

Pathak V. Rendon IS. Atrash S. *et al.* (2012) Comparing outcome of HIV versus non-HIV patients requiring mechanical ventilation. Clinical Medicine and Research 10. 57–64.

Post JS. (2018). Pneumocystis jirovecii pneumonia. Available at: http://hivmanagement. ashm.org.au/index.php/clinical-manifestations-of-hiv/key-opportunistic-infections/ pneumosystis-jirovecii-pneumonia#.

Taegtmeyer M. Weigel R. Dedicoat M. (2014). Chapter 13: HIV infection and disease in the tropics. In: Beeching N. Gill G. (eds). Tropical medicine: lecture notes. 7th Edition. Chichester, West Sussex: Wiley Blackwell.

Thornhill J. Mandersloot G. Bath R. Orkin C. (2014). Opt-out HIV testing in adult critical care units. The Lancet. 383. 1460.

Timsit JF. (2005). Open the intensive care unit doors to HIV infected patients with sepsis. Critical Care. 9. 6. 629–630.

United Nations. (2017). Goal 3: Ensures healthy lives and promote wellbeing for all at all ages. Available at: www.un.org/sustainabledevelopment/health/.

United Nations. (2019). Global HIV & AIDS statistics — 2018 fact sheet. Available at: www.unaids.org/en/resources/fact-sheet.

World Health Organization. (2017). HIV/AIDS Fact Sheet. Available at: www.who.int/ mediacentre/factsheets/fs360/en/.

23 Tuberculosis

Tuberculosis (TB) is the most common infectious disease in the world (Mandal *et al.*, 2004). TB is caused by the *Mycobacteria tuberculosis* (MTB) complex, given the genetically similar bacteria, and includes *M. tuberculosis, M. bovis* and *M. africanum* (Squire, 2014). TB often co-exists with other diseases including HIV. There should be a high degree of suspicion for dual infection with HIV-infected patients (Bisanzo *et al.*, 2016). Protection against TB includes effective diagnosis, treatment of patient with active infections and prevention of the transmission of TB to others (Centers for Disease Control and Prevention, 2003). The commonest cause of TB is pulmonary, accounting for 85% of presentations. Less common causes include extrapulmonary TB (lymphadenitis, genitourinary, miliary and bone, and meningeal and peritoneal TB) (Bisanzo *et al.*, 2016; Squire, 2014). TB presentation varies, and immunosuppressed patients may not present with 'classic' signs and symptoms (Bisanzo *et al.*, 2016).

Signs and symptoms include:

- general signs: fever, night sweats, fatigue, anorexia, weight loss;
- pulmonary TB: cough >2 weeks, haemoptysis, chest pain, difficulty in breathing, crepitation, wheeze, clubbing;
- extrapulmonary TB: dependent on location, e.g. abdominal TB may present with abdominal pain and ascites;
- Multidrug-Resistant TB: this should be considered in any patient with TB recurrence after treatment or treatment failure.

(Bisanzo *et al.*, 2016)

The indication of the infectiousness of TB patients may include:

- presence of a cough;
- cavity in lungs;
- Acid-Fast Bacilli (AFB) on sputum smear;
- TB disease in lungs, airway or larynx;
- patient not covering their mouth and nose when coughing;
- not receiving adequate treatment;

- positive sputum;
- undergoing cough-inducing procedures.

(Centers for Disease Control and Prevention, 2016)

Investigations include:

- pulmonary TB: sputum smears with culture for sensitivity testing;
- extrapulmonary TB: fluid or tissue biopsy with adenosine deaminase and culture and stain;
- molecular testing: e.g. Xpert, MTB/RIF; nucleic acid and amplification;
- HIV testing for all TB patients;
- imaging: chest X-ray, CT chest.

(Bisanzo *et al.*, 2016)

Critical care considerations

Effective barrier nursing

- If no specialist air-conditioning is available, windows should be kept open to promote cross ventilation, especially in waiting areas, examination rooms, when taking sputum specimens and on wards/critical care.
- Patients with suspected or confirmed TB infection should be isolated. High-risk groups include HIV-infected, prior TB, malnourished, smokers, diabetics, drug users, infants, elderly and those living in crowded conditions, e.g. prisons, hostels, refugee camps) or those with significant contact with TB patients, e.g. healthcare workers.
- Good hand hygiene using soap and water.
- Staff and visitors should have access to personal protective equipment including approved respiratory masks, which have been fit tested, particularly when nursing Multidrug-Resistant TB (MDR-TB) or Extensively Drug-Resistant TB (EXD-TB). This includes appropriate training and maintaining a register of those who have been tested.
- Staff should ensure they have had the appropriate vaccinations.
- Self-ventilating patients should be asked to wear face masks as appropriate, e.g. during transfer for investigations.

Airway

- Care when handling sputum, e.g. tracheal suctioning, chest physiotherapy.
- 'Cough etiquette' explained to self-ventilating patients. This includes covering mouth and nose with tissues when coughing, appropriate disposal of tissues and use of sputum pots.
- Patients may experience haemoptysis (occasionally massive) due to a Rasmussen aneurysm. Emergency suction must be available at the bedside.
- Airway obstruction may be caused by laryngeal or retropharyngeal TB.

Breathing

- Administration of oxygen to treat hypoxia; care should be taken as use of oxygen and nebulisers will result in aerosolization. Oxygen saturations should be maintained >95%.
- Endo-bronchial TB may result in wheezing or cough.
- Patients may develop respiratory failure due to tuberculous bronchopneumonia leading to collapse and consolidation. In consequence they may require intubation and mechanical ventilation. When intubating patients, staff should have access to appropriate PPE.
- When ventilating a patient with pulmonary TB, specialist precautions include trying to prevent breaks in the ventilator circuits, as this may aerosolise and spread TB within the unit. If available, closed suction catheters should be used.
- Patients may develop pleural effusions and empyema in acute TB infections.
- Abdominal TB may result in ascites; this may affect respiratory function due to a distended abdomen and splinting of the diaphragm resulting in hypoxia.
- Therapeutic thoracentesis (to a maximum of 1.5litres) or paracentesis may be considered to improve shortness of breath.

Circulation

- Patients may present with fever and night sweats. Initially this may be pyrexia of unknown origin until a TB diagnosis is confirmed. Anti-pyretics (paracetamol) should be administered.
- Cardiac monitoring and observation for cardiogenic shock. This may be caused by a massive pericardial effusion.
- Renal and liver function should be monitored regularly. Renal and liver failure may be due to TB or the effects of drug regimens.
- Haematuria, frequency and dysuria may be present.
- Monitoring of renal function and fluid balance will prevent AKI. In addition, drug regimens may cause renal damage.
- Hepatosplenomegaly may present in approximately 25% of military TB cases.
- Disseminating Intravascular Coagulation (DIC) may be caused by miliary TB.

Neurological

- TB to the central nervous system may present in the form of meningeal disease. Disease progression includes changes in mental and personality. Progressive drowsiness, meningism, cranial nerve palsies (particularly 3rd and 6th), focal long-tract signs and eventual coma. Hyponatraemia is common.
- Cerebral TB may cause pituitary apoplexy or stroke.
- Bone TB can present in the spine. Patients may present with chronic back pain involving the lower thoracic and lumbar regions. Spinal instability and spinal cord compression is an emergency and will require immediate care.

Nursing care

- TB patients are often malnourished and nutritional support is required. Specialist dietician input will be required with anorexic or malnourished patients.

Specialist input

- Input from specialist teams, particularly as patients may be on multiple drug regimens for other conditions, e.g. HIV, diabetes, and these regimens may interact.
- Counselling and testing for HIV.

(Bisanzo *et al.*, 2016; Centers for Disease Control and Prevention, 2003; TB Coalition for Technical Assistance, 2015; Hagan & Nathani, 2013; Mandal *et al.*, 2004)

Treatment

TB treatment therapies are complex, lasting months and determined by national TB control programme guidelines (Bisanzo *et al.*, 2016; Mandal *et al.*, 2004). Treatments may include isoniazid and rifampicin for six months. In addition, pyrazinamide and ethambutol is taken for the first two months (Mandal *et al.*, 2004; WHO, 2017).

References

Bisanzo M. Gema F. Wangoda R. (2016). Part 4: Infectious diseases. Chapter 131: Tuberculosis. In: Wallis LA. Reynolds TA (eds). African Federation of Emergency Medicine handbook of acute and emergency care. 3rd Edition. Oxford: Oxford University Press.

Centers for Disease Control and Prevention. (2003). Morbidity and mortality weekly report. 52. FP–11. Available at: www.cdc.gov/mmWR/PDF/wk/mm5206.pdf.

Centers for Disease Control and Prevention. (2016). Fact sheet: infection control in healthcare settings. Available at: www.cdc.gov/tb/publications/factsheets/prevention/ichcs.htm.

Hagan G. Nathani N. (2013). Clinical review: tuberculosis on the intensive care unit. Critical Care. 17. 240.

Mandal BK. Wilkins EGL. Dunbar EM *et al.* (2004). Chapter 14: Tuberculosis. In: Mandal BK. Wilkins EGL. Dunbar EM. Mayon-White R (eds). Lecture notes on infectious diseases. 6th Edition. Blackwell Publishing.

Squire B. (2014). Chapter 12: Tuberculosis. In: Beeching N. Gill G. (eds). Tropical medicine: lecture notes. 7th Edition. Chichester, West Sussex: Wiley Blackwell.

Tuberculosis Coalition for Technical Assistance. (2015). Implementing the WHO policy on TB infection control. Available at: www.tbcare1.org/publications/toolbox/tools/ic/TB_IC_Implementation_Framework.pdf.

World Health Organization. (2017). Tuberculosis. Available at: www.who.int/tb/en/.

24 Tetanus

Tetanus is a preventable disease caused by Gram-positive anaerobe bacillus called *Clostridium tetani*. Effective immunisation programmes in HIC have eradicated this disease, whereas in low-income settings tetanus remains a significant cause of mortality (Askoy *et al.*, 2014). The WHO (2018a) aimed to eradicate maternal and neonatal tetanus (MNT) by 2015 and, apart from 18 countries, this has been achieved (WHO, 2018b). In other groups the overall incidence is gradually reducing globally. In 2015, the WHO reported 10,301 cases worldwide respectively (WHO, 2018c), compared to an annual incidence exceeding 110,000 in 1980 (Rodrigo *et al.*, 2014). Challenges to providing vaccination programmes include inadequate cover in national vaccination programmes due to geographical spread of population, individuals missing vaccinations due to limited access to trained healthcare workers and facilities. Conflict or disaster may result in a vaccination programme being stopped or sporadic in cover (Carter & Viveash, 2017).

The spore-forming bacillus is found in the bowels of herbivorous animals and distributed in soil. Examples of tetanus prone wounds include those contaminated with manure, soil or rusty metal, via an umbilical cord cut with a non-sterile instrument, burns, frostbite, puncture wounds and high-velocity missile injuries (WHO, 2003, 2018b; Aksoy *et al.*, 2014). In approximately 20% of cases the entry site cannot be identified, and the cause is unknown (Gibson *et al.*, 2009).

Once the bacteria enter the body, in the presence of an anaerobic environment, spores develop. Toxins are transported via the blood and lymphatic system. Once the toxin reaches the central nervous system, it affects the peripheral motor end plates, spinal cord, brain and sympathetic nervous system. The toxin interferes with neurotransmitters, blocking impulses, leading to tetanospasmin, an exotoxin (Centers for Disease Control and Prevention, 2018). Once the tetanospasmin reaches the central nervous system, it causes involuntary contraction (rigidity) and brief periods of muscle contraction (spasms). There are four types of tetanus:

* neonatal (affecting children under 1 month);
* cephalic (affecting the head);
* generalised (commonest type seen within critical care);
* local (Berger, 2015; Lalloo, 2014).

The incubation period of tetanus is 2–20 days. Signs and symptoms of generalised tetanus are outlined in Box 24.1. There are no specific laboratory tests to diagnose tetanus and diagnosis is based on clinical history and findings, e.g. muscle contraction. Differential diagnosis is limited, but includes dental abscesses, strychnine poisoning, dystonic reactions, hypocalcaemia and seizures in adults (Lalloo, 2014).

Box 24.1   Signs and symptoms of generalised tetanus (Berger, 2015)

- Trismus (locked jaw).
- *Risus sardonicus* – severe facial muscle spasms.
- Abdominal wall rigidity.
- Spasms in the arms and legs.
- Severe pain.
- Spasms triggered by sensory stimulus.
- Possible airway obstruction or respiratory compromise due to participation of the diaphragm in general contractions.
- Autonomic instability.
- Rhabdomyolysis and renal failure.

Men are deemed higher risk as they tend to be economically active, involved in manual labour and higher risk of injury, whereas women are routinely vaccinated during pregnancy (Muteya *et al.*, 2013). However, anyone who is not vaccinated is at risk and the incidence may increase due to overcrowding, a lack of personal hygiene, lack of knowledge/health promotion, limited access to primary healthcare, ineffective vaccination programmes and lack of shoes resulting in injuries to lower limbs. Often wounds to lower limbs are the cause of infection; for example, a study conducted by Muteya *et al.* (2013) identified the point of entry was found in 71.5% of cases, with 61.9% localised in lower limbs.

In cases of severe tetanus, critical care admission is appropriate; however, mortality rates can be high. Ajose and Odusanya (2009) reported mortality of 70% from generalised tetanus in one hospital in Nigeria. Muteya *et al.* (2013) reported tetanus accounted for 2.5% of all admissions and had a mortality of 52.4% within the tetanus cohort in critical care admissions in the Democratic Republic of Congo.

Critical care considerations include:

Airway

- The airway in a tetanus patient could become compromised due to reduced level of consciousness due to sedation given to control seizures or trismus.
- Patients may also experience *risus sardonicus*, a distorted, abnormal facial expression, commonly associated with tetanus. Glottal and laryngeal spasms may result in fluid (saliva) being aspirated into the airway and the patient being unable to

maintain a patent airway. Atropine can be administered to prevent antisialagogue and aspiration. Emergency bedside suction must be available.

- An emergency airway plan should be agreed and immediate access to emergency equipment and difficult airway equipment is required (Box 24.2).
- Tetanus patients may have complicated airway and a situation of 'unable to intubate and unable to ventilate' may present. An emergency tracheostomy or crichothyroidotomy may be required, and difficult airway equipment must be immediately available. Close observation and early detection of airway compromise will ensure an appropriately skilled team is available.

Box 24.2   Example emergency airway management plan (Carter & Viveash, 2017)

In the event of an emergency intubation:

- call surgeons/Ear Nose and Throat (ENT) immediately.

Plan A:
  Either:

- Awake/asleep nasal or oral fibre-optic intubation if competent.
- Consider Atropine as an antisialagogues.

Or:

- Direct laryngoscopy and oral intubation.
- If unsuccessful, go to plan B.

Plan B:

- Oropharyngeal airway and two nasopharyngeal airways and bag, valve mask ventilation.
- If unsuccessful, go to plan C.

Plan C:

- Insertion of a laryngeal mask airway (LMA).
- If unsuccessful, go to plan D.

Plan D:

- Surgical cricothyroidotomy.
- Scalpel, bougie and tracheostomy tubes to be at bedside always.

Breathing

- Sudden laryngospasm can be life-threatening.
- Spasms of laryngeal and respiratory muscles cause respiratory failure. In consequence, patients may require mechanical ventilation.
- Observation for signs of respiratory failure. Oxygen therapy should be provided to maintain oxygen saturations >95%.

Circulation

- Cardiac monitoring for signs of cardiac arrhythmias and invasive blood pressure monitoring is indicated.
- Maintaining haemodynamic stability, hypotension should be treated with IV fluid boluses.
- Complications of using magnesium to control seizures may result in hypocalcaemia, cardiac instability due to autonomic stimulation of the central nervous system, rapid deterioration including bradycardia, hypotension or hypertension. Daily serum magnesium levels and physiological monitoring to assist with early detection and identification of trends in physiological observations is required.
- Control of autonomic instability, e.g. verapamil for hypertension, atropine for bradycardia.
- Monitoring of renal function and fluid balance to prevent AKI.
- Observation for signs of rhabdomyolysis and potential complications, e.g. hyperkalaemia.

Neurological care

- Control muscle spasms/seizures (diazepam, magnesium infusion, anaesthetic agents, e.g. propofol). The use of these drugs may result in respiratory depression and require mechanical ventilation (Rodrigo et al., 2014).
- The choice of pharmacological methods to control seizures in tetanus remains unclear. In 2004, a Cochrane Systematic Review on the efficacy of diazepam concluded using diazepam resulted in improved survival rates in children, when compared to a combination of phenobarbitone and chlorpromazine (Okoromah & Lesi, 2004). Rodrigo et al. (2014) suggested midazolam may be more effective than diazepam, when used in conjunction with muscle relaxants, anaesthetic agents and magnesium sulphate. However, both studies identified that there remains a paucity of evidence into the most appropriate pharmacological method to control spasms in tetanus.
- Magnesium is an accepted intervention when dealing with seizures in eclampsia; however, the evidence for the use in tetanus remains limited. Rodrigo et al. (2012) reported there is minimal research available into the use of this drug and concluded from the studies available, magnesium does not reduce mortality. When using magnesium infusions there are potential complications.

Wound care

- Wounds debridement and irrigation is essential.

  o Infected wounds should not be closed and regular surgical debridement until the wound is completely clean may be required.

- Antibiotics (500mg metronidazole every eight hours is the antibiotic of choice. Benzylpenicillin 0.6–1.2g every six hours can be given).
- Neutralise toxin:

  o human hyperimmune globulin or equine anti-tetanus globulin;
  o tetanus vaccine.

Nursing care

- Tetanus patients should be nursed in a quiet and darkened room, as any light or noise can worsen the spasms and cause convulsions.
- Supportive treatments include:

  o a naso-gastric tube and enteral feeding: may be required in patients with dysphagia, fluctuating conscious level, trismus and the risk of aspiration;
  o DVT prophylaxis;
  o pressure area prevention.

(WHO, 2018d; Carter & Viveash, 2017; Bisanzo *et al.*, 2016; Lalloo, 2014; Berger, 2015; Okoromah & Lesi, 2004)

References

Ajose F. Odusanya O. (2009). Survival from adult tetanus in Lagos, Nigeria. Tropical Doctor. 39. 1. 39–40.

Askoy M. Celik EC. Ahiskalioglu A. Karakaya A. (2014). Tetanus is still a deadly disease: a report of six tetanus cases and reminder of our knowledge. Tropical Doctor. 44. 1. 38–42.

Berger S. (2015). Tetanus: global status. Epidemiology, pp 7–8. Los Angeles, CA: Gideon Informatics Inc.

Bisanzo M. Gema F. Wangoda R. (2016). Chapter 127: Malaria. In: Wallis LA. Reynolds TA (eds). African Federation of Emergency Medicine handbook of acute and emergency care. Oxford: Oxford University Press.

Carter C. Viveash S. (2017). Nursing a critically ill tetanus patient in an intensive care unit in Zambia. British Journal of Nursing. 25. 20. 1123–1128.

Centers for Disease Control and Prevention. (2018). Tetanus: for clinicians: pathogenesis. Available at: www.cdc.gov/tetanus/clinicians.html.

Gibson K. Bonaventure Uwineza J. Kirviri W. Parlow J. (2009). Tetanus in developing countries: a case series and review. Canadian Journal of Anesthesia. 56. 307–315.

Lalloo D. (2014). Chapter 37. Tetanus, pp 259–261. In: Beeching N. Gill G (eds). Tropical medicine – lecture notes. Chichester, West Sussex: Wiley Blackwell.

Muteya MM. Kabey AK. Lubanga TM *et al.* (2013). Prognosis of tetanus patients in the intensive care unit of Provincial Hospital Jason Sendwe, Lubumbashi, DR Congo. Pan African Medical Journal. 14. 93.

Okoromah CAN. Lesi AFE. (2004). Diazepam for treating tetanus. Available at: www.cochrane.org/CD003954/NEONATAL_diazepam-for-treating-tetanus.

Rodrigo C. Fernando D. Rajapakse S. (2014). Pharmacological management of tetanus: an evidence-based review. Critical Care. 18: 217. Available at: www.ncbi.nlm.nih.gov/pmc/articles/PMC4057067/.

Rodrigo C. Samarakoon L. Fernando SD. Rajapakse S. (2012). A meta-analysis of magnesium for tetanus. Anaesthesia. 67. 1370–1374.

World Health Organization. (2003). Surgical care at the district hospital. Available at: www.who.int/surgery/publications/en/SCDH.pdf?ua=1.

World Health Organization. (2018a). Maternal and neonatal tetanus elimination. Available at: www.who.int/immunization/diseases/MNTE_initiative/en/.

World Health Organization. (2018b). Tetanus. Available at: www.who.int/immunization/diseases/tetanus/en/.

World Health Organization. (2018c). Tetanus (total) cases reported. Available at: http://apps.who.int/immunization_monitoring/globalsummary/timeseries/tsincidencettetanus.html.

World Health Organization. (2018d). Prevention and management of wound infection. Available at: www.who.int/hac/techguidance/tools/guidelines_prevention_and_management_wound_infection.pdf?ua=1.

25 Viral haemorrhagic fevers

Viral haemorrhagic fevers (VHF) are a broad group of viral illnesses that share similar clinical characteristics and pathophysiology (Bisanzo *et al.*, 2016). VHF are zoonotic and transmitted from vertebrate animals to humans by bites of infected ticks or mosquitoes, from infected bats and rodents (Hidalgo *et al.*, 2017). VHF include 30 different viruses and are classified into 4 groups:

- Filoviridae (Ebola and Marburg);
- Arenaviridae (Lassa fever, Junin and Machupo);
- Bunyaviridae (Crimean-Congo haemorrhagic fever, Rift Valley fever, Hantaan haemorrhagic fevers);
- Flaviviridae (yellow fever, dengue, Omsk haemorrhagic fever, Kyasanur Forest disease).

(Leligdowicz *et al.*, 2016; WHO, 2017a)

VHF are often severe and fatal, resulting in serious febrile illness, microvascular damage and increased vascular permeability (WHO, 2017b: Bisanzo *et al.*, 2016; Leligdowicz *et al.*, 2016). Initial presentation includes generalised malaise and fever common with other tropical diseases including malaria, leptospirosis, typhoid or influenza. There may be petechiae and episodes of minor bleeding like epistaxis and bleeding gums (Hidalgo *et al.*, 2017). VHF should be suspected in any patients with unexplained bleeding from mucous membranes (gums, nose, vagina), skin (e.g. puncture sites), conjunctiva or gastro-intestinal tract, or any patient with a fever who has had contact with unexplained death, febrile illness or bleeding within three weeks (Bisanzo *et al.*, 2016).

Personal protective equipment

Regular training of healthcare workers to deal with a VHF outbreak is required. Patients should be immediately isolated in suspected, probable and confirmed areas (WHO, 2016). To control an outbreak the following areas will need to be identified:

- large area with isolation rooms;
- rooms/areas for donning and doffing protective clothing;
- observation areas;
- dedicated equipment in each area includes diagnostic equipment including X-ray, ultrasound and point of care laboratory equipment;
- management of waste including soiled linen; in many cases this will need to be incinerated.

(Richards *et al.*, 2018)

VHF are a major cause of concern and during an outbreak pose a hazard to healthcare staff. Healthcare staff must have access to sufficient personal protective equipment (PPE) (scrubs, gowns, aprons, two pairs of gloves, mask, head cover, eyewear and rubber boots). In addition, healthcare workers need to be trained to use this equipment; this includes practical aspects, such as practising wearing and working in PPE. Topics for training include donning and doffing PPE, infection prevention strategies (including environmental cleaning and care of the dead) and supportive treatment strategies.

Wearing of PPE in a non-climate-controlled environment has been identified as a significant challenge for healthcare workers dealing with VHF. Challenges include the following:

- PPE could not be worn for longer than 45–60 minutes.
- Tight-fitting goggles tended to fog.
- Heat and humidity affected 'duck billed' N-95 masks making them ineffective.
- Face shields did not provide full face coverage.

These challenges can result in individuals performing unsafe practices, e.g. readjusting fogged goggles with contaminated hands, heat illness and increasing the risk when performing interventions, e.g. insertion of a cannula due to poor visibility, tiredness and heat (Leligdowicz *et al.*, 2016). Additional challenges include communicating with patients when wearing PPE, documentation of observations and care provided in the 'dirty zone' and psychological care.

Provision of critical care in a VHF outbreak

Providing critical care within a resource limited environment during a VHF outbreak will be a challenge due to limited infrastructure, lack of resources, trained healthcare staff and limited evidence into treatment strategies (Dünser *et al.*, 2012). The numbers infected will determine the type of critical care provided. With large numbers of patients, care may focus on supportive care and intensive nursing only; however, as cases decrease or if there are few cases initially it may be possible to provide more aggressive treatment including non-invasive ventilation, mechanical ventilation, monitoring, renal replacement, etc. (Rees *et al.*, 2015; Paterson & Callahan, 2015).

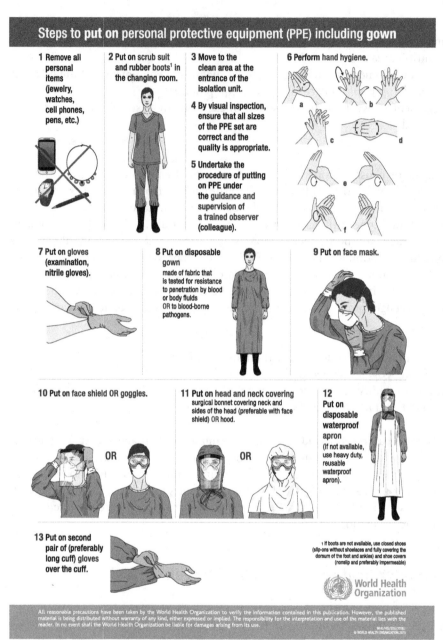

Figure 25.1 Steps to put on PPE including gown

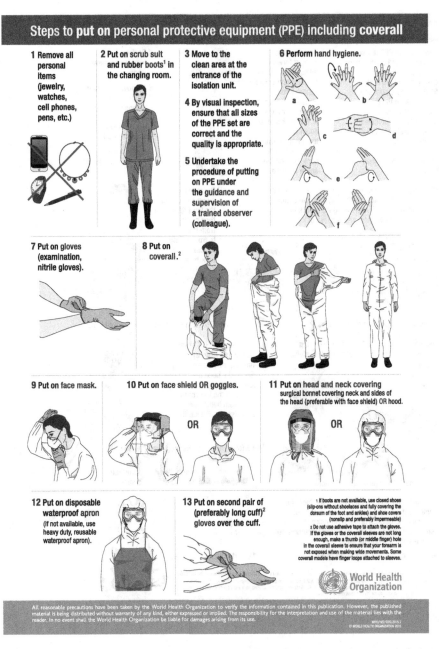

Figure 25.2 Steps to put on PPE including coverall

Steps to **take off** personal protective equipment (PPE) including **gown**

1 Always remove PPE under the guidance and supervision of a trained observer (colleague). Ensure that infectious waste containers are available in the doffing area for safe disposal of PPE. Separate containers should be available for reusable items.

2 Perform hand hygiene on gloved hands.[1]

3 Remove apron leaning forward and taking care to avoid contaminating your hands. When removing disposable apron, tear it off at the neck and roll it down without touching the front area. Then untie the back and roll the apron forward.

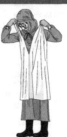

4 Perform hand hygiene on gloved hands.

5 Remove outer pair of gloves and dispose of them safely.
Use the technique shown in Step 17

6 Perform hand hygiene on gloved hands.

7 Remove head and neck covering taking care to avoid contaminating your face by starting from the bottom of the hood in the back and rolling from back to front and from inside to outside, and dispose of it safely.

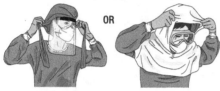

OR

8 Perform hand hygiene on gloved hands.

9 Remove the gown by untying the knot first, then pulling from back to front rolling it from inside to outside and dispose of it safely.

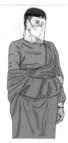

10 Perform hand hygiene on gloved hands.

11 Remove eye protection by pulling the string from behind the head and dispose of it safely.

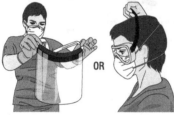

OR

12 Perform hand hygiene on gloved hands.

13 Remove the mask from behind the head by first untying the bottom string above the head and leaving it hanging in front; and then the top string next from behind head and dispose of it safely.

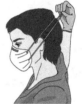

14 Perform hand hygiene on gloved hands.

15 Remove rubber boots without touching them (or overshoes if wearing shoes). If the same boots are to be used outside of the high-risk zone, keep them on but clean and decontaminate appropriately before leaving the doffing area.[2]

16 Perform hand hygiene on gloved hands.

17 Remove gloves carefully with appropriate technique and dispose of them safely.

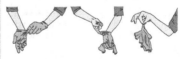

18 Perform hand hygiene.

[1] While working in the patient care area, outer gloves should be changed between patients and prior to exiting (change after seeing the last patient)
[2] Appropriate decontamination of boots includes stepping into a footbath with 0.5% chlorine solution (and removing dirt with toilet brush if heavily soiled with mud and/or organic materials) and then wiping all sides with 0.5% chlorine solution. At least once a day boots should be disinfected by soaking in a 0.5% chlorine solution for 30 min, then rinsed and dried.

World Health Organization

Figure 25.3 Steps to take off PPE including gown

Steps to **take off** personal protective equipment (PPE) including **coverall**

1 Always remove PPE under the guidance and supervision of a trained observer (colleague). Ensure that infectious waste containers are available in the doffing area for safe disposal of PPE. Separate containers should be available for reusable items.

2 Perform hand hygiene on gloved hands.[1]

3 Remove apron leaning forward and taking care to avoid contaminating your hands.
When removing disposable apron, tear it off at the neck and roll it down without touching the front area. Then untie the back and roll the apron forward.

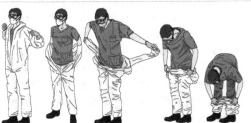

4 Perform hand hygiene on gloved hands.

5 Remove head and neck covering **taking care** to avoid contaminating your face by starting from the bottom of the hood in the back and rolling from back to front and from inside to outside, and dispose of it safely.

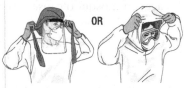

OR

6 Perform hand hygiene on gloved hands.

7 Remove coverall and outer pair of gloves:
Ideally, in front of a mirror, tilt head back to reach zipper, unzip completely without touching any skin or scrubs, and start removing coverall from top to bottom. After freeing shoulders, remove the outer gloves[2] while pulling the arms out of the sleeves. With inner gloves roll the coverall, from the waist down and from the inside of the coverall, down to the top of the boots. Use one boot to pull off coverall from other boot and vice versa, then step away from the coverall and dispose of it safely.

8 Perform hand hygiene on gloved hands.

9 Remove eye protection by **pulling the string** from behind the head and dispose of it safely.

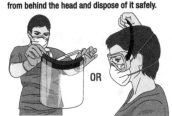

OR

10 Perform hand hygiene on gloved hands.

11 Remove the mask from behind the head by first untying the bottom string above the head and leaving it hanging in front; and then the top string next from behind head and dispose of it safely.

12 Perform hand hygiene on gloved hands.

15 Remove gloves carefully with appropriate technique and dispose of them safely.

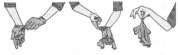

13 Remove rubber boots **without touching them** (or overshoes if wearing shoes). If the same boots are to be used outside of the high-risk zone, keep them on but clean and decontaminate appropriately before leaving the doffing area.[3]

14 Perform hand hygiene on gloved hands.

16 Perform hand hygiene.

[1] While working in the patient care area, outer gloves should be changed between patients and prior to exiting (change after seeing the last patient)
[2] This technique requires properly fitted gloves. When outer gloves are too tight or inner gloves are too loose and/or hands are sweaty, the outer gloves may need to be removed separately, after removing the apron.
[3] Appropriate decontamination of boots includes stepping into a footbath with 0.5% chlorine solution (and removing dirt with toilet brush if heavily soiled with mud and/or organic materials) and then wiping all sides with 0.5% chlorine solution. At least once a day boots should be disinfected by soaking in a 0.5% chlorine solution for 30 min, then rinsed and dried.

World Health Organization

Figure 25.4 Steps to take off PPE including coverall

Reproduced with kind permission from the World Health Organization.

Yellow fever

There are two forms of yellow fever, urban and jungle presentation (Hidalgo *et al.*, 2017). Transmission is by mosquitoes:

- The Aedes aegypti mosquito causes urban yellow fever.
- Haemagogus and other forest canopy mosquitoes acquire the virus from wild primates causing jungle yellow fever and then transmit the virus to humans through bites.

The disease is classified according to the clinical presentation: inapparent (<48hours of fever and headache), mild, severe and malignant. Incubation period ranges from three to six days, followed by sudden onset fever of 39°C to 40°C, tachycardia (and later bradycardia, Faget's sign (fever with bradycardia), facial flushing, conjunctival injection, red tongue with central furring, nausea, vomiting, constipation, headache, muscle pain, severe prostration, restlessness and irritability (Hidalgo *et al.*, 2017). Mild cases end at this stage after one to three days. As the disease progresses to moderate, severe and malignant stages, the fever falls after two to five days and a remission of several hours or days follows. Then the signs and symptoms re-occur with the 'classic triad' of jaundice, extreme albinuria and epigastric tenderness with haematemesis occur (Hidalgo *et al.*, 2017). Oliguria or anuria, petechiae and mucosal haemorrhage is common. The patient continues to deteriorate and become confused, unconscious and seizures are common.

Treatment is supportive and directed towards treating the symptoms. Good nursing care is essential, and correction of fluid and electrolyte imbalance and management of haemorrhage are priorities in treatment (Hidalgo *et al.*, 2017).

Lassa fever

Lassa fever occurs in West Africa; however, there is also a risk of travellers transporting the virus to other countries. The virus is transmitted to humans via contact with food or household items contaminated with rodent urine or faeces, or person-to-person infections, particularly in hospitals lacking effective infection prevention and control procedures (WHO, 2017a).

The incubation period is between 6 and 24 days, with a gradual onset of symptoms (Hidalgo *et al.*, 2017). Symptoms include fever, general weakness and malaise, headache, sore throat (white or yellow exudate may appear on the tonsils and coalesce into a pseudo-membrane), muscle, chest and abdominal pain, nausea, vomiting, diarrhoea, cough. In severe cases there is facial swelling, pulmonary oedema, bleeding from mucous membranes. Protein may be noted in the urine. As the disease progresses, hypovolaemic shock, seizures, tremor, disorientation and coma may occur. Deafness occurs in 25% of patients who survive the disease, but can partially return after one to three months. Transient hair loss and gait disturbance may occur during recovery (WHO, 2017b; Hidalgo *et al.*, 2017).

Treatment involves isolation, supportive care provided by effective and advanced infection prevention and control measures including negative pressure room with no air circulation and positive pressure filtered air respirator. Mortality can be as high as 50%; if ribavirin is given within six days at onset, mortality can be reduced tenfold (Hidalgo et al., 2017; WHO, 2016).

Ebola virus disease

Ebola virus disease (EVD) (previously termed Ebola haemorrhagic fever) can cause fatal haemorrhagic fever (Molus & Bush, 2015). Clinical signs and symptoms are not dissimilar to other VHFs (Richards et al., 2018). The incubation period for EVD is 2 to 21 days and people are not infectious until they develop symptoms; early signs include fever, rash (maculopapular), sore throat, myalgia and arthralgia, malaise and severe headaches. Late signs include severe watery diarrhoea, vomiting, abdominal pain, petechiae rash, hypovolaemic shock and haemorrhagic manifestations, for example mucosal or gastrointestinal bleeding (Molus & Bush, 2015; WHO, 2017b). Potential differential diagnosis includes: malaria, enteric fever, Gram-negative bacterial sepsis, staphylococcal or streptococcal infection, meningococcemia, plague, leptospirosis or viral hepatitis. In consequence, anyone suspected with EVD must be isolated until a diagnosis is confirmed (Bisanzo et al., 2016).

Patients are highly infectious, as person-to-person transmission occurs through mucous membrane contact with bodily fluids with someone who is infectious and symptomatic or from the infected dead (Leligdowicz et al., 2016). Subsequently strict isolation, wearing of PPE and use of infection prevention control practices, including decontamination of equipment and personnel, need to be followed.

Critical care focuses on supportive care and is based on the severe sepsis principles and includes:

Airway

- Airway protection if the patient has a reduced level of consciousness or massive upper gastrointestinal bleed.
- Performing airway interventions including intubation may be difficult when wearing PPE.
- Patients vomiting or coughing aerosolises the virus and increases the risk of contamination to healthcare staff.

Breathing

- Supplementary oxygen may be required to maintain oxygen saturations >95%.
- Respiratory failure may be caused by shock, fatigue, metabolic acidosis, secondary bacterial infection and iatrogenic complications, for example transfusion associated lung injury.

Circulation

- Fluid resuscitation should be used to maintain adequate perfusion. To achieve this, wide bore access in the ante-cubital fossa or central venous access will be required.
- Hydration targets include:

  - HR <100/min;
  - urine output > 0.5ml/kg/hr;
  - SPB >90mmHg;
  - other markers of perfusion:

    - capillary refill <3 seconds;
    - absence of skin mottling;
    - easily palpable peripheral pulses;
    - warm, dry extremities;
    - improved mental status.

  - Hydration should also include replacement of electrolytes.

- Blood and blood products should be administered in an actively haemorrhaging patient.

  - A target Hb of >7g/dL is recommended; however, if blood losses are expected to be significant and ongoing, a higher target of 9g/dL may be used.
  - Platelets should be administered if platelet count is <20 × 10^9/L. If surgical procedure is planned, platelets should be administered if <50 × 10^9/L.
  - An INR >2 fresh frozen plasma or prothrombin complex concentrate should be administered.
  - Low fibrinogen levels and significant haemorrhaging despite correcting the INR and administration of platelets, cryoprecipitate should be transfused.

- Fever should be treated with paracetamol; a lower dose is required in hepatic dysfunction. Non-steroidal anti-inflammatory drugs (NSAID) should be avoided due to the platelet-inhibiting and renal effects.

Neurological/pain

- Pain management includes:

  - opiates titrated to effect, e.g. fentanyl, morphine;
  - NSAIDs, aspirin, anti-coagulants and intramuscular injections should be avoided.

Nutrition

- Nausea and vomiting should be treated with anti-emetics.
- Consider naso-gastric tube and suction.
- Consider enteral nutrition; if not tolerated, parental nutrition should be used.

(Richards *et al.*, 2018; Bisanzo *et al.*, 2016;
Molus & Bush, 2015; WHO, 2016)

Treatment

There is currently no licensed treatment available and epidemics focus on prevention and containment. Therapeutic agents include EVD – ZMapp, a cocktail of three human-mouse chimeric anti-EBOV monoclonal antibodies. GS-5734, a prodrug of nucleoside viral RNA polymerase inhibitor and Brincidofovir an oral nucleotide analogue that has shown in laboratory trials antiviral activity against DNA viruses. However, none of these have shown conclusive benefit (Richards *et al.*, 2018).

Given the generalised signs and symptoms which may overlap with other infections, empirical antibiotic therapy with broad-spectrum antibiotics may be appropriate if there is a risk of secondary bacterial infections. Antibiotics and other treatments, e.g. anti-malarias, should be discontinued once diagnosis is confirmed, symptoms improve or without other indication to continue (WHO, 2016).

References

Bisanzo M. Gema F. Wangoda R. (2016). Chapter 127: Malaria. In: Wallis LA. Reynolds TA (eds). African Federation of Emergency Medicine handbook of acute and emergency care. Oxford: Oxford University Press.

Dünser MW. Festic E. Dondorp A *et al.* (2012). Recommendations for sepsis management in resource-limited settings. Intensive Care Medicine. 38. 4. 557–574.

Hidalgo J. Richards GA. Jimenez JIS. Baker T. Amin P. (2017). Viral haemorrhagic fever in the tropics: report from the task force on tropical disease by the World Federation of Societies of Intensive and Critical Care Medicine. Journal of Critical Care. 42. 366–372.

Leligdowicz A. Fischer WA. Uyeki TM *et al.* (2016). Ebola virus disease and critical illness. Critical Care. 20. 217. DOI: doi.org/10.1186/s13054-016-1325-2.

Molus L. Bush P. (2015). Ebola – critical care considerations. World Federation of Societies of Anaesthesiologists. Tutorial 315. Available at: www.wfsahq.org/images/wfsa-documents/Tutorials_-_English/315_-_Ebola_-_Critical_Care_considerations_1.pdf.

Paterson ML. Callahan CW. (2015). The use of intraosseous fluid resuscitation in a paediatric patient with Ebola virus disease. Journal of Emergency Medicine. 49. 6. 962–964.

Rees PS. Lamb LE. Nicholson-Roberts TC *et al.* (2015). Safety and feasibility of a strategy of early central venous catheter insertion in a deployed UK military Ebola virus disease treatment unit. Intensive Care Medicine. 41. 5. 735–743.

Richards GA. Baker T. Amin P *et al.* (2018). Ebola virus disease: report from the task force on tropical diseases by the World Federation of Societies of Intensive and Critical Care Medicine. Journal of Critical Care. 43. 352–355.

World Health Organization. (2016). Clinical management of patients with viral haemorrhagic fever: A pocket guide for front-line health workers. Available at: http://apps.who.int/iris/bitstream/10665/205570/1/9789241549608_eng.pdf?ua=.

World Health Organization. (2017a). Haemorrhagic Fevers, Viral. Available at: www.who.int/topics/haemorrhagic_fevers_viral/en/.

World Health Organization. (2017b). Fact sheet: Ebola virus disease. Available at: www.who.int/mediacentre/factsheets/fs103/en/.

26 | Cholera and typhoid

Cholera

Cholera is a Gram-negative bacterial infection caused by *Vibrio cholerae 01* and *V. cholerea 0139*. Incubation period is from less than one day to five days and causes an acute intestinal infection, profuse watery diarrhoea and vomiting. Symptoms include profuse, painless, severe watery diarrhoea, and sometimes vomiting, leading to severe dehydration and loss of electrolytes (WHO, 2017; Bisanzo *et al.*, 2016). It is spread from person to person via the faecal-oral route, or by infected food or water (Shears, 2014; Mandal *et al.*, 2004). It can be spread quickly by poor hand hygiene and infection control practices (Mandal *et al.*, 2004).

The incubation period is two to three days (Mandal *et al.*, 2004), and individuals may present with sudden onset vomiting and profuse watery diarrhoea with abdominal cramps. Fever is absent (Mandal *et al.*, 2004). Stools are white-yellow with mucous flecks ('rice-water'). This leads to rapid dehydration leading to hypovolaemic shock (Mandal *et al.*, 2004). Due to the large numbers of patients involved, many critically and acutely ill patients may present, which may overwhelm critical care and acute care services. The size of the outbreak will determine resources available and how patients will be treated. In this situation, critical care nurses may best utilise their skills by supervising groups of healthcare staff who have limited experience of dealing with severe hypovolaemic shock and electrolyte imbalances. Mortality rates can reach 50% in previously unaffected or unprepared countries, with appropriate response mortality can be <1% (Mandal *et al.*, 2004; Bisanzo *et al.*, 2016). There is little information published on nursing a patient with cholera in critical care.

Isolation and infection prevention control principles

- Patients need to be isolated and implementation of strict infection prevention control procedures to reduce the risk of spread.
- Healthcare facilities will need to:

- o provide sufficient water to facilitate hand hygiene;
- o appropriately dispose of human faeces.
- Provide adequate supply of safe drinking water.

Airway

- Airway patency may be lost in patients with reduced level of consciousness and vomiting. Emergency suction should be immediately available, and patients placed in the three-quarters prone/recovery position to protect their airway.
- Depending on the resources available, in the event of a compromised airway, endotracheal intubation may be appropriate.

Breathing

- Patients should be monitored for signs of respiratory failure.
- In the event of respiratory failure, mechanical ventilation may be appropriate, but will be dependent on the resources and experienced staff available.
- Supplementary oxygen as required to maintain oxygen saturations >95%.

Circulation

- Cholera is easily treatable if individuals receive prompt oral or intravenous fluid resuscitation. If the patient can take fluids, they should be encouraged to drink oral rehydration solution (ORS) and a glucose-electrolyte solution. A moderately dehydrated patient can require up to six litres of ORS on the first day. As a guide, one glass of ORS for every diarrhoeal stool in adults and ORS equal volume to diarrhoeal volume in children. Table 26.1 provides a guide for the use of ORS with no or limited dehydration.
- Severely dehydrated and shocked patients should be treated with rapid administration of intravenous fluids. Treat with 30ml/kg over three minutes, followed by 70ml/kg over two to three hours. Once perfusion and mental status has improved, patients should be transferred over to ORS. However, patients may require both oral and IV fluids to keep up with fluid loses. A 70kg patient will require up to 7litres of IV fluids, in addition to ORS (WHO, 2017).
- Fluid balance including urine output should be recorded hourly. Maintenance fluids will be required once the patient has been adequately fluid resuscitated. This includes combining the volume of urine and faecal matter lost, plus 500ml added for insensible losses.
- Depending on the number of patients, admission to critical care may not be possible. Basic monitoring should be established, and fluid resuscitation may be guided by the return of a radial pulse (equivalent to a systolic blood pressure of 90mmHg) and improved urine output (>0.5ml/kg/hr).

- Hypovolaemic shock will cause AKI and is a significant cause of deaths. Aggressive fluid resuscitation, monitoring of renal function and fluid balance will help prevent the risk of AKI.
- Anti-emetics should be administered as indicated. NSAIDs should be avoided in severe dehydration and evidence of an AKI.

Antibiotics

- Antibiotics as per local guidelines should also be administered. Common antibiotics used include tetracycline, doxycycline and furazolidone. These have been shown to reduce the volume and duration of diarrhoea, but have also been shown to be developing resistance in Africa.
- Pregnant or nursing women and children: Azithromycin 20mg/kg (max. 1g) orally once daily or erythromycin 500mg six-hourly for three days.
- Antibiotics are an adjunct to fluid resuscitation and reduce the duration and bacterial excretion. They should only be administered in severe cases, to prevent antimicrobial resistance.

(WHO, 2017; Bisanzo *et al.*, 2016; Shears, 2014; Mandal *et al.*, 2004)

Typhoid

Typhoid is also termed 'enteric fever', caused by Gram-negative bacteria *Salmonella enterica*. Typhoid is transmitted through food or water contaminated by faeces and urine of a patient or carrier. Direct 'case to case' spread is not common (Mandal *et al.*, 2004). The incubation period is 10–21 days. Patients present with fever and abdominal pain and predominately diarrhoea, although constipation is more common in children (Bisanzo *et al.*, 2016). Untreated typhoid has an estimated mortality of 20%, but is negligible when individuals receive treatment early (Mandal *et al.*, 2004). The reason for admission to critical care may be due to a complication, for example post-operatively following an emergency laparotomy for perforation or gastro-intestinal bleeding.

Critical care considerations:

Airway

- The patient's airway may become compromised due to:
  - reduced level of consciousness;
  - upper gastro-intestinal bleed;
  - vomit in the airway.
- Patients should be nursed in an area where they can be observed, and any deterioration immediately acted on. Emergency suction should be at the bedside.

Table 26.1 Dehydration and ORS

Evidence of some dehydration and ORS to be administered within first four hours

<4 months (<5kg)	200–400ml
4–11 months (5–7.9kg)	400–600ml
1–2 years (8–10.9kg)	600–800ml
2–4 years (11–15.9kg)	800–1200ml
5–14 years (16–29.9kg)	1200–2200ml
>14 years (>30kg)	2200–4000ml
No dehydration: ORS	
Children <2years	50–100ml Up to 500ml/day
Children 2–9 years	100–200ml Up to 1000ml/day
Patients >9years	2000ml/day

Source: Bisanzo *et al.*, 2016

Breathing

- Complications include pneumonia. Oxygen therapy should be provided to maintain oxygen saturations >95%.
- In the event of respiratory failure, intubation and mechanical ventilation may be required.

Circulation

- Once the organism has entered the intestinal mucosa it travels to the regional glands and multiplies. The organisms then enter the bloodstream in large numbers resulting in fever. Fever may be caused by perforation and peritonitis.
- During the second to third week of illness, the organism causes damage to the Peyer's patch of the ileum. This leads to ulceration, causing haemorrhage and perforation.
- Hepatosplenomegaly occurs in approximately 75% of cases leading to complications.
- The patient may present with signs of sepsis and should be treated accordingly.
- Continuous cardiac monitoring should be established and observation for bradycardia. Bradycardia should be treated with atropine.
- Patients should be closely monitored for signs of gastro-intestinal bleeding.
- Nausea and vomiting.
- Constipation may be present during week one, and progress to diarrhoea during weeks two and three. Diarrhoea is described as 'pea-soup like'.

- Fluid balance monitoring and replacement fluids are important to prevent AKI.
- Other complications include cholecystitis, cholangitis, hepatitis, pancreatitis. Abscesses in spleen, bone or ovary.

Pain/neurological

- Typhoid encephalopathy may lead to delirium and confusion.
- Steroids should be used in severe disease or encephalopathy only.
- Patients may complain of abdominal pain. Appropriate analgesia should be given and the effects monitored.

Exposure

- Development of 'rose spots' (pale pink/salmon macules on trunk and abdomen) occur in approximately 30% of patients.

Surgical intervention

- In the event of perforation surgical intervention is required.
- Cholecystectomy should be performed only when symptoms of gall bladder disease is present.

Antibiotics

- Antibiotics: in severe cases ceftriaxone and uncomplicated cases fluroquinolone. Although local guidelines should be followed due to increasing antibiotic resistance in some areas.

(Bisanzo *et al.*, 2016; WHO, 2015; Mandal *et al.*, 2004)

References

Bisanzo M. Gema F. Wangoda R. (2016). Chapter 135: Cholera and Typhoid. In: Wallis LA. Reynolds TA (eds). African Federation of Emergency Medicine handbook of acute and emergency care. Oxford: Oxford University Press.

Mandal BK. Wilkins EGL. Dunbar EM (eds). (2004). Chapter 9: Infections of the gastrointestinal tract. In: Mandal BK. Wilkins EGL. Dunbar EM (eds). Lecture notes on infectious diseases. 6th Edition. Hoboken, NJ: Blackwell Publishing.

Shears P. (2014). Chapter 21: Cholera. In: Beeching N. Gill G (eds). Tropical medicine: lecture notes. 7th Edition. Chichester, West Sussex: Wiley Blackwell.

World Health Organization. (2015). Typhoid. Available at: www.who.int/immunization/diseases/typhoid/en/.

World Health Organization. (2017). Cholera. Available at: www.who.int/topics/cholera/en/.

27 Influenza

Influenza causes severe respiratory illnesses, which often require admission to hospital and critical care. The WHO (2017) identifies the incidence and mortality relating to severe influenza is increasing each year, with an estimated 650,000 deaths in 2017. The WHO (2018b) identifies three types of influenza:

- seasonal;
- pandemic;
- zoonotic or variant.

Potential differential diagnosis to influenza includes community acquired pneumonia, hospital acquired pneumonia, severe acute respiratory infection, exacerbation of chronic lung disease, e.g. asthma or chronic obstructive pulmonary disease, sepsis, encephalopathy, encephalitis, transverse myelitis, meningitis, Guillain-Barré syndrome, myocarditis and rhabdomyolysis (Public Health England, 2017).

Diagnosis of influenza is predominately clinically; however, tracheal secretions can be sent for laboratory testing. Rapid influenza diagnostic tests (RIDTs) are available but have a lower sensitivity than other methods and reliability is determined by the conditions in which they are used (WHO, 2018a).

Severe influenza can result in severe pneumonia, complicated by ARDS, septic shock and multi-organ failure, with a rapid deterioration (WHO, 2013). There is also a significant risk to healthcare workers, particularly those working in critical care with ventilated patients; for example, if using open suction systems, breaking the ventilator circuits results in particles being aerosolised (WHO, 2018a; Public Health England, 2017).

Seasonal influenza

Seasonal influenza circulates and cause diseases every year. Infection occurs:

- directly by inhaling virus-infected particles, e.g. by sneezing or coughing;
- indirectly by touching contaminated objects or surfaces then introducing the virus by rubbing eyes, sucking fingers, etc.

(Meunier, 2014)

Incubation is between one and five days and severity varies. At-risk groups include pregnant women, the young, elderly and those immunocompromised (WHO, 2018a). This type of influenza is continually evolving resulting in people getting infected several times throughout their life. There are three types of seasonal influenza: A, B, C:

- Influenza type A is sub-divided according to the variety and combination of two proteins on the surface of the virus, the hemagglutinin 'H' protein and neuraminidase 'N' protein. Examples include Influenza A (H1N1) and A (H3N2).
- There are two types of Influenza type B. They were named after where they were first identified: Victoria lineage and Yamagata lineage.
- Type C causes mild, sporadic cases and minor localised outbreaks (WHO, 2017).

Pandemic influenza

Pandemic influenza are viruses which are not previously circulating amongst humans and to which most people do not have immunity. The virus causes a large outbreak to occur, normally outside of influenza season. Influenza type A (H1N1) was first identified in 2009 and spread across the world causing a pandemic. The virus is now established in humans and it is classed as a seasonal influenza (WHO, 2018a). Pandemic influenza is a concern for critical care, as it can affect large numbers of people. This will put a significant strain on already stretched critical care services, resources and staff. Hospitals should have major incident and escalation plans to respond to outbreaks which are not trauma in origin.

Zoonotic or variant influenza

These are influenza viruses that are routinely circulating in animals that transfer to humans. They tend to be named after their host, for example include swine influenza, avian influenza (WHO, 2018b). They do not easily transfer from animals to humans and occur through direct or indirect contact. The most recent novel coronavirus, reported in 2012, is the Middle East respiratory syndrome coronavirus (MERS-CoV).

Impact on critical care services and staff

Patients with suspected or confirmed influenza could transmit the pathogen to healthcare workers. Recent outbreaks have affected healthcare workers resulting in further burden on critical care resources and a reduction in trained staff who can look after critically ill patients (Al-Dorzi et al., 2016; Rankin, 2006; Loeb et al., 2004). Unfortunately, influenza outbreaks have highlighted deficiencies in healthcare systems including lack of PPE and resources (Rankin, 2006).

During the SARS outbreak in Canada, the workplace was deemed a 'very dangerous place to work' and resulted in healthcare workers not coming to work (Rankin, 2006). With limited information, the fear of transmitting the pathogen to colleagues, family and friends led to social isolation. At work staff reported boredom and loneliness as they were 'quarantined' and not allowed to go to other areas of the hospital, e.g. staff canteen.

With few healthcare workers trained to look after critically ill patients, nurses will be required to work long hours with few breaks. This can lead to fatigue and exhaustion, which increases the risk of mistakes or failing to follow IPC measures (Rankin, 2006).

The pressure across the healthcare system on an influenza outbreak should not be underestimated. Even in HIC the demand for hospital and critical care services will often exceed availability. During the SARS outbreak in Ontario, 72% of total hospital capacity was required for influenza patients; at the peak demand for critical care beds was 171% and 118% of ventilator capacity. All elective procedures were cancelled and additional critical care areas were established, but lacked experienced staff and ventilators, etc. (Christian *et al.*, 2006). This lead to difficult triage and treatment decisions having to be made by healthcare professionals who were faced with the realities of a lack of resources and patients who had a potentially reversible condition.

Recognition of influenza

Influenza can be a common reason for admission to critical care in seasonal epidemics (Roa *et al.*, 2012). Early and rapid detection of these patients is necessary to initiate prompt treatment and isolate patients. Influenza is a respiratory illness with a wide range of signs and symptoms. It is characterised by sudden onset of fever and cough, with other common symptoms including chills, headache, sore throat and aching muscles and joints (Department of Health, 2009).

Treatment of influenza

When a patient presents with a suspected severe acute respiratory infection (SARI), key treatment principles involve (WHO, 2015):

- early recognition of patients with SARI;
- implementation of infection prevention control procedures;
- collection of specimens for laboratory diagnosis and antimicrobial therapy;
- management of severe respiratory distress, hypoxemia and ARDS;
- management of septic shock;
- prevention of complications;
- experimental versus specific therapeutics;
- management of high-risk patients, e.g. pregnant.

Isolation and infection prevention control measures

Infection prevention control measures include the following:

- Prompt identification of influenza cases.
- Isolating suspected and confirmed influenza patients.

- Immunisation should be available for key healthcare workers.
- Education of healthcare workers, patients and visitors regarding the importance of good respiratory and hand hygiene.
- Visitors to patients with influenza should be limited.
- Healthcare staff not well should be advised to stay at home.
- Appropriate environmental cleaning and waste disposal.
- Adequate ventilation.
- Use of PPE and hand hygiene.

(Department of Health, 2009)

Personal protective equipment

All patients triaged, and any suspect SARI cases should be isolated, by giving them a medical mask and placing them in a separate area. When admitted there should be at least one to two metres between patients and those not wearing PPE. Ideally, patients should be nursed in single rooms which are adequately ventilated. If the patient is self-ventilating, patients should be encouraged to perform good respiratory hygiene (e.g. covering mouth and nose during coughing, and sneezing into a tissue, which should be disposed of immediately). Cohorting of suspected and confirmed influenza together is not recommended. Once diagnosed if there are insufficient rooms, it may be appropriate to cohort patients to reduce transmission to other patients and limit the number of staff entering the dirty area (WHO, 2015).

Healthcare workers will need to wear personal protective equipment (PPE); this includes specialised masks or respirators. Sufficient PPE including masks must be available and not re-used. Prior to wearing specialist masks and respirators they normally need to be fitted to the individual and specific training provided. The procedure for donning and doffing PPE is as follows:

- Identify hazards and manage risks.
    - Gather the PPE required.
    - Plan where you are going to put on/take off PPE.
    - Do you have a 'buddy' or mirror to check you are correctly wearing PPE?
    - Do you know how to deal with waste generated?
- Put on gown.
- Put on particulate respirator or medical mask. Perform user seal check if using a respirator.
- Put on eye protection, e.g. face shield or goggles. Consider using anti-fog or fog-resistant goggles. Caps are optional; if worn, they should be applied after eye protection.
- Put gloves on, ensuring they cover the cuffs of the gown.

To remove PPE, avoid contamination of self, others and the environment by removing the most contaminated items first.

- Remove gown and gloves – peel off gown and gloves and role inside out, dispose of gloves and gown safely.
- Perform hand hygiene.
- Remove cap (if worn).
- Remove goggles from behind. Place them in a separate container for re-processing.
- Remove respirator from behind.
- Perform hand hygiene.

(Public Health England, 2017)

High-risk procedures

Certain procedures have been identified as potentially increasing the risk of transmitting influenza to others (Department of Health, 2009). Many of these procedures may be carried out in critical care increasing the exposure to critical care staff. Procedures include:

- intubation, extubation and related airway procedures, e.g. manual ventilation and open suctioning;
- cardiopulmonary resuscitation;
- bronchoscopy;
- surgery and post-mortem procedures in which high-speed devices are used;
- non-invasive ventilation (NIV), e.g. Bilevel Positive Airway Pressure ventilation (BiPAP) and Continuous Positive Airway Pressure ventilation (CPAP);
- high-frequency oscillating ventilation (HFOV);
- induction of sputum.

If you are involved in any of these procedures, they should be carried out in well-ventilated single rooms with the doors shut. Only healthcare workers who are critical to the procedure should be present and full PPE including a gown, gloves, eye protection and an FFP3 respirator should be worn by those undertaking these procedures and by those in the same room (Department of Health, 2009).

Critical care considerations

Nursing a critically ill patient there are specific infection control measures you should consider the following:

- Close observation of patients, as they may deteriorate rapidly. Conservative fluid management should be followed if there is no evidence of shock.
- Blood cultures and upper airway respiratory tract secretions should be taken. Empirical antibiotics should not be delayed and in the presence of sepsis should be given in one hour of presentation.
- Airborne precautions should be taken in the following situations:

o   High-flow oxygen, nebulisers and non-invasive ventilation has the potential to generate aerosols.

o   When intubating or undertaking any airway procedures, e.g. suctioning, changing ventilator circuits, e.g. to replace HMEs, insert a sputum trap; open suctioning due to a lack of closed suction systems may aerosolise particles.

- Mechanical ventilation should be initiated early. Lung-protective ventilation strategies including low volume (6ml/kg), low pressure (plateau airway pressure of <30cmH$_2$O) should be adopted. To reach lung protection ventilation:

o   Permissive hypercapnia.

o   To reach target SpO$_2$ PEEP should be used.

o   Deep sedation may be required to provide adequate ventilation.

o   Ventilator should not be disconnected due to the loss of PEEP and lung collapse.

o   In severe ARDS:

o   Prone positioning may be used to improve oxygenation (PaO$_2$/FiO$_2$ <15). Evidence has shown this should be implemented early and for at least 16 consecutive hours. Care should be taken when turning patient.

o   Neuromuscular blockade for initial 48 hours.

o   Use of higher PEEP in moderate to severe ARDS (PaO$_2$/FiO$_2$<200).

o   Conservative fluid management for ARDS patients who are not in shock.

- Septic shock should be managed with crystalloid fluid challenges and vasopressors if hypotension continues despite adequate/aggressive fluid resuscitation.
- IV hydrocortisone (up to 200mg/day, 1mg/kg six-hourly for children) or prednisolone (up to 75mg/day) to patients with persistent shock and requiring increasing doses of vasopressors. This should be tapered once the shock resolves.
- High-risk patients should have specialist input, e.g. obstetricians, midwives, etc.
- The use of experimental virus-specific drugs will be determined by the type of influenza; these may be experimental and will be guided by infection control specialists.

(Public Health England, 2017; Department of Health, 2009)

References

Al-Dorzi H. Aldawood AS. Khan R *et al*. (2016). The critical care response to a hospital outbreak of Middle East respiratory syndrome coronavirus (MERS-CoV) infection: an observational study. Annals of Intensive Care. 6. 101. DOI: https://doi.org/10.1186/s13613-016-0203-z.

Christian MD. Hawryluck L. Wax RS *et al*. (2006). Development of a triage protocol for critical care during an influenza pandemic. Canadian Medical Association Journal. 175. 11. 1377–1381.

Department of Health. (2009). Pandemic (H1N1) 2009 Influenza: A summary of guidance for infection control in healthcare settings. London: HMSO. Available at: https://assets.publishing.service.gov.uk/government/uploads/system/uploads/attachment_data/file/361997/Pandemic_influenza_guidance_for_infection_control_in_critical_care.pdf.

Loeb M. McGeer A. Henry B *et al*. (2004). SARS among Critical Care Nurses, Toronto. Emerging Infectious Diseases. 10. 2. 251–255.

Meunier YA. (2014). Tropical diseases. A practical guide for medical practitioners and students. New York: Oxford University Press.

Public Health England. (2017). Seasonal influenza: guidance for adult critical care units. Version 1.0. July. Available at: https://assets.publishing.service.gov.uk/government/uploads/system/uploads/attachment_data/file/635596/adult__seasonal_influenza_critical_care_guidance.pdf.

Rankin J. (2006). Godzilla in the corridor: The Ontario SARS crisis in historical perspective. Intensive and Critical Care Nursing. 22. 130–137.

Roa PL. Rodriguez-Sanchez B. Catalan P *et al*. (2012). Diagnosis of influenza in intensive care units: lower respiratory tract samples are better than nose–throat swabs. American Journal of Respiratory and Critical Care. 186. 929–930.

World Health Organization. (2013). Clinical management of severe acute respiratory infections when novel coronavirus is suspected: What to do and what not to do. Available at: www.who.int/csr/disease/coronavirus_infections/InterimGuidance_Clinical Management_NovelCoronavirus_11Feb13u.pdf.

World Health Organization. (2017). Up to 650 000 people die of respiratory diseases linked to seasonal flu each year. Available at: www.who.int/mediacentre/news/releases/2017/seasonal-flu/en/.

World Health Organization. (2018a). Influenza (seasonal). Available at: www.who.int/mediacentre/factsheets/fs211/en/.

World Health Organization. (2018b). Influenza virus infections in humans (February 2014). Available at: www.who.int/influenza/human_animal_interface/virology_laboratories_and_vaccines/influenza_virus_infections_humans_feb14.pdf?ua=1.

28 Malaria

Malaria is a parasitic infection caused by the genus *Plasmodium*. Malaria is common in tropical countries in Africa, Asia, Oceania and South and Central America (Karnad *et al.*, 2018). Malaria affects approximately 5% of the world's population (Mahajan *et al.*, 2014). In 2015, an estimated 212 million malaria cases were diagnosed (WHO, 2017), which resulted in 1–2.5 million deaths annually (Mahajan *et al.*, 2014). Malaria is spread by the female anopheles mosquito, and is preventable. Five species affect humans (Fletcher & Beeching, 2013):

- *Plasmodium falciparum*;
- *Plasmodium vivax*;
- *Plasmodium ovale*;
- *Plasmodium malariae*;
- *Plasmodium knowlesi*.

Plasmodium falciparum is the commonest form, responsible for 60% of infections, and the rest of infections are caused by P. vivax. P. ovale, P. malariae and P. knowlesi (WHO, 2015). Specific syndromes seen with Plasmodium including:

- P. falciparum: cerebral malaria, hypoglycaemia, renal/respiratory failure, severe anaemia, shock;
- P. vivax, P. ovale: anaemia, hypersplenism, relapse up to five years after acute infection;
- P. malariae: chronic asymptomatic parasitaemia, nephrotic syndrome;
- potential mixed infections.

(WHO, 2017; Bisanzo *et al.*, 2016)

Diagnosis

Malaria can be uncomplicated or severe. Uncomplicated malaria is characterised by high spiking fevers, usually accompanied by chills and rigors. Other signs include headaches, muscular ache, vague abdominal discomfort, lethargy, malaise and loss of appetite (Karnad *et al.*, 2018). If untreated, the illness may progress to severe malaria and cerebral malaria. Signs of severe malaria include unconsciousness, prostration, seizures, acute renal failure, metabolic acidosis, hypoglycaemia, anaemia, jaundice, acute pulmonary oedema, shock and hyperparasitemia (WHO, 2015).

The gold standard for testing for malaria is microscopy, which identifies the species and quantities of parasites in the blood. This takes time and is now being replaced by Rapid Diagnostic Tests (RDTs). RDTs detects P. falciparum only and are dependent on storage, use and interpretation. Potential differential diagnosis includes influenza, viral hepatitis, meningitis, septicaemia, pneumonia, gastroenteritis, typhoid, tick fever, viral haemorrhagic fever and acute HIV (de Wit *et al.*, 2016; Bisanzo *et al.*, 2016; Cox *et al.*, 2016). In the event of negative smear or RDT repeat tests should be performed until the patient improves or diagnosis is confirmed.

Bell and Lalloo (2014) identify that patients with HIV and malaria co-exist in many countries. The immunosuppression caused by HIV results in symptomatic malaria and increased chance of developing severe disease and potential malarial treatment failure. In consequence, it may be appropriate to perform a HIV test in a patient with an unknown HIV status, to ensure patients receive appropriate treatments.

Prevention

While malaria is preventable, within the hospital environment transmission can continue between patients and staff due to overcrowding and a lack of nets; this allows mosquitoes to continue to bite patients (Carter & Mukonka, 2017; Shepherd *et al.*, 2010). Subsequently, in malaria season, spray wards, doors and windows covered with nets and, if available, every bed should have a mosquito net. Sufficient bed nets must be available to allow them to be changed between patients, as this may in turn become an infection risk.

Management

Severe and cerebral malaria may require admission to critical care. Severe malaria from P. falciparum accounts for approximately 1% of infections (Karnad *et al.*, 2018). The fundamental principles in the management of malaria are similar to sepsis and septic shock (Karnard *et al.*, 2018). The following provides an overview of the general principles of nursing a critically ill malaria patient and highlights specific treatment interventions.

- Patients should be managed in an area where they can be observed, especially if the patient has a reduced level of consciousness and risk of fitting.
- RDTs completed to confirm diagnosis.
- Good nursing care is an essential part of the care of a critically ill malaria patient. This will help prevent errors in diagnosis and treatment (Table 28.1).

Table 28.1 Potential errors in diagnosis and treatment in malaria

Diagnosis	Treatment

Failure to:
 	
• consider a diagnosis of malaria either typical or atypical;
• elicit a history of exposure (including travel history);
• do a thick blood film;
• identify P. falciparum in a dual infection with P. vivax;
• recognise and treat hypoglycaemia;
• diagnose alternative or associated infections (bacterial, viral);
• recognise malaria due to similarity in other infections, e.g. influenza, hepatitis, viral haemorrhagic fever;
• recognise respiratory distress;
• recognise the severity in the patient's condition;
• conduct ophalmoscopic examination for the presence of papilloedema and malaria retinopathy;
• correctly identify severe malaria.
	• Delays in starting treatment.
	• Inadequate nursing care.
	• Incorrect calculation of anti-malarial medications.
	• Inappropriate administration of anti-malarial medications.
	• IM into the buttock, particularly of quinine, which can damage the sciatic nerve.
	• Failure to switch patients from parenteral to oral therapy after 24 hours, or as soon as they can take and tolerate oral medication.
	• Failure to:
	
	  o review antimalarial treatment for a patient whose condition is deteriorating;
	  o re-check blood glucose concentration in a patient who develops seizure or deepening coma;
	  o recognise and treat minor ('subtle') convulsions;
	  o recognise and manage pulmonary oedema;
	  o recognise and treat minor seizures;
	  o give antibiotics to treat possible meningitis presumptively if a decision is made to delay lumbar puncture;
	  o avoid fluid bolus resuscitation in children who are not dehydrated.
	
	• Delays in starting renal replacement therapy.

Source: WHO, 2012

Airway

• Reduced level of consciousness due to cerebral malaria, shock or hypoglycaemia may result in a loss of airway patency and protective mechanisms. Unconscious patients should be nursed in the three-quarters prone position or recovery position and never left unattended. Airway opening procedures and airway adjuncts leading to intubation may be required.

Breathing

- Respiratory complications in P. falciparum malaria include pulmonary oedema due to the rapid administration of fluids and Acute Respiratory Distress Syndrome (ARDS). The same strategies to treat and prevent ARDS due to other causes are applicable to malaria (Chapter 14). Malaria ARDS is associated with a high mortality.
- There is an overlap between sepsis, pneumonia and malaria. Therefore, the threshold for starting antibiotics should be low.

Circulation

- Initial aggressive fluid resuscitation in children with severe malaria is controversial. The WHO (2015) advise against rapid fluid boluses of colloids or crystalloids in children.
- In adults haemodynamic monitoring is essential as excessive fluid resuscitation may result in pulmonary oedema, while inadequate volume replacement will lead to acute kidney injury and worsening metabolic acidosis. Fluid resuscitation should be provided in boluses of 10–20ml/kg and monitored continuously with regular re-assessment to determine the effect.
- Shock occurs in approximately 10% of patients. Vasopressors may be required; however, adrenaline should be avoided as this may increase lactate production.
- Lactate acidosis is common and a marker of poor prognosis. A high lactate level is caused by anaerobic glycolysis in under-perfused tissues, due to microcirculation obstruction by parasitised erythrocytes. Other factors include hepatic and renal impairment.
- Blood cultures should be taken on admission and antibiotics started early and de-escalated or discontinued if bacterial infection is ruled out.
- Thrombocytopenia is common in severe malaria; however, spontaneous bleeding is not common.
- Haemolysis can cause acute, severe anaemia. The recommended threshold for transfusion in adults is 7g/dl as for other critically ill patients. For children it has been recommended a Hb of 4–6g/dl is acceptable.
- Leukocyte counts can be normal, which may be useful in differentiating between bacterial infections that imitate malaria.
- In approximately 10% of cases Disseminating Intravascular Coagulopathy (DIC) occurs. It is a late sign, associated with multi-organ failure and poor outcome.
- Exchange transfusion (Chapter 29) may be appropriate with patients with a high parasite count.
- Actively treat pyrexia (>39°C) by administering paracetamol as an antipyretic. Tepid sponging and fanning may make the patient comfortable. Except for P. vivax malaria, three stages of fever have been identified: the cold stage, during which the patient has rigors and temperature increases; the hot stage, whereby the patient is flushed, has a rapid pulse and pyrexia for a few hours; and the sweating stage, when the patient sweats significantly and the temperature falls for a period.

- Acute kidney injury can occur due to volume depletion, shock, microcirculation obstruction. In P. falciparum haemoglobinuria (brown or black urine), sometimes termed blackwater fever, occurs due to severe renal failure. Although the term 'blackwater fever' is an obsolete term, it can still be used by some clinicians to describe this condition. Strict fluid balance monitoring, one-hourly urine measurement and urea and electrolyte blood tests should be monitored. Haemodialysis or RRT may be required in up to 35% of patients.
- Observe the patient and record observations. This may help identify complications including metabolic acidosis, pulmonary oedema, hypovolaemic shock.
- If available perform arterial blood gases and other routine bloods to assess renal function, glucose, electrolytes and anaemia.

Neurological

- Check hourly blood glucose level of hypoglycaemia. Hypoglycaemia may be due to impaired hepatic gluconeogenesis, glucose consumption by the parasites and the effects of quinine stimulating pancreatic insulin secretion. Hypoglycaemia should be treated with intravenous glucose (5ml/kg 10% dextrose). In the event of no access to glucose monitoring empirical dextrose containing IV fluid (e.g. 5% dextrose) should be given and in the event of evidence of hypoglycaemia (e.g. reduced consciousness, fitting) administration of buccal or IV dextrose should be given. In addition, a naso-gastric tube can be inserted to provide nutrition and sugar. Hypoglycaemia is common in children, pregnant women and those treated with intravenous quinine.
- Observe for other sources of reduced level of consciousness, e.g. meningitis.
- Seizures should be treated with a benzodiazepine, e.g. intravenous diazepam, midazolam or lorazepam. If seizures continue, phenytoin or phenobarbitone may be required.
- In an unconscious patient, perform neurological observations and observe for deterioration. Apply neurological protection principles if concerned about cerebral malaria or increased intra-cranial pressure.
- Neurological outcome is better in adult survivors, whereas in children cerebral malaria includes hemiplegia, spasticity, blindness and impaired learning. Neurological care includes:

  o fever control;
  o elevating head of the bed;
  o effective treatment of seizures;
  o osmotic therapy;
  o hyperventilation specifically targeted to raised intracranial pressure.

- High dose dexamethasone can be harmful and is associated with prolonged duration of coma.
- If trained to do so, examine the optic fundi. Retinal whitening, vascular changes or haemorrhages, if present, will assist in confirming diagnosis. Papilloedema is rare, and if seen a lumbar puncture is contra-indicated.

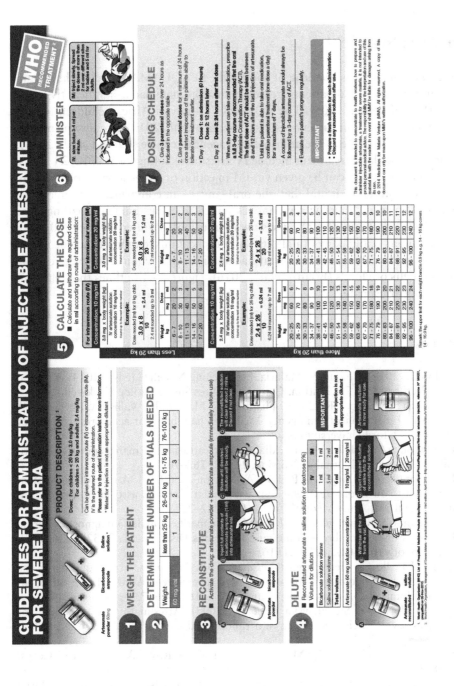

Figure 28.1 Example artesunate treatment regimen

Reproduced with kind permission from Medicines for Malaria Venture.

(Karnad *et al.*, 2018; Carter & Mukonka, 2017; Bisanzo *et al.*, 2016; Bell & Lalloo, 2014; WHO, 2012, 2015; Taylor, 2012; White *et al.*, 2014)

Anti-malaria treatment

Up until 2005, quinine was the drug of choice; the SEAQUAMAT study, a large randomised control trial, found patients treated with artesunate had a significantly lower mortality (Dondorp *et al.*, 2005). The AQUAMAT study of African children treated with artesunate showed comparable results (Dondorp *et al.*, 2010). In consequence, IV artesunate replaced quinine as the anti-malarial agent of choice (Karnad *et al.*, 2018).

In complicated malaria treatment include IV artesunate 2.4mg/kg at 0, 12, 24 hours. If no IV access, artesunate can be given via IM injection or suppositories for children. Once the patient can take an oral diet, the oral course can commence. An alternative is IV quinine; however, there is regional resistance. If using quinine, loading dose 20mg/kg in 5% dextrose over four hours (slow IV infusion). Maintenance dose 10mg/kg IV every eight hours until taking oral. Potential complications to quinine include risk of QT prolongation, therefore continuous cardiac monitoring is required. Hypoglycaemia monitor blood glucose levels (Bisanzo *et al.*, 2016). Figure 28.1 outlines the treatment of malaria using artesunate.

References

Bell D. Lalloo D. (2014). Chapter 9: Malaria. In: Beeching N. Gill G (eds). (2014). Tropical medicine: lecture notes. 7th Edition. Chichester, West Sussex: Wiley Blackwell.

Bisanzo M. Gema F. Wangoda R. (2016). Chapter 127: Malaria. In: Wallis LA. Reynolds TA (eds). African Federation of Emergency Medicine: handbook of acute and emergency care. Oxford: Oxford University Press.

Carter C. Mukonka P. (2017). Malaria: diagnosis, treatment and management of a critically ill patient. British Journal of Nursing. 26. 13. 762–767.

Cox AT. Schoonbaert I. Trinick T. Phillips A. Marion D. (2016). A case of an avoidable admission to an Ebola treatment unit with malaria and an associated heat illness. Journal of the Royal Army Medical Corps. 162. 222–225.

de Wit E. Falzarano D. Onyango C. *et al.* (2016). The merits of malaria diagnostics during an ebola virus disease outbreak. Emerging Infectious Diseases. 22. 2. 323–326. DOI: https://dx.doi.org/10.3201/eid2202.151656.

Dundorp AN. Fanello CI. Hendriksen IC *et al.* (2010). Artesunate versus quinine in the treatment of severe falciparum malaria in African children (AQUAMAT): an open-labelled, randomized control trial. The Lancet. 376. 1647–1657.

Dundorp AN. Nosten F. Stepniewska K *et al.* (2005). Artesunate versus quinine for treatment of severe falciparum malaria: a randomised control trial. The Lancet. 366. 717–725.

Fletcher TE. Beeching NJ. (2013). Malaria. Journal of the Royal Army Medical Corps. 159. 158–166.

Karnad DR. Mat Nor MD. Richards GA *et al.* (2018). Intensive care in severe malaria: report from the task force on tropical diseases by the World Federation of Societies of Intensive and Critical Care Medicine. Journal of Critical Care. 43. 356–360.

Mahajan SK. Kaushik M. Rains R. Thakur P. (2014). Scrub typhus and malaria co-infection causing severe sepsis. Tropical Doctor. 44. 1. 43–45.

Shepherd P. Shepherd H. Mueller S. 2010. Treating surgical wounds in rural south-western Uganda. Wounds International. 1. 4. 11–14.

Taylor WR. Hanson J. Turner GD. White NJ. Dondrop AM. (2012). Respiratory manifestations of malaria. Chest. 142. 492–505.

White NJ. Pukrittayakamee S. Hien TT. Faiz MA. Mokuolou OA *et al.* (2014). Malaria. The Lancet. 383. 723–735.

World Health Organization. (2012). Management of severe malaria. 3rd Edition. Available at: https://apps.who.int/iris/bitstream/handle/10665/79317/9789241548526_eng.pdf; jsessionid=41AD29859A7006EDD569E84E03AC5498?sequence=1.

World Health Organization. (2015). Guidelines for the treatment of Malaria. 3rd Edition. Available at: https://apps.who.int/iris/bitstream/handle/10665/162441/9789241549127_eng.pdf?sequence=1.

World Health Organization. (2017). Malaria. Available at: www.who.int/malaria/en/.

29 | Sickle cell disease

Sickle cell disease (SCD) is an inherited haemoglobin disorder that affects how the oxygen is transported within the blood. Individuals with sickle cell trait (SCT) are generally asymptomatic and may be diagnosed accidently, for example from blood investigations prior to surgery or antenatal care (Brown, 2012). SCT is prevalent in parts of the world where malaria is endemic and is known to provide protection against *Plasmodium falciparum* malaria (Brown, 2012).

The term 'SCD' is an umbrella term for sickle cell anaemia and thalassemia; the terms 'SCD' and 'sickle cell anaemia' can be used interchangeably, and although linked they are different conditions (Livesay & Ruppert, 2012; Brown, 2012). SCD is described as a syndrome including any abnormal haemoglobin which combines with a sickle haemoglobin (HbS). Combinations include sickle cell anaemia (HbSS), sickle cell disease (HbSS) and sickle/beta thalassemia (HbS/Beta).

SCD is characterised by a change in the shape of red blood cells. In SCD when red blood cells are oxygenated, they retain the normal cell shape. However, when they become deoxygenated they polymerise causing them to change shape and become long fibres and 'stick' together, causing them to become sickle in shape (Brown, 2012). When the cell becomes oxygenated again it returns to a biconcave shape. This continual change in shape causes the cell to become irreversibly sickle shaped and haemolysed, resulting in a shortened life span of 10–20 days, instead of the normal life span of a red blood cell of 120 days. The excessive haemolysis leads to chronic haemolytic anaemia (Brown, 2012). The misshaped cell lacks plasticity and can block small blood vessels, reducing blood flow (Thachil & Bates, 2014).

Reasons for admission to critical care may be sickle cell disease (SCD) related or SCD-unrelated events (Cecchini *et al.*, 2014). The clinical spectrum of SCD-related conditions can range from simple pain to multi-organ failure (Cecchini *et al.*, 2014); conditions include (Table 29.1):

- vaso-occlusive crises (VOC);
- acute chest syndrome (ACS);
- fever or sepsis;

- shock;
- acute cor-pulmonale;
- pulmonary oedema;
- acute kidney injury;
- hyperhaemolysis transfusion reactions;
- medullary necrosis;
- erythroblastopenia;
- splenic sequestration;
- splenic sequestration;
- aplastic crises;
- stroke;
- posterior reversible encephalopathy syndrome;
- SCD-related cerebral vasculopathy (seizures and strokes);
- opiate overdose;
- priapism.

(Checkett & Mfinanga, 2016; Cecchini *et al.*, 2014)

In addition, people with SCD are living longer and may develop morbidities such as pulmonary hypertension, hepatic (liver) and renal dysfunction. These conditions may exacerbate acute VOC episodes (Brown, 2012).

Vaso-occlusive crises (VOC)

Vaso-occlusive crises (VOC) often result in hospital admission. VOC occurs when the sickle-shaped cells occlude blood vessels, preventing oxygen and nutrients reaching tissues; this leads to tissue hypoxia, tissue necrosis and severe pain. VOC is the commonest form of sickle cell crises, but others include:

- sequestration crisis: pooling of blood in an organ (spleen in children, liver in adults and lungs in both children and adults);
- aplastic crisis: bone marrow stops or reduces function for a brief period. This can be triggered by infection (Parvovirus B19) or folic acid deficiency;
- haemolytic crises: caused by a rapid drop in haemoglobin levels.

(Brown, 2012)

The underlying cause of VOC is often infection, therefore the cause should be identified and appropriately treated (Livesay & Ruppert, 2012). Causes may also include temperature changes, dehydration and trauma (Checkett & Mfinanga, 2016). Signs of VOC may include pain in chest, back, hips, shoulders, proximal arms and legs. Stroke is a significant complication of VOC, with children more likely to experience an acute stroke than adults. The incidence of ischaemic stroke decreases as patients get older and haemorrhagic stroke becomes more common. However, adults with SCA are at increased risk of ischaemic risk than the general population (Livesay & Ruppert, 2012).

Table 29.1 Potential conditions associated with sickle cell

Condition	History	Potential causes
Vaso-occlusive crises (VOC)	Pain in chest, back, hips, shoulder, proximal arms, legs	Infection Temperature change Dehydration Trauma
Acute chest syndrome	Infiltrate on chest X-ray PLUS Cough, fever, tachypnoea, chest pain, wheezing	Pulmonary infarction triggered by infection, thromboembolism Differential diagnosis: • fat embolism; • myocardial Infarction; • pulmonary embolism; • pneumonia.
Fever	Fever and any systemic symptoms of sepsis	Sickle cell patients are at risk of sepsis due to functional asplenia (absence of normal spleen function).
Splenic sequestration	Acute, painful enlargement of spleen with decrease in Hgb and platelets	Sequestration of sickled red blood cells in the spleen Differential diagnosis: • malaria; • thalassemia; • haemolytic anaemia.
Aplastic crisis	Acute, severe drop in Hb, white cells and platelets	Infection Folate deficiency Marrow necrosis
Stroke	Sudden onset neurological symptoms	VOC crises in the brain Differential diagnosis: • non-occlusive ischaemic or haemorrhagic stroke.
Priapism	Painful erection lasting >4 hours	Penile VOC

Source: Checkett & Mfinanga, 2016

Acute chest syndrome

Acute chest syndrome (ACS) is defined as the combination of a new pulmonary infil-trate on chest X-ray with chest pain, fever, tachypnoea, wheezing and cough. ACS is a frequent cause of vaso-occlusive event (VOE) leading to critical care admission and respiratory support (Cecchini *et al.*, 2014). Differential diagnosis includes fat embolism, myocardial infarction, pulmonary embolism or pneumonia (Checkett & Mfinanga, 2016).

The severity of lung injury caused by ACS varies, with severe cases leading to ARDS. The cause of the lung injury is not clear, but believed to result from bacterial or viral infection, fat embolism from bone infarction and necrosis, vaso-occlusion of the pulmonary vasculature or a combination (Livesay & Ruppert, 2012).

Blood transfusion

Therapeutic target for blood transfusions in patients with VOC remains controversial (Livesay & Ruppert, 2012). Types of blood transfusion include:

* 'top-up' transfusion, which adds to the donor's blood without removing any of the recipient's blood;
* 'exchange' transfusion whereby donor blood replaces recipient's blood. This can either be full exchange of the patient's whole blood volume or partial/limited exchanges, when smaller volumes are used (Christie, 2016).

Transfusions should only be used when there is a clinical indication, for example to correct symptomatic anaemia, end-organ failure because of hypoxia, acute stroke and ACS (Cecchini *et al.*, 2014; Checkett & Mfinanga, 2016; Thachil & Bates, 2014). Cross-matching may take longer in SCD patients as sickle cell patients must undergo an extended cross-match for atypical antibodies (Patil *et al.*, 2017).

Surgical care

ACS is more common in SCD patients undergoing operative procedures requiring general anaesthesia and abdominal surgical procedures (Livesay & Ruppert, 2012). This requires patients to be appropriately optimised prior to surgery which may be difficult if the surgical intervention is an emergency, for example due to trauma or an emergency caesarean section.

Electively, perioperative blood transfusion may be indicated to replace sickle cells with normal red blood cells to reduce operative complications including stroke and ACS due to increased blood viscosity (Christie, 2016). However, transfusion poses additional risks including access to safe, screened blood and sufficient quantities. Intra-operatively, if available blood conserving techniques should be used, for example the use of cell-savers (Patil *et al.*, 2017).

Other complications include hypothermia. Temperature can cause VOC; therefore, patients' temperature should be monitored and actively warmed while in theatre and during the post-operative period. All fluids should be warmed prior to administration.

Pregnancy

Common conditions affecting SCD pregnant women include VOC, ACS, thromboembolic events, anaemia and increased risk of infection (Patil *et al.*, 2017). SCD pregnant women are also at higher risk of pre-eclampsia, eclampsia and HELLP (haemolysis, elevated liver enzymes and low platelets). Three major causes of death in pregnancy SCD include ACS, sepsis and multi-organ failure (Howard *et al.*, 1995). Specific considerations include:

- *Monitoring.* SCD pregnant women may need to be admitted and monitored to detect any early signs of deterioration. Care includes monitoring, hydration (including encouraging oral fluids), avoiding excessive starvation with ketosis, strict fluid balance monitoring and keeping the patient warm.
- *Pain management.* The use of pethidine (meperidine or Demerol) should be avoided as this can increase the risk of pethidine-associated seizures in SCD. In addition, non-steroidal anti-inflammatory drugs (NSAIDs) should be avoided in pregnancy between 12 and 18 weeks (Patil *et al.*, 2017). Epidurals may be useful for VOC in lower limbs during labour and deemed safer than spinals. Epidurals allow a slow incremental block to be achieved.
- *Delivery.* A prolonged second stage of labour should be avoided and minimise the risk for an emergency delivery or caesarean section.
- *Infection.* Common causes include urinary tract infections (UTI).

(Patil *et al.*, 2017)

Critical care admission and management

Many patients are first admitted to general wards from emergency departments with an isolated VOC and deteriorate often due to ACS. Ward-based care includes aggressively managing VOC and involves (Cecchini *et al.*, 2014; Livesay & Ruppert, 2012):

- supplementary oxygen;
- aggressive IV hydration;
- folate supplementation;
- analgesia;
- transfusion of packed red cells as necessary;
- Bed-rest.

Monitoring and observation for deterioration is critical in all SCD patients, to prevent a vaso-occlusive event leading to ACS and acute deterioration. During a severe sickle cell crisis and acute deterioration patients may require admission to critical care units. The reversible nature of many conditions associated with SCD justifies the admission of these young patients to critical care, and poor outcome is associated with a delayed critical care admission (Cecchini & Fartoukh, 2015). A team approach including physiotherapists and haematology is required. Management may include the following.

Airway

- Observation for signs of airway obstruction due to reduced level of consciousness.

Breathing

- Supplementary oxygen should be administered to keep oxygen saturations >95%. Use supplemental oxygen irrespective of saturations when using opioids.
- Splinting of diaphragm may lead to respiratory failure and hypoxia.
- Mechanical ventilation may be required due to respiratory failure. Neuromuscular blockade may be required to improve oxygenation. Paralysing agents should only be used when sedation alone does not reduce the work of breathing, ventilator dyssynchronous and hypoxia.
- Ventilation prevention strategies should be used to prevent ARDS.

Circulation

- All patients should be monitored for signs of arrhythmias. This includes cardiac monitoring and one-hourly observations.
- Establishing IV access may be difficult, as SCD patients may have had multiple hospital admissions, invasive lines and potentially exchange transfusions. If central access is required a vas-cath may be more appropriate than a traditional central line as this will allow quick transfusions and exchange transfusions to be undertaken.
- IV fluids to prevent dehydration and careful fluid monitoring particularly in chest crises.
- In ongoing shock, vasopressors may be required.
- Haemoglobin and haematocrit should be closely monitored every 12 hours. Transfusion should only be used if there is clinical indication. A haemoglobin decrease of 1% combined with continued hypoxaemia may indicate the need for red blood cell transfusion and possibly exchange transfusion. The procedure to undertake an exchange transfusion is outlined in Box 29.1.
- When giving blood transfusion or exchange transfusion observe for signs of complication. Delayed haemolytic transfusion reactions (DHTR) can occur from 24 hour to 21 days after a transfusion.
- Folic acid and iron supplementation.
- Sickle cell patients are at risk of sepsis due to functional asplenia (absence of normal spleen function). The source of sepsis should be identified and treated. Antibiotics should be prescribed if sepsis suspected or confirmed.
- Temperature should be monitored, with the aim of keeping the patient's core temperature >36°C. Patients should be kept warm and actively warmed.
- Fluid balance should be monitored.
- Acute kidney injury (AKI) is a significant risk. Careful cardiovascular assessment for signs of volume depletion should be observed. Damage to glomerular filtration may result in low or low-normal serum creatinine levels. In consequence, the patter and rate of serum creatinine change should be considered rather than the absolute value of creatinine. These subtle signs may be the only indicators of AKI.

Box 29.1   Procedure for an exchange transfusion (Patil *et al.*, 2017)

Step 1: Baseline blood tests:

- HbS percentage;
- urea and creatinine;
- calcium;
- magnesium;
- liver function tests;
- cross-match (if not already done).

Step 2: Cross-match six to eight units of packed red blood cells (PRBC).

- Blood will need to be fully cross-matched and include Rh and Kell antigens.
- Liaise with haematology and laboratory staff to ensure no alloantibodies are present.

Step 3: Assemble equipment:

- infusion pump;
- giving set;
- scales/transfusion bags to collect venesected blood;
- blood warmer;
- thermometer;
- blood pressure, ECG, saturation monitor;
- sterile gloves;
- Patent vas-cath or central line.

Step 4: Assemble drugs:

- calcium chloride/gluconate;
- packed red cells;
- Five to eight 500ml normal saline bags.

Step 5: Process:

- Warm blood using blood warmer.
- Start infusion of saline 500ml bag over 30 minutes.
- Venesect 500ml over 30 minutes.
- Once 500ml saline given, venesect volume of first unit of PRBC.
- Start first unit of PRBC over 40 minutes.
- Venesect volume of second unit once first unit has been transfused.

- Transfuse second PRBC unit over one hour.
- Venesect volume of third unit once second unit has been transfused.
- Transfuse third unit over two hours.
- Re-check full blood count and HbS.

If HB <8g/dl transfuse first use while performing second venesection.

Target HBS <30%

Target final Hb will be determined by condition, e.g. pregnancy final Hb 10–11g/dl. Hb >11g/dl should be avoided due to hyperviscosity risk.

Monitor for signs of hyperkalaemia and hypocalcaemia – check venous blood gas intermittently and cardiac monitoring for signs for ECG changes.

Neurological

- Pain is caused during VOC and caused by sickled blood flowing through small capillary beds. Stress and anxiety can also exacerbate pain. Analgesia (opioids) should be given and assessed for its effectiveness.
- Pain management can be complicated due to opioid tolerance and pain secondary to VOC. Opioid overdose leading to respiratory compromise and reduced level of consciousness is a risk. Analgesia should not be denied to a patient in pain and individualised pain management plans need to be agreed.
- Observation for signs of neurological complications including stroke, seizures, headaches and neuropathy.

Potential complications:

- Chronic anaemia, haemolysis and intermittent acute VOCs result in progressive organ damage, leading to multi-organ failure.
- Complications of bed-rest, e.g. pressure sores, DVT, PE, pneumonia.

(Patil et al., 2017; WHO, 2017; Checkett & Mfinanga, 2016; Thachil & Bates, 2014; Livesay & Ruppert, 2012; Cecchini et al., 2014; Gardner et al., 2010; Cecchini & Fartoukh, 2015)

References

Brown M. (2012). Managing the acutely ill adult with sickle cell disease. British Journal of Nursing. 21. 2. 90–96.

Cecchini J. Fartoukh M. (2015). Sickle cell disease in the ICU. Current Opinion in Critical Care. 21. 569–575.

Cecchini J. Lionnett F. Djibré M *et al*. (2014). Outcomes of adult patients with sickle cell disease admitted to the ICU: A case series. Critical Care Medicine. 42. 1. 1629–1639.

Checkett K. Mfinanga J. (2016). Chapter 115: Sickle cell disease. In: Wallis LA. Reynolds TA (eds). (2016). African Federation of Emergency Medicine: handbook of acute and emergency care. Oxford: Oxford University Press.

Christie J. (2016). Preoperative blood transfusions for sickle cell disease: A Cochrane review summary. International Journal of Nursing Studies. 64. 137–138.

Gardner K. Bell C. Bartram JL *et al*. (2010). Outcome of adults with sickle cell disease admitted to critical care – experience of a single institution in the UK. British Journal of Haematology. 150. 610–613.

Howard RJ. Tuck SM. Pearson TC. (1995). Pregnancy in sickle cell disease in the UK: results of a multi-centre survey of the effects of prophylactic blood transfusion on maternal and foetal outcome. British Journal of Obstetrics and Gynaecology. 102. 947–951.

Livesay S. Ruppert SD. (2012). Acute chest syndrome of sickle cell disease. Critical Care Nurse Quarterly. 35. 2. 183–195.

Patil V. Ratnayake G. Fastovets G. (2017). Clinical 'pearls' of maternal critical care part 2: sickle-cell disease in pregnancy. Current Opinion in Anaesthesiology. 30. 3. 326–334.

Thachil J. Bates I. (2014). Chapter 56: Haemoglobinopathies and red cell enzymopathies. In: Beeching N. Gill G. (eds). Tropical medicine: lecture notes. 7th Edition. Chichester, West Sussex: Wiley Blackwell.

World Health Organization. (2017). Sickle cell disease and other haemoglobin disorders. Geneva: World Health Organization.

<table>
<tr><td>30</td><td></td></tr>
</table>

30   Poisoning

Acute poisoning is a common medical emergency (Leach, 2004). Poisoning can lead to organ dysfunction and metabolic derangements, which can lead to critical care admission (Jayakrishnan *et al.*, 2012). Poisoning may be self-poisoning (e.g. recreational drug use, attempted suicide), homicidal, industrial, warfare or terrorism (Nolan *et al.*, 2011). Drug toxicity can be caused by inappropriate dosing and drug reactions. General principles and management of poisoning are based on clinical features, examination, resuscitation and investigations (Wood & Wyncool, 2014). Common types of poisoning requiring critical care admission include:

- organophosphate poisoning;
- opioid;
- cocaine toxicity;
- benzodiazepines;
- tricyclic antidepressants;
- paracetamol.

Early critical care admission can influence outcome following poisoning (Jayakrishnan *et al.*, 2012). The priorities of treatment include decontamination, limiting the absorption of ingested poisons, enhancing elimination or the use of antidotes (Nolan *et al.*, 2011). Hospitals must have access to a drug/poisons database to help identify treatment plans. General critical care considerations when nursing a poisoning patient include the following:

- Personal safety and access to personal protective equipment must be used.
- Patients may require decontamination; this includes removal of clothing. Care should be taken as drugs may be absorbed into clothing, and when handled PPE should be worn.
- Patients should be assessed and closely monitored for signs of deterioration.

Airway

- Airway obstruction and respiratory arrest are secondary to decreased level consciousness.
- Early intubation can decrease the risk of aspiration. In the presence of chemicals such as cyanide, hydrogen sulphide, corrosives and organophosphates, use caution when performing airway management procedures, as there is risk of inhalation of chemicals.
- In the event of vomiting, emergency suction must be immediately available.
- An unconscious or semi-conscious patient should be positioned in the three-quarters prone or recovery position and not left unattended.

Breathing

- Self-ventilating patients should be given supplementary oxygen and oxygen saturations maintained >95%.
- Continuous pulse oximetry.
- Mechanical ventilation is required in respiratory failure and hypoxia.
- Measure arterial blood gases and correct acidosis.
- Bronchoconstriction using nebulised salbutamol or ipratropium bromide.

Circulation

- Patients must have continuous cardiac monitoring. Many drugs result in arrhythmias. Tachyarrhythmias may require cardioversion.
- Perform 12 lead ECGs.
- Regular blood pressure monitoring, either invasive or non-invasive. If using NIBP, the frequency should be set to five-minute intervals.
- Monitor electrolytes, particularly potassium level.
- Drug-induced hypotension should be managed with IV fluids. Vasopressors may be required.
- Measure the patient's temperature as hypo- or hyperthermia can occur after drug overdose.
- Strict fluid balance charting should be followed.

Disability (neurological)

- Monitor Glasgow Coma Scale and pupil size and reaction.
- Measure blood glucose levels and treat hypoglycaemia.
- Observe and treat seizures.

Exposure

- Examination of the patient may reveal clues, for example odours, needle marks or signs of corrosion of the mouth.
- Measure temperature.

Antidotes

- Routine use of gastric lavage for gastrointestinal decontamination is not recommended.
- Laxatives and emetics are not recommended in the management of acutely poisoned patients.
- Activated charcoal absorbs certain drugs; however, its efficacy decreases over time following ingestion and there is little evidence that treatment with activated charcoal improves clinical outcome. Charcoal should only be given if the patient has an intact or protected airway. Dose may be single or multiple depending on the poisoning. Multiple doses may be indicated in life-threatening poisoning with carbamazepine, dapsone, phenobarbital, quinine and theophylline.
- Urine alkalisation (urine pH >7.5) by IV sodium bicarbonate is indicated for moderate to severe salicylate poisoning in those who do not need haemodialysis.
- Specific antidotes include:
  - o paracetamol overdose: acetylcysteine;
  - o organophosphate, sodium nitrate, sodium thiosulfate, hydroxocobalamin poisoning: high dose atropine;
  - o cyanides: amyl nitrate.

(Nolan *et al.*, 2011)

The use of gastric lavage has limited effect and delays the use of activated charcoal if indicated. Activated charcoal is a treatment for many acute poisonings, and works by absorbing toxins. Exceptions include elemental metals, pesticides, alcohol including ethanol, strong acids and alkaline and cyanide. Activated charcoal should be given within one hour of the overdose for the maximum effect. Care must be taken to protect patients airway, in a semi-/unconscious patient due to the risk of vomiting (Leach, 2004).

Organophosphate poisoning

Organophosphate is a widely used pesticide in LICs. It is widely accessible, and poisoning may occur due to accidental, occupational or attempted suicide (Soltaninejad & Shadnia, 2014). Organophosphates have also been used as nerve agents in chemical weapons. Organophosphate poisoning (OPP) can be divided into the following categories:

- Muscarinic effects.

  o Hypersecretion (increased sweating, salivation and bronchial secretions), constricted pupils, bradycardia, hypotension, bronchoconstriction, vomiting, diarrhoea, urinary incontinence.

- Nicotinic effects.

  o Skeletal and respiratory muscular weakness, fasciculations.

- Central nervous system (CNS) effects.

  o Restlessness, anxiety. Headaches, seizures, unconsciousness.

  (Katz *et al.*, 2016; Olson & van Hoving, 2016a)

Critical care considerations

- Healthcare professionals are at risk of secondary exposure/contamination when in direct contact and handling patients or by 'off-gassing'.
- Cardiac monitoring observing for arrhythmias (QT interval or PVCs).
- Fluid resuscitation to treat hypotension; inotropes may be required to maintain a MAP >70mmHg.
- Observations for respiratory failure, treat hypoxia and bronchoconstriction using nebulised salbutamol or ipratropium bromide. Mechanical ventilation as indicated.
- Treatment of seizures using IV benzodiazepines.
- Antidotes:

  o Muscarinic effects: IV atropine.

    o Test dose 1mg atropine in adults.
    o 2–4mg every 15 minutes until full atropinisation (control of excessive bronchial and oral secretions).
    o Maintenance continuous infusion 0.05mg/kg/hr.
    o Observe the patient for atropine toxicity (similar signs to OPP CNS effects).
    o As condition improves, reduce atropine gradually over 24 hours.

  o Nicotinic effects: cholinesterase reactivator, e.g. obidoxime.

    o Effects may be limited if given >24 hours after exposure.
    o Contra-indications: carbamate poisoning.
    o Dose: 250mg (3–5mg/kg) IV or IM every five minutes after the first atropine dose. If appropriate response, additional one to two doses can be given every two hours.

Opioid poisoning

Opioid poisoning causes respiratory depression, which can rapidly lead to hypoxia, respiratory arrest and if left untreated death. Acute signs of opioid poisoning include respiratory depression (respiratory rate <8/min or apnoeic), pinpoint pupils and reduced level of consciousness. Specific treatment includes the following:

- Administer high-flow oxygen. Ventilate using a self-inflating bag and mask (Ambu bag) if breathing inadequate or apnoeic.
- Antidote: naloxone (Narcan)
    - Naloxone can be given intravenously (IV), intramuscularly (IM), subcutaneously (SC), intranasally (IN).
    - Initial adult doses are 400mcg (IV), 800mcg (IM, SC) or 2mg IN.
    - Additional boluses should be titrated to effect. Large opioid overdoses can require doses of 6–10mg.
    - Naloxone is short-acting 45–70 minutes, but respiratory depression can occur 4–5 hours after overdose. Therefore, patients should be monitored and observed in critical care.
    - Acute withdrawal from opioids can cause pulmonary oedema, ventricular arrhythmias and severe agitation. If the cause of the overdose was iatrogenic, the patient will be in immediate pain as all the analgesic effects will have been removed. In opioid dependence, the patient will be in acute withdrawal. Specialist input will be required.

Cocaine toxicity

Cocaine abuse and dependence is a global epidemic (Shanti & Lucas, 2003). Cocaine overdose may be complicated by alcohol and other emergency situations, for example being involved in accidents and trauma situations. Cocaine toxicity results in a multi-system response which can result in organ failure. Common symptoms and signs includes sympathetic overstimulation including agitation, tachycardia, hypertensive crisis, hyperthermia and myocardial ischaemia and angina (Nolan et al., 2011). Specific treatment include:

- small doses of IV benzodiazepines (midazolam, diazepam, lorazepam);
- glycerine trinitrate and phentolamine, which can reverse cocaine-induced coronary vasoconstriction.

Benzodiazepines

Benzodiazepine overdose includes respiratory depression, hypotension and unconsciousness. Specific treatment includes administration of the antidote flumazenil. Flumazenil should be used when there is no risk or history of seizures. Rapid reversal can cause toxicity (seizures, arrhythmias, hypotension and withdrawal syndrome in patients with dependence).

Tricyclic antidepressants

Drugs include: amitriptyline, despiramine, imipramine, nortriptyline, doxepin and clomipramine. For the first six hours following ingestion the patient is at most risk. Signs of overdose include:

- hypotension;
- life-threatening arrhythmias – widening QRS complex, heart block, lengthening PR interval;
- seizures;
- unconsciousness;
- anticholinergic effects (mydriasis, fever, dry skin, delirium, tachycardia, ileus, urinary retention).

Specific treatment includes the following:

- Cardiac monitoring and 12 lead ECG.
- Optimisation of electrolytes (potassium, sodium).
- Sodium bicarbonate for tricyclic induced ventricular conduction abnormalities. Aim for blood pH to be between 7.45 and 7.55.
- Treat seizures with IV benzodiazepines, followed by phenobarbitone or Propofol. Avoid phenytoin as it may worsen cardiac arrhythmias (Olson & van Hoving, 2016b).

Paracetamol

Paracetamol overdose depletes glutathione stores resulting in a build-up of hydroxy-lamine metabolites which damages the liver and kidneys. Management includes gastric lavage and activated charcoal within the first four hours of ingestion. If paraceta-mol levels at four hours remain elevated or >10g has been ingested, N-acetylcysteine (NAC) should be administered to increase glutathione levels. NAC is most effective within 12 hours of ingestion. Patients must be monitored as hepatic damage can be evident after 24 hours, peak at 3–4 days and recovery phase lasts approximately 8 days (Leach, 2004).

References

Jayakrishnan B. Al Asmi A. Al Qassabi A. Nandhagopal R. Mohammed I. (2012). Acute drug overdose: clinical profile, etiologic spectrum and determinants of duration of intensive medical treatment. Oman Medical Journal. 27. 6. 501–504. Doi: 10.5001/omj.2012.120.

Katz KD. Brooks DE. Tarabar A. Kirkland L. (2016). Organophosphate toxicity clinical presentation. Available at: https://emedicine.medscape.com/article/167726-clinical.

Leach R. (2004). Acute and critical care at a glance. 2nd Edition. Chichester, West Sussex: Wiley-Blackwell.

Nolan J. Soar J. Lockley A et al. (2011). Advanced life support. 6th Edition. London: Resuscitation Council (UK).

Olson KR. Van Hoving DJ. (2016a). Chapter 275: Organophosphate poisoning. In: Wallis LA. Reynolds TA (eds). African Federation of Emergency Medicine: handbook of acute and emergency care. Oxford: Oxford University Press.

Olson KR. Van Hoving DJ. (2016b). Chapter 254: Toxic effects of antidepressants. In: Wallis LA. Reynolds TA (eds). African Federation of Emergency Medicine: handbook of acute and emergency care. Oxford: Oxford University Press.

Shanti CM. Lucas CE. (2003). Cocaine and the critical care challenge. Critical Care Medicine. 31. 6. 1851–1859.

Soltaninejad K. Shadnia S. (2014). Chapter 2: History of the use and epidemiology of organophosphorus poisoning. In: Balali-Mood M. Abdollahi M (eds). Basic and clinical toxicology of organophosphorus compounds. London: Springer-Verlag. DOI: 10.1007/978-1-4471-5625-3_2.

Wood, DM Wyncool DL. (2014). Chapter 88: Management of acute poisoning. In: Bersten AD. Soni N (eds). OH's Intensive Care Manual, 7th Edition. Oxford: Elsevier.

31 Diabetes mellitus

Today, diabetes and its associated conditions is a global concern, with a significant increase in the prevalence of diabetes. This has become a concern for LICs, as healthcare systems adapt and respond to this new chronic disease (WHO, 2017; Gill et al., 2014). An estimated 10% of healthcare budgets in African countries is spent on diabetes care; this demonstrates the impact of this disease and the resources required (Beran et al., 2015).

Diabetes mellitus is a chronic, metabolic disease characterised by deranged blood glucose levels, characterised by hyperglycaemia, resulting from defects in insulin secretion, insulin action or both (Gill & Mbanya, 2013). Chronic complications of diabetes include retinopathy, nephropathy, coronary artery disease, peripheral vascular disease and cerebrovascular disease. Diabetes mellitus is classified as either type I or type II. Type I diabetes occurs when the pancreas fails to produce insulin, whereas type II diabetes occurs when the pancreas does not produce enough insulin or the body's cells do not respond to the insulin. Type II diabetes is common in low-income settings due to urbanisation, changes in dietary quality, overweight and obesity, reduced physical activity and use of anti-retroviral drugs (Gill & Mbanya, 2013). Additional challenges in the provision of diabetic services may include low or intermittent supplies of insulin in rural areas. This may lead to diabetic patients under dosing to make supplies last longer, which leads to poor control, weight loss and increased chances of complications (Gill & Mbanya, 2013).

Acute complications which may require critical care admission include hypoglycaemia, diabetic keto-acidosis and hyperosmolar hyperglycaemic states (HHS). However, the impact of diabetes on patients requiring surgical care, or developing gestational diabetes or having malnutrition-related diabetes mellitus may also require critical care input or be at increased risk of deterioration.

Blood glucose testing

In critical care blood glucose testing can be measured by either a drop of capillary blood and placing this on a test strip which is read by blood glucose meter or from an arterial blood gas. Results can be measured in either mmol/l or mg/dl.

To correctly monitor a capillary blood glucose level you will require the following equipment:

- blood glucose meter;
- test strips;
- control solution;
- single-use safety lancets;
- gloves;
- Cotton wool/gauze;
- sharps box.

(Rutledge & Nesbitt, 2016)

To measure a blood glucose:

- Check the equipment. Test strips are in date, monitor and test strips have been calibrated and internal quality control measures have been carried out and documented in accordance with hospital and manufacturers' guidelines.
- Explain the procedure to the patient.
- Wash hands and put on personal protective equipment.
- Take a single-use lancet device. The most common site for taking blood is from a fingertip. Repeated use of the same site can lead to damage to the nerve ending and the site becoming less sensitive. When taking blood, the outer aspect of the finger is deemed less painful. The thumb and forefinger should be avoided, and sites must be rotated to prevent infection, reducing pain and the skin becoming toughened.
- The finger may require 'milking' from palm of the hand towards the finger to gain a sufficient amount of blood for the test.
- Insert the test strip into the glucose meter and apply the blood to the test strip. Check the type of test strips as some require the blood to be applied from the side (hydrophilic) instead of being dropped onto the strip.
- Dispose of the lancet immediately.
- Place gauze or cotton wool over puncture site. Observe for signs of continued bleeding.
- Document the result and act on your findings.

(Rutledge & Nesbitt, 2016; Dougherty & Lister, 2011)

Hypoglycaemia

Hypoglycaemia is a common metabolic complication and is a common cause of unconsciousness in hospitalised patients (Odell, 2013). The symptoms and blood glucose level at which complications occur is variable (Becker & Kabeza, 2016). Blood glucose level are considered low when <4mmol/l (70mg/dl) in adults or <3.5mmol/l in children (Becker & Kabeza, 2016).

The management of hypoglycaemia includes the following:

- Assess the patient using the A–E approach. A semi-conscious or unconscious patient is at risk of airway obstruction and should be managed in the three-quarters prone or recovery position.

- Check blood glucose levels.
- If the patient can eat, give them food/drink.
- IV dextrose:

  o Infants/children 5ml/kg 10% dextrose. Then commence dextrose containing maintenance fluids.
  o Adults 25–50ml 50% dextrose or 125–250ml 10% dextrose. Then commence 5–10% dextrose maintenance.

- If IV access is difficult, consider IO, IM Glucagon 1mg, naso-gastric or rectal glucose.
- If no IV access give 10% sucrose solution (1 rounded teaspoon of sugar in 3.5 tablespoons of water) orally.
- If patient has persistent hypoglycaemia, give continuous IV dextrose infusions (5% to 10%). In children, the fluid must have added electrolytes.
- On recovery, give a long-lasting carbohydrate snack.
- Attempt to identify the cause of hypoglycaemia and correct it.
- If hypoglycaemia is due to sulphonylureas, put up a slow IV dextrose infusion (5–10%) for 12–24 hours.

(Gill & Mbanya, 2013; Becker & Kabeza, 2016)

Diabetic keto-acidosis

Diabetic keto-acidosis (DKA) is an acute complication of diabetes hyperglycaemia. It is often the presenting feature of type I diabetes and most cases occur in established patients. Presentation includes ketones in urine, acidosis and severe dehydration. In all presentations, a source of infection (pneumonia, urinary tract, skin, malaria, etc.), should be investigated. Challenges when dealing with DKA include:

- late presentation;
- low and irregular food supply;
- lack of insulin and oral agents;
- absence of dieticians and podiatrists;
- lack of monitoring equipment;
- limited laboratory support.

Effective management requires laboratory support (including arterial blood gas monitoring, electrolytes, renal function and glucose monitoring). The situation and resources will determine interventions; all patients should have the following:

- Admit to critical care.
- Assess using the A–E approach and manage accordingly. This includes invasive monitoring (central line and arterial line if available).
- Arterial blood gas monitoring to monitor acidosis and potassium.
- Dipstick urine for ketones.
- Take bloods for urea and electrolytes (U&E).

- Urinary catheter and fluid balance monitoring.
- One-hourly blood glucose monitoring.
- Look for source of infection (perform Malaria RDT if appropriate).
- Consider naso-gastric tube for administration of nutrition and drugs.

DKA management with all resources available:

- Aggressive fluid resuscitation. Give 500ml 0.9% saline quickly, then 500ml hourly for four to six hours.
- Insulin. Soluble insulin 50 units in 50ml normal saline IV (1ml = 1unit). Start dose at four to six units/hr.
- Potassium. If initial potassium level normal, start potassium chloride (KCL) added to saline at 10–30mmol/hr. Titrate according to electrolyte results.
- Bicarbonate should only be used if the patient is critically ill. Give 50 mmol dilute (do not use 8.4%) NaCHO3 by IV slowly.
- Monitoring to include:
  - initial blood gases, blood glucose levels and U&E;
  - hourly blood glucose monitoring;
  - laboratory blood glucose monitoring and U&E two-hourly.
- When blood glucose <15mmol and patient has improved stop IV insulin and saline. Convert to glucose, potassium infusion 100ml/hr, alternating insulin and KCL content according to laboratory results. When patient is conscious and able to eat, convert to subcutaneous insulin.

In a resource-limited environment, DKA can be managed as follows:

- Fluids. 500ml 0.9% saline quickly, then 500ml hourly for four to six hours. If not available use Hartmann's (Ringer's infusion) or Darrow's solution. In primary healthcare clinics awaiting transfer to hospital give subcutaneous or rectal fluids at a slower rate.
- Insulin. Soluble 20 units IM stat and 10 units IM hourly. If no soluble insulin, use lente or isophane 20 units IM stat and 15 units IM hourly.
- Potassium. None for first hour, then 20mmol/hr for three hours and 10mmol/hr for two hours.
- Bicarbonate. Bicarbonate is only administered in patients who are critically ill and not improving. The dose is 50mmol NaCHO3 (not 8.4%) given slowly IV. Repeat if necessary only once.
- Monitoring. Hourly blood glucose monitoring and four-hourly urine ketones.
- When blood glucose <15mmol/l convert to IV fluids 5% glucose 500ml two-hourly for four to six hours. Then 500ml for four hours. Continue with IM insulin. When patient can eat, change to subcutaneous insulin.
- Arrange for urgent transfer to hospital/critical care unit.

(Becker & Kabeza, 2016;
Gill & Mbanya, 2013; Gill et al., 2014)

Hyperosmolar hyperglycaemic states (HHS)

Hyperosmolar hyperglycaemic state (HHS) requires accurate laboratory support to measure initial urea, electrolyte and glucose. This allows for the serum osmolarity to be calculated (Gill & Mbanya, 2013):

Osmolarity = (2 (Sodium + Potassium) + Urea + Glucose (all levels in mmol/L)

Patients with HHS tend to be elderly and severely dehydrated. Severe dehydration maybe caused by infection or recent diuretic therapy. HHS has a high mortality and thrombolytic complications due to dehydration is common. In consequence, heparin treatment is usually included in treatment protocols. Other management includes the following:

- Larger volumes of fluids are required; however, because of advanced age, rate of fluid resuscitation tends to be slower.
- 0.9% saline is used, unless the patient is hypernatraemic (Na >150mmol/l), half-normal (0.45%) saline should be considered until plasma Na <150mmol/l.
- Potassium replacement is less aggressive.
- Bicarbonate is never given.
- Insulin requirements are often lower.

(Gill & Mbanya, 2013)

Malnutrition-related diabetes mellitus

Malnutrition-related diabetes mellitus (MRDM) is a sub-type of diabetes, which is also termed 'tropical diabetes' or 'tropical pancreatic diabetes'. Patients tend to be young males who have either had or present with malnutrition. It is believed malnutrition leads to pancreatic damage, which may be evident with pancreatic radiological calcification, abdominal pain and steatorrhoea. Patients often require insulin and may be insulin resistant but are not insulin dependent or ketosis prone (Gill & Mbanya, 2013).

Gestational diabetes

Gestational diabetes mellitus (GDM) is a new diagnosis of diabetes during pregnancy and post-partum the mother returns to normal glucose tolerance, although there is an increased risk of type II diabetes later in life. Risk factors include obesity, past medical history of GDM, family history of diabetes and a history of large babies (>4kg) (Gill & Mbanya, 2013). Dangers of GDM include:

- foetal macrosomia;
- eclampsia;
- foetal growth retardation;

- birth difficulties;
- neonatal hypoglycaemia;
- neonatal respiratory distress.

Management of GDM includes the following:

- Tight glycaemic control to reduce maternal and foetal complications.
- Type I diabetics may need to increase the frequency of insulin.
- Type II diabetes may need to convert to insulin.
- Close neonatal care, with preparation for a caesarean section (at 36–38 weeks).

(Gill & Mbanya, 2013)

Diabetes and surgical care

Poorly controlled diabetes is associated with poor surgical outcomes. Surgery causes an increase in an individual's stress response leading to increased blood glucose levels up to six to eight times higher than normal (Dunning, 2014). This leads to osmotic diuresis, increased hepatic glucose output, lipolysis and insulin resistance. Unless controlled this increases the risk of a diabetic patient developing diabetic keto-acidosis (DKA), hyperosmolar hyperglycaemic states (HHS), lactic acidosis and infection (Dunning, 2014). Certain types of surgery can increase the risk of diabetic complications, for example cardiac bypass surgery is associated with a greater risk of HHS. In addition, anaesthesia causes a release in counter-regulatory hormones and glucagon leading to insulin resistance, glycogenesis, hyperglycaemia and neutrophil dysfunction which inhibits wound healing. The stress response leads to gastro-intestinal instability resulting in nausea and vomiting resulting in increased risk of dehydration which will exacerbate fluid loss (Dunning, 2014).

Nursing care will be determined by the type of procedure and if it is an urgent, emergency or elective procedure. Key points include the following:

- Urinalysis and electrolytes recorded pre-operatively and available as part of the pre-anaesthetic assessment.
- Prioritise the patient for first on the surgical list, to prevent prolonged fasting and potential counter-regulatory hormone release that leads to hyperglycaemia.
- When fasting record check blood glucose levels two-hourly then one hour prior to surgery. If hyperglycaemic, consider glucose/insulin/potassium regimen. Aim to prevent hyperglycaemia as this reduces the risk of adverse outcome in diabetic patients, often with the use of a sliding scale insulin regimen pre-, intra- and post-operatively.
- Avoid hypoglycaemia as this inhibits white cell function and increases the risk of bleeding, resulting in complications such as sepsis, acidosis, hypotension and hypovolaemia. All patients should be monitored for signs of hypovolaemia and dehydration; additional IV fluids may be required.
- A persistent hyperglycaemia may be an indication of underlying infection, surgical or metabolic complication and severe pain (Dunning, 2014).

- Obtain specialist diabetic input to guide care.
- Observe for AKI, particularly if using radiologic contrast.
- Administration of IV potassium supplements requires cardiac monitoring.
- Diabetic patients' pressure areas must be monitored regularly due to the increased risk of neuropathic feet and pressure area damage.

(Berhe *et al.*, 2017; Dunning, 2014)

Insulin administration

In hospitals insulin errors are common (James & Diggle, 2016). Errors can occur during the prescribing and administration due to:

- dosage errors;
- illegibility of prescriptions;
- incomplete prescriptions;
- Errors in dosing intervals, e.g. during international transfers and time differences;
- incorrect insulin formations being used;
- lack of understanding between the link with the mealtime and insulin administration relationship;
- failure to change prescriptions when patient's dietary requirements change, e.g. NBM, parental feeds;
- drug interactions;
- transcription errors;
- the term 'u' being written for units and mistaken for an extra '0';
- insufficient pumps to administer insulin infusions;
- poorly stored insulin, e.g. lack of refrigerators, not temperature regulated/checked.

(Grant, 2011)

To mitigate the risk of insulin errors include the following:

- Obtain accurate medical history including name, strength, dose and timing of each insulin dose. Depending on the situation encourage patients or their families to bring insulin vials for correct identification and dose validation.
- Avoid using abbreviations such as 'u' to indicate the number of units.
- Avoid verbal orders unless a medical emergency. Care should be taken to write the verbal order down and have it confirmed with another registered practitioner.
- Correctly store insulin, particularly if there is a risk of packaging being mistaken for other medications.
- Use an independent double checker to check all insulin doses.
- Education of staff relating to best practice and risks.
- Monitor patients' response and condition, e.g. acutely ill patients may not have had the opportunity to eat a regular meal or take their insulin as they normally would, potentially leading to complications.

(Paparella, 2006)

Table 31.1 Example glucose insulin potassium regime when no insulin pump available

Start intravenous infusion of 5% or 10% dextrose (500ml bag) over five hours and add insulin and potassium chloride (KCL) to each 500ml bag as below.

Change bag according to blood sugar level. Flow rate 100ml/hr.

Blood glucose level		Insulin (units/bag)	Serum potassium (mmol/L)	KCL (mmol/bag)
mg/dl	*mmol/L*			
<72	3.9	No	<3	20
72–108	4–5.9	5	3–5	10
109–180	6–9.9	10	>5	No
181–360	10–19.9	15		
>360	>20	20		

Source: Berhe *et al.*, 2017

Variable rate insulin infusion

Critically ill diabetic patients often require continuous infusions of insulin. The term 'sliding scale insulin' has been replaced with the term 'variable rate insulin infusion' (VRII) (Rickard *et al.*, 2016). All VRII should be administered via a syringe pump; however, in a resource limited environment specialist pumps may not be available. Rickard *et al.* (2016) conducted a study exploring the variations in intravenous fluid and electrolyte management during VRII. The study reported there were wide variations in fluid prescription and often lacked potassium supplementation; this could lead to hypokalaemia and other potential complications. Berhe *et al.* (2017) outline the glucose, insulin, potassium regime when an infusion pump is not available (Table 31.1).

References

Becker JU. Kabeza AB. (2016). Chapter 157: Diabetic ketoacidosis. In: Wallis LA. Reynolds TA (eds). African Federation of Emergency Medicine: Handbook of Acute and Emergency Care. Oxford: Oxford University Press.

Beran D. Yudkin TS. De Carter M. (2015). Access to care for patients with insulin requiring diabetes in developing countries. Care Studies of Mozambique and Zambia. Diabetes Care. 28. 2136–2140.

Berhe YW. Gebregzi AH. Endalew NS. (2017). Guideline on peri-operative glycaemic control for adult patient with diabetic mellitus: resource limited areas. International Journal of Surgery Open. 9. 1–6.

Dougherty L. Lister S (eds). (2011). The Royal Marsden Hospital Manual of Clinical Nursing Procedures. 8th Edition. Oxford and Ames, IA: Wiley Blackwell.

Dunning T. (2014). Care of people with diabetes: A manual of nursing practice. 4th Edition. Chichester, West Sussex: John Wiley & Sons Ltd.

Gill G. Mbanya JC. (2013). Chapter 58: Diabetes Mellitus. In: Mabey D. Gill G. Parry E. Weber MW. Whitty CJM (eds). (2013). Principles of medicine in Africa. 4th Edition. Cambridge: Cambridge University Press.

Gill G. Wilkinson M. Mortimer K. (2014). Chapter 59: Non-communicable diseases. In: Beeching N. Gill G (eds). Tropical medicine: lecture notes. 7th Edition. Chichester, West Sussex: Wiley Blackwell.

Grant P. (2011). A multi-system approach to reducing insulin errors. Clinical Risk. 17. 180–187.

James J. Diggle J. (2016). Insulin error: is there a new kid on the block? Journal of Diabetes Nursing. 20. 6. 200–201.

Odell M. (2013). Chapter 3: Recognizing and managing the critically ill and 'at risk' patient on a ward. In: Mallett J. Albarran JW. Richardson A (eds). Critical care manual of clinical procedures and competencies. Chichester, West Sussex: Wiley Blackwell.

Paparella S. (2006). Avoiding errors with insulin therapy. Journal of Emergency Nursing. 32. 4. 325–327.

Rickard LJ. Cubas V. Ward ST *et al*. (2016). Slipping up on the sliding scale: fluid and electrolyte management in variable rate intravenous insulin infusions. Practical Diabetes. 35. 5. 159–165.

Rutledge K. Nesbitt I. (2016). Chapter 8: Assessment and support of hydration and nutrition status and care. In: Mallett J. Albarran JW. Richardson A (eds). Critical care manual of clinical procedures and competencies. Chichester, West Sussex: Wiley Blackwell.

World Health Organization. (2017). Diabetes programme. Available at: www.who.int/diabetes/en/.

32 Hypertension and acute stroke

Hypertension is a global concern, contributing to the burden of heart disease, stroke and kidney failure and premature death and disability. In this chapter, the practical management of hypertension which may be undiagnosed or inadequately controlled leading to stroke is outlined. Hypertension is a significant concern for low- to low-middle income countries, in addition to poorly diagnosed or inadequately controlled hypertension; by 2020 an estimated 1.15 billion hypertensive patients in low-income settings will require healthcare (Gill *et al.*, 2014; Mittal & Singh, 2010). Causes of hypertension may be due to:

- malignant hypertension due to neurological and/or cardiovascular decompensation;
- pregnancy;
- elderliness;
- diabetes;
- renal disease.

(Walker & Edwards, 2013)

The cause of the hypertension will determine the treatment, for example hypertension due to pregnancy will be managed differently to sub-arachnoid haemorrhage with decompensation. The long-term effects of uncontrolled hypertension may result in admission to critical care due to:

- stroke;
- left ventricular hypertrophy;
- renal failure;
- coronary artery disease;
- hypertensive retinopathy;

Issues surrounding under-diagnosis and poor management may result in hypertensive patients only being identified during crises or acute conditions.

Management of acute stroke

Stroke can be caused by either ischaemia or intracranial haemorrhage (Table 32.1). Diagnosis requires neuroimaging to determine the cause and treatment options (Table 32.2). Within low-income settings, access to computed tomography (CT) scanning can be limited and the associated transfer to the scanner is also an increased risk for deterioration. The availability of CT scanners within low-income settings has been estimated as 0.32 per 1 million people (Berkowitz, 2016). CT scans provide information on the size and location of stroke; presence of bleeding; possible degree of reversibility; cerebral haemodynamic status; status of intracranial and extracranial vasculature (Figueroa *et al.*, 2015).

Table 32.1 Types of stroke, potential causes and associated risk factors

Type	Causes	Risk factors
Ischaemia	Thrombosis or embolic	Hypertension Diabetes Hypercholesterolaemia renal disease Smoking Hypercoagulable status Heart disease Atrial fibrillation HIV infection and therapy may be associated with increased risk of stroke
Intracranial haemorrhage	Intracerebral or subarachnoid bleed	Hypertension Bleeding disorders CNS infection Stroke syndromes (underlying lesions, tumours, toxoplasmosis, brain abscess and other space-occupying lesions)

Table 32.2 Treatment for ischemic and haemorrhagic stroke

Type	Key treatments
Ischemic stroke	Aspirin Anticoagulants Thrombolysis Decompressive hemicraniectomy
Cerebral haemorrhage	Reduction in blood pressure as tolerated Reversal of anticoagulants if the cause of the stroke; this is based on each individual cases and benefit v. harm. Neurosurgical intervention to remove haematoma

Co-ordinated care starts from the point of injury, continues through the emergency department until rehabilitation. In consequence, critical care interventions should be provided when and where they are needed, and should not be delayed until a critical care bed becomes available.

Critical care considerations involve timely restoration of cerebral perfusion, limiting the secondary effects of neural injury and preventing/treating neurological and non-neurological complications. Other critical care interventions include:

Airway

- Intubation may be required if the patient's Glasgow Coma Score <8, to prevent aspiration and loss of airway patency.

Breathing

- Supplementary oxygen should be given to keep oxygen saturation s>95%.
- Hypoxia may be caused by partial airway obstruction, hypoventilation, aspiration and atelectasis.
- Mechanical ventilation may be required to treat hypoxia and respiratory failure.

Circulation

- Cardiac assessment – observing for cardiovascular or haemodynamic compromise, e.g. atrial fibrillation (AF), murmurs, absent pulses, carotid bruit.
- Additional complications with left ventricular hypertrophy and hypertensive heart failure may complicate weaning from mechanical ventilation or fluid resuscitation.
- Ischaemic stroke:

  - Determine the potential causes: cerebral embolism, herpes zoster, infective endocarditis.
  - Maintain cerebral perfusion.
  - Hypertension should not be treated unless a candidate for thrombolysis, malignant hypertension or other medical reason, e.g. aortic dissection.
  - Thrombolytic therapy is used to restore blood flow. Removal of the occlusive thrombus may be through pharmacological intravenous thrombolysis or mechanical methods.

- Haemorrhagic stroke:

  - Discontinue anticoagulants and anti-platelet therapy.
  - Consider reversing anticoagulants.
  - BP management using labetalol, nicardipine, esmolol, enalapril, hydralazine, nitroprusside, nitro-glycerine and monitoring.

- Hyperthermia and hypothermia should be actively treated and prevented. Hyperthermia enhances oxygen free radical production, exacerbates the blood-brain barrier breakdown and exacerbates cytoskeletal proteolysis.
- Potential complications include dehydration. Monitor fluid intake and ensure adequate fluids are provided (oral, naso-gastric or intravenously).
- Chronic renal disease may be further exacerbated by period of hypotension resulting in poor renal perfusion.

Neurological

- Glasgow Coma Scale monitoring and pupil assessment should be performed a minimum of every hour unless indicated. Specific problems may include:

    o motor deficit: paresis or paralysis;
    o sensory deficit: decreased sensation;
    o aphasia;
    o ataxia;
    o visual loss;
    o dysphagia;
    o unawareness of weakened side.

- Treatment of seizures.
- Monitoring of blood glucose levels. Both hypo- and hyperglycaemia have negative effects. Hyperglycaemia damages brain tissue through free radical production, injury to the blood-brain barrier and causes a lactic acidosis, whereas hypoglycaemia has a negative effect and impacts of ischaemic brain and infarct growth.
- Observe for signs of pain and look for a treatable cause.

Other considerations

- Swallow assessment and the provision of adequate hydration and nutrition. Patients may require a naso-gastric tube and enteral feeding.
- Prevention of deep vein thrombosis (DVT) by using DVT prophylaxis and early mobilisation.
- Prevention of complications of bed-rest.

    o Constipation or faecal incontinence:

        o Monitor bowel movements.
        o Maintain fibre and fluid intake.

- Prevention of contractures by passive limb movements and involvement of physiotherapists.
- Prevention of pressure sores by regular position changes.
- Careful repositioning to prevent injuries and 'painful shoulder':

- o   Use pillows to support flaccid arm.
- o   Ensure limbs do not become trapped in bedrails etc. during turns.
- o   Do not pull on arms when repositioning.

- During the rehabilitation stage:

- o   Observe for depression/emotional issues. Involve the patient in decisions and their care. Consider psychological support and medication for depression.
- o   Avoid indwelling catheters if possible; use incontinence pads or intermittent catheterisation.
- o   Early mobilisation.
- o   Input from specialist physiotherapist and neurological teams.

(Chandra *et al.*, 2016; Berkowitz, 2016; Figueroa *et al.*, 2015; Gill *et al.*, 2014; Walker & Edwards, 2013; Connor & Bryer, 2013)

Management of hypertension following acute ischaemic stroke

Following acute ischaemic stroke patients may be hypertensive. The cause may be due to stress response, chronic hypertension, increased intra-cranial pressure or activation of neuroendocrine system. Blood pressure tends to normalise over 24–48 hours. Severe hypertension may cause cerebral oedema, intracerebral haemorrhage and breakdown of the blood-brain barrier. Intervening and reducing the patient's blood pressure may be detrimental as the increasing blood pressure is necessary for maintaining cerebral perfusion. Unless patients have received thrombolytic therapy whereby control of hypertension to maintain a blood pressure <180/105mmHg in the first 24 hours is indicated. In other situations, the evidence is unclear for reducing blood pressure immediately. Most guidelines suggest not using anti-hypertensives, unless the systolic blood pressure >220 mmHg and diastolic blood pressure is >120 mmHg, or if the patient is at risk for acute heart failure or aortic dissection (Figueroa *et al.*, 2015).

Management of hypertension following acute intracranial haemorrhage

Following acute intracranial haemorrhage, the lowering of systolic blood pressure (SBP) is recommended. The target SBP is unclear; however, below 140mmHg appears safe. Following ischaemic stroke, BP can be allowed to autoregulate unless thrombolytic therapy is administered. With limited access to CT scanning, determining the cause of the acute stroke is difficult, therefore it is appropriate to consider lowering SBP to below 180mmHg for all patients with unknown aetiology. It is rare for patients with unknown aetiology for their condition to worsen when BP is lowered. The patient should be monitored and if any adverse effects are noted, BP can be increased with a bolus of IV crystalloid and then allowed to autoregulate (Berkowitz, 2016).

The use of aspirin in acute intracerebral haemorrhage is associated with increased risk of death. With no CT scans, healthcare workers may not administer aspirin to patients with unknown aetiology. It has been suggested initiating aspirin 24–48 hours post-acute stroke of unknown aetiology could minimise the risk of acute intracerebral haemorrhage while maximising the benefit for those with acute ischaemic stroke (Berkowitz, 2016).

References

Berkowitz AL. (2016). Perspectives: managing acute stroke in low-resource settings. Available at: www.who.int/bulletin/volumes/94/7/15-162610/en/.

Chandra A. Kestler A. Richards. D. (2016). Chapter 178: Acute stroke. In: Wallis LA. Reynolds TA (eds). African Federation of Emergency Medicine: handbook of acute and emergency care. Oxford: Oxford University Press.

Connor M. Bryer A. (2013). Chapter 60: Stroke. In: Mabey D. Gill G. Parry E. Weber MW. Whitty CJM (eds). Principles of medicine in Africa. 4th Edition. Cambridge: Cambridge University Press.

Figueroa SA. Zhao W. Aiyagari V. (2015). Emergency and critical care management of acute ischaemic stroke. CNS Drugs. 29. 17–28.

Gill G. Wilkinson M. Mortimer K. (2014). Chapter 59: Non-communicable diseases. In: Beeching N. Gill G. (eds). Tropical medicine: lecture notes. 7th Edition. Chichester, West Sussex: Wiley Blackwell.

Mittal BV. Singh AK. (2010). Hypertension in the developing world: challenges and opportunities. American Journal of Kidney Diseases. 55. 3. 590–598.

Walker RW. Edwards R. (2013). Chapter 59: Hypertension. In: Mabey D. Gill G. Parry E. Weber MW. Whitty CJM (eds). Principles of medicine in Africa. 4th Edition. Cambridge: Cambridge University Press.

33 | Snake and scorpion bites

Snake bites

There are many venomous snakes throughout the world. With an estimated 5.4 million people bitten each year and approximately 2.7 million envenomations (WHO, 2017). Around 95% of cases snake envenomation takes place in LICs or LMICs and involve the poorest and those who live in rural communities. With most bites affecting farm workers, women and children in rural communities, this makes it difficult to access healthcare services (Buckle & Hirshon, 2016a). For African and Asian countries envenomation is a considerable public health concern (Chippaux, 1998). Epidemiological data in countries with venomous snakes is variable making it difficult to establish the true extent of the problem. From the evidence available the incidence of snake bite envenomation is a global issue and has been re-classified as a Neglected Tropical Disease by the WHO (Chippaux, 2017). From approximately 81,000 to 138,000 people die annually; however, the number of people who are permanently disabled or have an amputation due to complications is significantly higher (WHO, 2017).

Many snake bites are not followed by severe envenomation; however, envenomation can be delayed and all patients who have been bitten should be assessed and monitored (Bellefleur & Chippaux, 2014). When envenomation occurs, challenges include the following:

- Delays in accessing care as often patients initially use traditional healers and remedies first. This results in a delay in receiving anti-venom and increased complications and costs (Chippaux, 2017).
- Quality and access to vaccines is variable. Shortages with anti-venom have been attributed to not bringing sustainable profits; in consequence, drug companies have difficulty in producing and developing new vaccines (Chippaux, 2017).
- Healthcare workers may have limited training in dealing with snake bites resulting in delays in care (Chippaux, 2017).

The WHO has developed specific resources for the prevention and clinical management of snake bites in Africa and South East Asia (WHO, 2010; Warrell, 2010). The following provides an overview of types of venomous snakes, initial first aid, diagnostic tests available and critical care considerations.

Venomous snakes can be divided into the following categories (Lalloo, 2014; Buckle & Hirshon, 2016a):

- vipers (long, hinged fangs, triangular shaped heads. Mainly nocturnal);
- elapids (smooth scales, round pupils, short, fixed fangs);
- Colubridae (rear fanged);
- sea snakes.

Twelve types of snakes are responsible for the majority of deaths worldwide. The types of venomous snakes present depends on the geographical location.

- Africa, Middle East and South Asia.

  - Saw-scaled or carpet vipers of the genus Echis (Picture 33.1).
  - Cobras of the genus Naja (Pictures 33.2 and 33.3).

- Africa and Arabian Peninsula.

  - Puff adders (Picture 33.4).

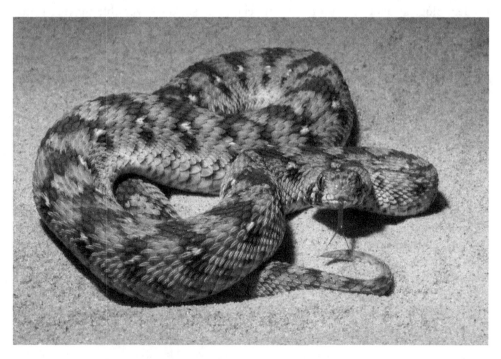

Picture 33.1 Echis ocellatus, a West African carpet viper from Niger

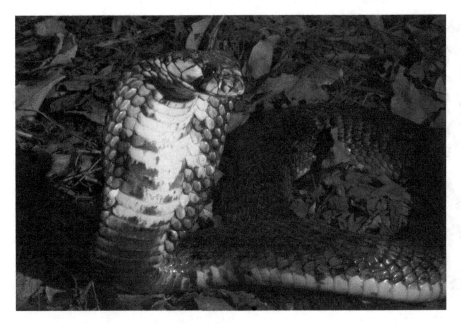

Picture 33.2 Naja haje, the Egyptian cobra

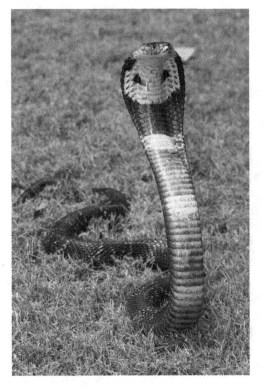

Picture 33.3 Naja kaouthia from Thailand

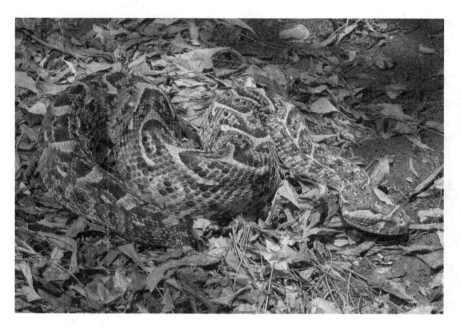

Picture 33.4 Bitis arietans

- Sub-Saharan Africa.
  - Mambas group of widely distributed venomous snakes with a neurotoxic venom (Picture 33.5).

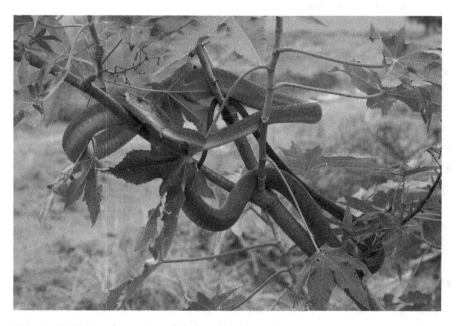

Picture 33.5 Dendroaspis polylepis (black mamba)

- Asia.

  o Russell's vipers' envenomation results in acute kidney injury often requiring haemodialysis. Two types of species: Daboia russelii in South Asia and Daboia siamensis (Siamese Russell's viper) (Picture 33.6).
  o Bungarus candidus. These snakes tend to enter houses at night, biting people who are sleeping unprotected on mats on the floor (Picture 33.7).

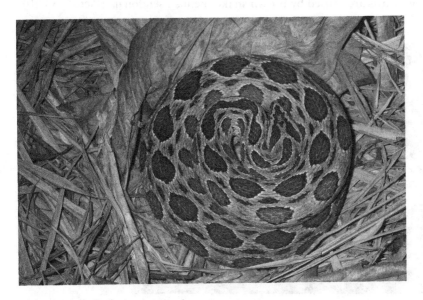

Picture 33.6 Daboia siamensis

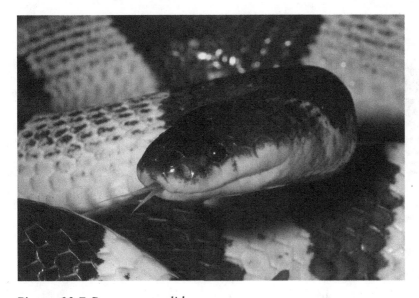

Picture 33.7 Bungarus candidus

- o Malayan pit viper Calloselasma rhodostoma. The snake remains motionless when approached and many victims are bitten after treading on it or near it. Often found in forests and plantations (Picture 33.8).

- Australasia.

  - o Papuan taipans (Oxyuranus scutellatus). Without anti-venom the case fatality rate after a bit is close to 100% (Picture 33.9).
  - o 50% of deaths are caused by brown snakes genus Pseudonaja (Picture 33.10).

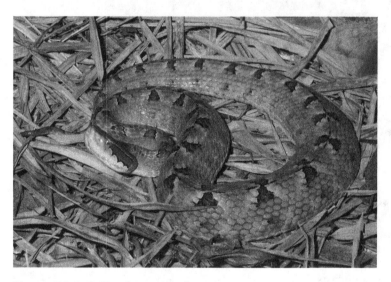

Picture 33.8 Calloselasma rhodostoma

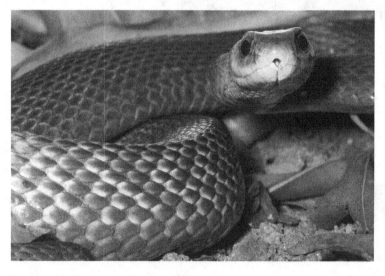

Picture 33.9 Oxyuranus scutellatus

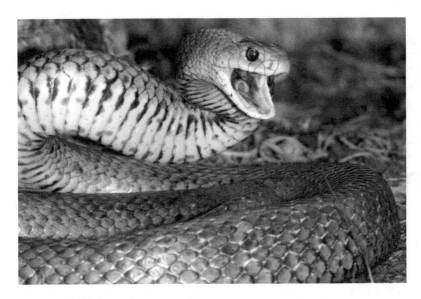

Picture 33.10 Pseudonaja textilis

- Americas.
    - o   Lancehead vipers of the genus Bothrops (Picture 33.11).
    - o   Rattlesnakes. There are many different species and bites are common (Picture 33.12).

(WHO, 2018a)

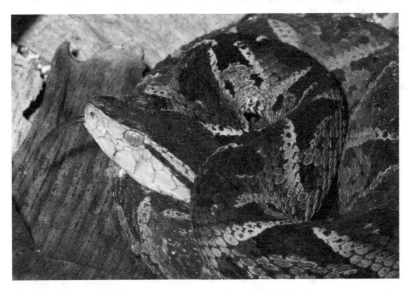

Picture 33.11 Bothrops asper from Costa Rica

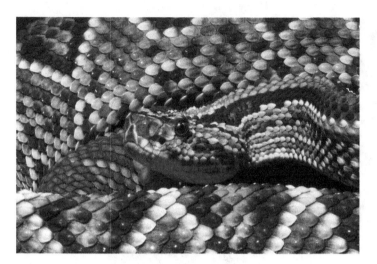

Picture 33.12 Crotalus durissus

The main clinical effects following a snake bite are either local or systemic and are outlined in Table 33.1. First aid includes the following (Lalloo, 2014; Buckle & Hirshon, 2016a):

- Reassurance.
- Immobilise the limb.
- Do not cut, do not use suction and do not use tourniquets.
- Consider a pressure bandage in regions where snake bites do not cause necrosis if there is a delay in transporting the casualty to hospital.
- Evacuate the casualty to hospital as soon as possible.
- If the snake has been killed, take it to the hospital with the casualty. Otherwise try to describe the snake and circumstances.

Critical care considerations include the following.

Table 33.1 The main clinical effects following a snake bite

Local effects	Systemic effects

• Pain
• Swelling
• Blistering
• Necrosis at the site of the wound
	• Non-specific symptoms (vomiting, headache, collapse)
	• Painful regional lymph nodes (this indicates absorption of venom)
	• Specific signs:
	  o non-clotting blood;
	  o bleeding from gums, old wounds, sores;
	  o neurotoxicity: ptosis, bulbar palsy and respiratory paralysis;
	  o rhabdomyolysis: muscle pains and black urine;
	  o shock: hypotension, usually resulting from hypovolaemia.

Source: Lalloo, 2014

Immediate actions

- Assess patient using the A–E approach to determine the severity of the envenomation. This is a medical emergency.
- Perform diagnostic testing either using a commercial diagnostic test or the 20-Minute Whole Blood Clotting (20MWBC).
- All patients should be admitted and observed for 12–24 hours.
- The patient should be closely observed, monitored and regular observations performed.
- Measure observations (pulse, blood pressure, respiratory rate and urine output). Observe for signs of shock or respiratory depression.

Diagnostic tests

Diagnostic tests may include the use of commercial diagnostic test, the 20-Minute Whole Blood Clotting test or using local algorithms and checklists which confirm the presence of important clinical signs and indicate the need for early treatment. There is currently only one commercial diagnostic test available. It works by confirming the type of venom present, by detecting the antibodies for specific types of venom produced by specific types of snakes (WHO, 2018b).

20-Minute Whole Blood Clotting *(20MWBC)*

Following envenomation spontaneous haemorrhage is an important clinical indicator for using anti-venom. Diagnosis can be supported by the use of the 20MWBC test to determine the clotting time of the patient (WHO, 2018b). One to two millilitres of blood is collected and added to clean, dry glass bottle or vial and left to stand at room temperature for 20 minutes. The bottle is then inverted and the presence or absence of a complete clot is recorded. If a blood clot forms then the test is negative, whereas if no clot forms and the blood remains liquid, the test is positive. A positive result indicates the presence of coagulopathy and the need for anti-venom. It is important that serial tests follow exactly the same procedure including uniformed glassware, sample volume and temperature to ensure consistency and accuracy (WHO, 2018b). The procedure is as follows:

Equipment required:

- PPE (gloves);
- tourniquet;
- stopwatch;
- syringe and needle;
- sharps box;
- a clean, dry glass bottle or vial.

Procedure:

- Assemble equipment and explain procedure to patient. Gain consent.
- Wash hands and apply PPE.
- Apply tourniquet and identify vein to draw blood.
- Clean site with antiseptic and allow to dry.
- Draw blood (one to two millilitres).
- Transfer blood to the clean, dry glass bottle and apply lid. Start the stopwatch.
- Dispose of syringe and needle in a sharps box immediately.
- Remove PPE and wash hands.
- Do *not* shake the bottle.
- After 20 minutes, turn the bottle upside down to see if a clot has formed.
- Dispose of glass bottle in accordance with local procedures.
- Document results.

Airway

- Observation for airway compromise and intubation in the event of loss of airway due to respiratory failure, neurotoxicity or reduced level of consciousness.
- The WHO (2018c) identified that many patients die on their way to hospital as result of being transported supine and having their airway obstructed by vomit or paralysis in the tongue. Until specialist help is available patients should be nursed on their side (recovery position), with access to suction and emergency airway equipment.
- Initiate oxygen in the evidence of respiratory distress and hypoxia.

Breathing

- Intubation and mechanical ventilation is indicated if the patient is unable to maintain their own airway and/or respiratory depression due to paralysis of diaphragm or intercostal muscles.

Circulation

- Establish continuous cardiac monitoring, to detect arrhythmias.
- Perform/repeat 20MWBC test or commercial test if available to determine coagulopathy and type of snake.
- Take bloods for:
    o haemoglobin, white cell count and platelet count;
    o prothrombin time, activated partial thromboplastic time, fibrinogen levels;
    o serum urea and creatinine;
    o Cross-match;

- Observe for non-clotting blood.
- Observe for signs of internal or external bleeding. Internal bleeding may include intracranial bleeding), external may be subtle, e.g. gums, injection sites.
- Transfusion of blood for haemorrhage.
- Transfusion of clotting factors for clotting disorders.
- Avoid intramuscular injections and invasive procedures in the coagulopathic patient.
- Fluid resuscitation as required to treat hypotension. Vasopressors may be required.
- Observation for the development of AKI. Insert urinary catheter and measure urine output hourly. Observation for signs of myoglobinuria.
- The effectiveness of systemic antibiotics remains unproven.

Disability

- Observe for signs of neurotoxicity (limb weakness, paralysis, difficulties in talking, swallowing or respiratory complications).

Exposure

- Carefully examine the limb for signs of necrosis, tracking and swelling.
- Observe for signs of compartment syndrome.
- Check for muscle tenderness and myoglobinuria in sea snake bites.
- Sloughy wounds should be removed using an appropriate dressing (Chapter 37).
- Strict asepsis should be maintained when cleaning wounds.
- Consider tetanus prophylaxis.

Anti-venom

- If signs of systemic or severe local envenoming, administer anti-venom. The response to the anti-venom should be monitored. Anaphylaxis may occur, therefore anaphylaxis drugs and emergency resuscitation equipment should be immediately available.
- Early administration is lifesaving, but also prevents the necrotic effects and other effects systemically.

Rehabilitation

- Snake bites cause skin and soft tissue injuries resulting in scarring. Deeper muscle damage may result in amputation or complex delayed wound healing. The severity of the damage caused will determine the patient's rehabilitation and recovery needs. Poor wound healing can lead to disfigurement, contractures and loss of function.
- Depends on the type of snake, for example spitting cobras can spray venom into eyes leading to conjunctivitis, corneal abrasions and blindness.

- AKI may result in the need for long-term haemodialysis or even kidney transplantation, which may be limited within the country.
- Depending on how long from the time of envenomation to the time of administration of anti-venom this may delay patients' recovery.
- Other effects of prolonged recovery and disability include the poverty caused by being unable to work due to prolonged hospital stay or travel to hospital for treatment; being ostracised from communities and being unable to return to work and contribute to the family and community is a serious long-term consequence of snake bite envenomation.

(WHO, 2018c; Bellefleur & Chippaux, 2014;
Lalloo, 2014; Buckle & Hirshon, 2016a)

Scorpion stings

In some areas of the world, scorpion stings are more common than snake bites and can be fatal (Lalloo, 2014). Envenoming effects can be either local or systemic; clinical features include:

- tachypnoea;
- excessive salivation;
- nausea and vomiting;
- lachrymation;
- sweating;
- abdominal pain;
- muscle twitches and spasms;
- hypertension;
- pulmonary oedema;
- cardiac arrhythmias (bradycardia or tachycardia);
- hypotension;
- respiratory failure;
- skin necrosis.

Management:

- Transfer the casualty to hospital urgently.
- Immobilise the limb and use cold compresses to slow absorption of the toxin.
- Victims should be admitted, observed, monitored and regular observations recorded for any deterioration.
- Patients should be assessed using the A–E approach.

Airway

- Observation for airway compromise. If excessive salivation, nurse the patient on their side (recovery position) and ensure suction is available at the bedside.

- Intubation may be required if the airway becomes compromised due to excessive secretions or trismus.

Breathing

- Observation for signs of respiratory distress, due to respiratory failure or pulmonary oedema.
- Continuous pulse oximetry and respiratory monitoring.
- Treat pulmonary oedema with diuretics.

Circulation

- Continuous cardiac monitoring to observe for signs of arrhythmias (Chapter 15).
- Treat bradycardias with 0.5mg atropine and assess response.
- Blood pressure monitoring and in the event of hypertensive crises treat with vaso-dilators (nitro-glycerine, nifedipine, hydralazine) as appropriate.
- Establish IV access and IV fluid resuscitation as required. Vasopressors may be required.

Disability (neurological)

- Assess Glasgow Coma Scale and pupils regularly one hourly.
- Agitation or any psychomotor symptoms treat with benzodiazepines.
- Observe for signs of fitting and treat accordingly.
- Assess pain level and administer pain relief (ideally opiates if available).

Anti-venom

- If appropriate, administer scorpion anti-venom. There is a risk of anaphylaxis (Chapter 12) and emergency resuscitation equipment and drugs to treat anaphylaxis must be immediately available.

Wound care

- Carefully examine the limb for local signs of necrosis or other complications, e.g. swelling.
- Observe for signs of compartment syndrome.
- Strict asepsis should be maintained when cleaning wounds and appropriate dressings used (Chapter 37).
- Consider tetanus vaccine.

(Lalloo, 2014; Buckle & Hirshon, 2016b)

References

Bellefleur JP. Chippaux JP. (2014). Snakebite envenoming. In: Leone M. Martin C. Vincent JL (eds). Cham, Germany: Uncommon diseases in the ICU. Springer.

Buckle C. Hirshon JM. (2016a). Chapter 91: Snake bites. In: Wallis LA. Reynolds TA (eds). African Federation of Emergency Medicine: handbook of acute and emergency care. Oxford: Oxford University Press.

Buckle C. Hirshon JM. (2016b). Chapter 90: Scorpion stings. In: Wallis LA. Reynolds TA (eds). African Federation of Emergency Medicine: handbook of acute and emergency care. Oxford: Oxford University Press.

Chippaux JP. (1998). Snakebite appraisal of the global situation. Bulletin of the World Health Organization. 76. 515–524.

Chippaux JP. (2017). Snakebite envenomation turns again into a neglected tropical disease. Biomed Central. 23. 38. DOI: https://doi.org/10.1186/s40409-017-0127-6.

Lalloo D. (2014). Chapter 58: Bites and stings. In: Beeching N. Gill G (eds). Tropical medicine: lecture notes. 7th Edition. Chichester, West Sussex: Wiley Blackwell.

Warrell D. (2010). Guidelines for the management of snake-bites. World Health Organisation. Available at: http://apps.who.int/iris/bitstream/10665/204464/1/B4508.pdf?ua=1.

World Health Organization. (2010). Guidelines for the prevention and clinical management of snakebite in Africa. Available at: http://apps.who.int/iris/bitstream/10665/204458/1/9789290231684.pdf?ua=1.

World Health Organization. (2017) Snakebite envenoming. Available at: www.who.int/mediacentre/factsheets/fs337/en.

World Health Organization. (2018a) Snake gallery. Available at: www.who.int/snakebites/resources/photo_gallery_snakes/en/.

World Health Organization. (2018b). Diagnostic tests and tools. Available at: www.who.int/snakebites/treatment/Diagnostic_tests_and_tools/en/.

World Health Organization. (2018c). Treatment. Available at: www.who.int/snakebites/treatment/en/.

Trauma care

In this chapter, the over-arching principles of trauma care from both a military and civilian perspective are outlined. In previous chapters we explored the provision of critical care services in both resource limited and military environments; the clinical environment and the resources available will determine how you can best apply the principles of trauma care outlined below.

Trauma or injury is defined as 'tissue damage resulting from transfer of different forms of energy, either intentionally or unintentionally' (Ayana *et al.*, 2012). Injuries can be caused by blunt or penetrating objects, a blast or a combination. Trauma is the leading cause of mortality worldwide, killing more people every year than HIV, TB and malaria combined (WHO, 2017). Injury remains the leading cause of death amongst males between 15 and 29 years (UN, 2017). The UN (2017) identified approximately 1.25 million people die from road traffic injuries, and road traffic deaths have increased by an estimated 13% globally since 2000. As part of the SDGs the aim is to halve the global number of deaths and injuries from road traffic accidents (RTA) by 2020. Within low- and middle-income countries trauma is the greatest burden of death and disability, accounting for approximately 90% of the total burden of injury (WHO, 2004). With timely interventions the WHO (2017) identified if 'fatality rates from severe injury were the same in low- and middle-income countries as in high-income countries, nearly 2 million lives could be saved every year'.

Prevention

With many traumatic injuries due to road traffic collisions, the first stage in trauma care is to prevent injuries, through safety initiatives including wearing of either helmets or seat belts (WHO, 2017). In conflict, preventative measures may include the wearing of body armour, ballistic glasses or fire-retardant clothes. Through the various prevention strategies, this may reduce the number of casualties or severity of injuries sustained and 'buy time' until help arrives or the individual makes it to a hospital.

When an injury occurs, the primary aim must to be prevent disability and ill health (WHO, 2017). After blast injuries many patients die immediately due to exsanguination. Within some organisations the trauma treatment paradigm has changed from the

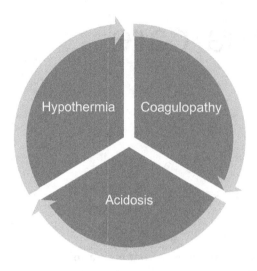

Figure 34.1 Lethal triad of trauma

Table 34.1 Potential life-threatening injuries

Catastrophic haemorrhage	Exsanguination
Airway	Airway obstruction
Breathing	Tension pneumothorax Open pneumothorax Flail chest
Circulation	Haemothorax Cardiac tamponade

traditional Airway (A), Breathing (B), Circulation (C) approach to <C>ABC (Edwards & Smith, 2016). Trauma results in blood loss, decompensation mechanisms due to hypothermia, coagulopathy and acidosis; this is termed the lethal triad of trauma (Figure 34.1) (Crossan & Cole, 2013). Until all three elements are appropriately managed a vicious cycle develops, which leads to increased mortality (Holcomb, 2005).

Life-threatening injuries

Potential life-threatening injuries due to trauma are outlined in Table 34.1.

Preparation

In preparation to receive a patient, your role and where you are working will determine how the unit responds and prepares to receive a trauma patient. The trauma and critical care team should consider the following:

- Assess the situation:
  - o What is the incident? Is it likely to involve multiple casualties or specific injuries, e.g. children, explosion causing burns, etc.?
  - o Are you and your team safe?
  - o Is this a major incident?
  - o Do you need to activate the major incident plan?
- Prepare:
  - o Prepare bed-spaces and allocate the team appropriately. Patients may need to be discharged sooner than expected in order to prepare bed-spaces.
  - o Are there any additional resources needed? For example, more IV fluids, drugs.
- Consider all eventualities:
  - o Are you expected to accept patients directly to critical care to stabilise before transferring them for definitive care? This will require additional resources and planning for departments outside of the emergency department.
  - o What happens if your staff are called to help in the emergency department? How will you prepare and manage patients already admitted?
  - o Make sure your staff are briefed and ensure they have access to refreshments and breaks as required.

On arrival a structured handover should be provided. Then the trauma team should complete both a primary and secondary survey (WHO, 2017) (Table 34.2) to help identify immediate and ongoing life-threatening problems. Organisations may have their own trauma documentation which can be used as part of the handover and act as an aide memoire for the team.

Table 34.2 Trauma Care Survey Checklist

Immediately after primary and secondary surveys:

Is further airway intervention needed? • GCS <8 • Hypoxaemia or hypercarbia • Face, neck, chest or any severe trauma	• Yes, done • No
Is there a _tension_ pneumothorax?	• Yes, chest drain inserted • No
Is the pulse oximeter placed and functioning?	• Yes • Not available
Large-bore IV placed and fluids started?	• Yes • Not indicated • Not available
Full survey for (and control of) external bleeding including:	• Scalp • Perineum • Back

Table 34.2 Continued

Assessed for pelvic fracture by:	• Exam • X-ray • CT
Is spinal immobilisation needed?	• Exam • Ultrasound • CT • Diagnostic peritoneal lavage
Neurovascular states of all 4 limbs checked?	• Yes
Is the patient hypothermic?	• Yes, warming • No
Does the patient need (if no contraindication):	• Urinary catheter • Chest drain • Nasogastric tube • None indicated

Before team leaves patient:

Has the patient been given:	• Tetanus vaccine • Analgesics • Antibiotics • None indicated
Have all tests and imaging been reviewed?	• Yes • No, follow-up plan in place
Which serial examinations are needed?	• Neurological • Abdominal • Vascular • None
Plan of care discussed with:	• Patient/family • Receiving unit • Primary team • Other specialists
Relevant trauma chart or form completed?	• Yes • Not available

Reproduced with kind permission from the WHO, 2017.

Haemorrhage control

To control massive haemorrhage improvised or commercial tourniquets may have been applied. Other forms of haemorrhage control include direct pressure, elevation, dressings, packing of wounds with gauze or use of novel haemostatics such as QuikClot or HemCon and splinting of long bone fractures and pelvis. On arrival if a patient has an improvised or commercial tourniquet in place, the tourniquet must be checked to confirm it is effective. The time of application is noted and every time the patient is moved the tourniquet effectiveness should be checked, for example after a log roll or moving from stretcher to trolley.

C-spine control and airway management

When managing an airway always assume a cervical spine injury and provide inline immobilisation, replacing with a well-fitting hard collar, sand-bags and tapes at the earliest opportunity (Hardcastle & O'Reilly, 2016). C-spine control should be considered when safe to do so and resources available; this may mean C-spine control is only applied once the patient arrives in the emergency department. C-spine should be assessed and continued to be managed at every stage of the patient pathway until it has been confirmed clear.

Care should be taken with cervical collars as they can reduce venous blood flow through internal jugular veins, which may affect cerebral blood flow in a head-injured patient. In an intubated and ventilated patient, with limited access to a CT scan it may not be possible to clear the C-spine immediately. Prolonged use of hard collars may cause problems including pressure sores and impede venous drainage and increase intra-cranial pressure.

Breathing

Life-threatening breathing conditions associated with trauma include blast lung, tension pneumothorax and flail chest.

Blast lung

Following an explosion, a proportion of people nearest the explosion will die immediately from blast lung. Those that survive may deteriorate over time and blast lung can be missed because there is little evidence of injury or external signs of trauma (Hardcastle & O'Reilly, 2016). Signs of blast lung include coughing, haemoptysis, hypoxia, chest pain, chest X-ray ('butterfly' pattern of bilateral patchy infiltrates), signs of air embolism, increasing oxygen requirements and development of respiratory failure. Treatment includes observation, oxygen and mechanical ventilation if required.

Tension pneumothorax

Tension pneumothorax in a self-ventilating patient may develop over a period, whereas in a ventilated patient it may be immediate. Signs include respiratory distress, asymmetrical chest movement, tracheal deviation (away from the affected side), reduced breath sounds, hypoxia, tachycardia, hypotension, cyanosis (Hardcastle & O'Reilly, 2016). Treatment includes immediate needle decompression, landmarks 2nd intercostal space, mid-clavicular line and placement of a chest drain.

Flail chest

Flail chest occurs when two or more fractures to ribs or the sternum occur resulting in a 'free segment' that causes paradoxical movements when breathing. This leads to hypoventilation and can lead to atelectasis. Flail chest is also associated with pain, an inability to cough and an inability to clear secretions.

Management of a flail chest may include early positive pressure ventilation in the event of respiratory failure, chest drain and analgesia (Hardcastle & O'Reilly, 2016). Splinting of the external chest wall with tape is of no benefit.

Circulation

Potential sources of haemorrhage include:

- chest: massive haemothorax, cardiac tamponade, tension pneumothorax;
- abdomen: hollow or solid organ injury;
- pelvis: fracture with vascular disruption;
- long bones: fracture with haemorrhage;
- peripheral vascular injury or other source of external injury;
- spinal trauma causing neurogenic shock.

(Hardcastle & O'Reilly, 2016)

Establishing intravascular access in trauma care is essential. This may be achieved using peripheral intravenous (IV) cannulas, central venous catheters (CVC) and/or intra-osseous (IO) access.

Damage control surgery

'Damage control surgery' is a term often used to aggressively manage the lethal triad of trauma (ICRC). The International Committee of the Red Cross (ICRC) recognises there is a place of DCS within resource limited environments and outlines its use in the War Surgery Manual (Giannou et al., 2013). If appropriate, DCS can be used to treat life-threatening abdominal, thoracic injures, limb and vascular injuries (Giannou et al., 2013). Although DCS tends to focus on the surgical control of haemorrhage, the post-operative care, including critical care, is equally important. Balogh et al. (2010) summarise the damage control principle 'as a treatment mode applied to severely-injured trauma patients with deranged physiology, to restore the physiology rather than the anatomy . . . it is all about physiology'. Continuing DCS interventions in critical care involves the following elements (Kisat *et al.*, 2016):

- Increased requirement of nurse to patient ratio during the critical post-operative period (2:1).
- Access to blood and blood products.
- Laboratory support.
- Ventilators with the ability to deliver advanced ventilation strategies.
- Access to equipment to facilitate re-warming, coagulation and acidosis correction.

For DCS to be successful a whole team approach to the management of the patient needs to be considered and recognised that it is more than the surgical intervention; care must be initiated immediately at the point of injury and continue until the patient is stabilised.

Hypothermia mitigation

Hypothermia in trauma is a poorly visible problem but a significant challenge; it can be either endogenous or accidental, but is associated with increased mortality and morbidity (Carter *et al.*, 2014). Even in hot climates, hypothermia is a significant concern (Aitken *et al.*, 2009). In trauma, even mild hypothermia leads to poor coagulation and impaired clotting and platelet dysfunction, with mortality rising significantly with patients with temperatures less than 35°C (Aitken *et al.*, 2009).

Hypothermia mitigation strategies include treatments at the point of injury; however, with varying pre-hospital and emergency care, patients may present hypothermic. Hypothermia mitigation strategies may include use of warming blankets, warmed fluids and blood and blood products, increasing the ambient temperature. Temperature should be recorded and hypothermia prevented, recognised and aggressively treated (Carter *et al.*, 2014).

Blood and blood products

Timely, affordable, screened blood is an essential component of surgical and trauma care (Jenny *et al.*, 2017). The Lancet Commission recommends at least 15 units of blood/1000 people/year; however, in LICs this can range from 4 to 11 units of blood/1000 people/year (Meara *et al.*, 2016). There are three guiding principles relating to the provision of blood and blood products for transfusions (Jenny *et al.*, 2017):

- Adequate volume of blood supply.
- Safe protocols for blood donation and transfusion.
- Appropriate regulation to provide sustainable distribution which is equitably and safe.

Provision of transfusion services can be centralised and/or de-centralised with volunteer organisations, NGOs and public and private blood banks all providing services.

The screening of blood can be variable due to a lack of resources to screen donations' in addition, lack of resources, including power for fridges, affect the quality of blood storage (Jenny *et al.*, 2017).

In a resource limited environment, understanding how to access blood for a trauma patient will determine the amount and availability of blood and blood products; for example, donations may come from relatives. Early communication with the hospital blood bank will mobilise what blood resources are available early. It is likely that decisions relating to ongoing care may be made due to the lack of adequate blood products.

Traumatic brain injury (TBI)

Traumatic brain injury (TBI) is a significant cause; Ayana *et al.* (2012) identified the majority of trauma patients seen in the emergency department in a rural hospital in Ethiopia had head and neck injuries (980/33%). There is little published on brain stem death testing in resource limited environments and there are no consensus guidelines for this area of practice. Within many countries the topic of brain death has many complications as socio-cultural, ethnic and religious diversity do not universally accept the concept of brain death (Waweru-Siika *et al.*, 2017; Mbakile-Mahlanza *et al.*, 2015; Turner, 1998; Tomlinson *et al.*, 2013). This presents significant challenges when trying to discuss withdrawal of treatment and refusal results in patients remaining ventilated for prolonged periods. Balancing futility in treatment, cultural sensitivities and allocation of limited resources will require understanding of the culture and communications skills (Tomlinson *et al.*, 2013).

Secondary survey/missed injuries

Polytrauma patients often have competing and conflicting injuries which pose challenges for critical care nurses (Crossan & Cole, 2013). With the priority on stabilising the patient and treating life-threatening injuries, there is a risk of missed injuries. Sae-Sia *et al.* (2012) identified that often limb and intra-abdominal injuries are missed. This may be due to other competing injuries, e.g. active bleeding or chest injuries, inadequate initial primary and secondary surveys, interventions including intubation may delay diagnosis. On admission to critical care a thorough assessment should be conducted to identify any missed injuries and given the severity of injuries it may be the first time there is an opportunity to review thoroughly what has happened. Thomson and Greaves (2008) highlight 40% of minor injuries are orthopaedic injuries and were missed in the Emergency Department.

Trauma in conflict

While advances in trauma care outlined above have resulted in the USA and the UK significantly reducing deaths in military trauma casualties in Iraq and Afghanistan (Kushner, 2017), transferring these successes to non-military organisations in resource limited environments is difficult (Chu *et al.*, 2010). This is due to a variety of reasons but could include that many of the healthcare facilities are damaged and healthcare workers fled or been killed (Attar & Gupta, 2017). Treatment will have commenced before the patient arrives to a field hospital (Jeffrey, 2012), whereas in the civilian sector patients will be self-triaged, due to the lack of pre-hospital care and long transport times to a hospital (Sinclair, 2017). Civilians of all ages are often the innocent casualties in war. Although the principles of trauma care remain the same, the resources available will determine the management. The following principles of care should be provided when dealing with a trauma patient:

- Triage: To prioritise patients who require immediate attention. Within a conflict situation healthcare services may already be overwhelmed and an additional influx of casualties or types of casualties, e.g. paediatrics or burns, may overwhelm the hospitals resources.
- First aid and basic medical care: To initially manage <C>ABC. This may be variable, and may involve improvisation of tourniquets and dressings. Patients may arrive by various modes of transport, e.g. cars, buses, at different healthcare facilities which may have limited trauma resources.
- Early surgical care saves lives and prevents long-term disability. Rehabilitation and ongoing pain management are equally important; this includes access to rehabilitative devices, e.g. prosthetics, crutches, wheelchairs.
- Is critical care appropriate? If there are no critical care services available, it may be appropriate to consider grouping sicker patients together in one location so they can be observed.

(SHPERE, 2013)

When dealing with traumatic wounds the following considerations should be applied:

- All wounds should be considered contaminated.
- All wounds, no matter how small or inaccessible, should be explored and debrided.
- Delayed closure following extensive cleaning and debriding.
- Within a resource limited environment, only the simplest of dressing changes should be conducted on the ward, due to the unsterile environment. All other dressings should be done in the operating theatres.
- Consideration for tetanus immunisation, particularly if there is a high index of suspicion the patient has not received this previously.
- Wounds can produce elevated levels of exudate, depending on the dressing used, e.g. gauze and bandage will become easily contaminated and cause odour, which can be unpleasant and embarrassing for the patient. The resources available will determine how best you will be able to manage this.
- Highly exudating wounds should be factored in when calculating the patient's overall fluid requirements.
- In the cases of suicide bombings, wounds may be further contaminated by foreign human material in the wound.
- All patients should receive regular appropriate doses of analgesia; this may include a peripheral nerve block, epidurals and patient-controlled analgesia if available.

Those who have sustained traumatic amputation should be started on pregabalin and/or amitriptyline as soon as possible to prevent neuropathic limb pain (Wyld-bore & Aldington, 2013).

- Factors which may prevent wound healing include:
  - o fungal and bacterial infection;
  - o massive transfusion, which may cause immunological compromise;
  - o poor nutrition and malnourishment.

(Attar & Gupta, 2017; Sinclair, 2017; SPHERE, 2013; Jeffrey, 2012)

Paediatric trauma in conflict

Conflicts affect all age groups, and weapons cause injury patterns not normally seen in practice (Inwald *et al.*, 2014). The challenge of providing care to severely injured children is of concern to both NGOs and military organisations (Sands, 2016; Pearce, 2015; Kenward *et al.*, 2004). Specific challenges may include limited availability of appropriately trained paediatric staff, treating children on adult wards and transferring children on to other facilities (Pearce, 2015; Kenward *et al.*, 2004). For military personnel this has been recognised as having additional challenges as the primary effort of many military healthcare facilities is to provide support to the military population at risk and they are resourced to deal with this. International humanitarian laws require emergency treatment to be provided to the indigenous population and captured persons, which may include children.

Similar challenges are also identified by nurses working with NGOs; due to the nature of NGO recruitment taking people on short-notice contracts or as volunteers means they may not always have experience in all fields (Sands, 2016). Often NGOS and military organisations arrange 'just in time training' to address potential shortfalls and meet the needs of the situation; this may include paediatric training and exposure.

Children decompensate later than adults, but deteriorate faster. In trauma injury patterns can be different due to 'resilient bones' meaning severe internal damage can occur without any overlying rib or skull fractures (Hardcastle & O'Reilly, 2016). Common management problems may include (Hardcastle & O'Reilly, 2016):

- over- or under-resuscitation;
- medication errors;
- failure to recognise and treat hypothermia;
- failure to recognise and treat hypoglycaemia.

Any seriously injured child should be assessed using the <C>ABC approach as outlined above. Additional information can be found in the paediatric section (Chapter 38), burns section (Chapter 35) and the transfer (Chapter 21).

Trauma in pregnancy

Any female trauma patient between 10 and 50 years should have a pregnancy test performed (Hardcastle & O'Reilly, 2016). The stage of pregnancy will determine the extent of the physiological changes associated with pregnancy and the foetal viability. In the third trimester, there is a risk for abruptio placentae, uterine rupture and premature labour (Hardcastle & O'Reilly, 2016). When dealing with pregnant women considerations are outlined in Chapter 39.

In summary, trauma is currently the leading cause of death amongst males aged between 15 and 29 years (UN, 2017). The wider impact on disability and death on families and communities is significant, as individuals affected are either unable to return to work and earn money or require ongoing long-term care. Trauma care requires the team to respond, adapt and prioritise treatment. Critical care nurses are often involved in the immediate and ongoing care of trauma patients and to achieve this sustainable and reliable resources, equipment, supplies and a healthcare workforce are essential (Dave & Gosselin, 2017). From both a military and a civilian perspective trauma is a time-critical emergency and the survival is determined by the interventions undertaken at the scene, how quickly the patient receives definitive care and the prevention of complications.

References

Aitken LM. Hendrikz JK. Dulhunty JM. Rudd MJ. (2009) Hypothermia and associated outcomes in seriously injured trauma patients in a predominately sub-tropical climate. Resuscitation. 80. 219–223.

Attar S. Gupta S. (2017). Chapter 2: A healthcare system destroyed: surgical care in Syria. In: Kushner AL. Operation crisis: surgical care in the developing world during conflict and disaster. Baltimore, MD: Johns Hopkins University Press.

Ayana B. Mekonen B. Lollino N. (2012). The 'hit by a stick' disease: an epidemiologic study of the cause of trauma in a non-profit hospital in rural Ethiopia. Tropical Doctor. 42. 1–4.

Balogh ZJ. (2010). In: Scannell BP. Waldrop NE. Sasser HC *et al*. Skeletal traction versus external fixation in the initial temporization of femoral shaft fractures in severely injured patients. The Journal of Trauma. 68. 633–640.

Carter C. Hughes W. Cumming J. Parker P. (2014). Nursing challenges with a severely injured patient in critical care: the importance of hypothermia mitigation. Nursing in Critical Care. 19. 1. 50.

Chu K. Trelles M. Ford N. (2010). Rethinking surgical care in conflict. The Lancet. 375. 9711. 262–263.

Crossan L. Cole E. (2013). Nursing challenges with a severely injured patient in critical care. Nursing in Critical Care. 18. 5. 236–244.

Dave DR. Gosselin RA. (2017). Chapter 6: Wounds and fractures: Orthopaedics after the Indian Ocean Earthquake. In: Kushner AL. Operation crisis: surgical care in the developing world during conflict and disaster. Baltimore, MD: Johns Hopkins University Press.

Edwards S. Smith J. (2016). Advances in military resuscitation. Emergency Nurse. 26. 6. 25–29.

Giannou C. Baldan M. Molde A. (2013). War surgery: Working with limited resources in armed conflict and other situations of violence. Volume 2. Available at: https://shop.icrc.org/la-chirurgie-de-guerre-travailler-avec-des-ressources-limitees-dans-les-conflits-armes-et-autres-situations-de-violence-volume-416.html.

Hardcastle T. O'Reilly G (2016). Chapter 279: Advanced trauma life support and principles of trauma management. In: Wallis LA. Reynolds TA (eds). AFEM Handbook of Acute and Emergency Care. Oxford: Oxford University Press.

Holcomb JB. (2005). The 2004 Fitts Lecture: current perspective on combat casualty care. The Journal of Trauma, Injury, Infection and Critical Care. 59. 4. 990–1002.

Inwald DP. Arul GS. Montgomery M. *et al.* (2014). Management of children in the deployed intensive care unit at Camp Bastion, Afghanistan. Journal of the Royal Army Medical Corps. 160. 236–240.

Jeffrey S. (2012). Challenges of treating military wounds. Nursing Standard. 26. 45. 63–68.

Jenny HE. Saluja S. Sood R *et al.* (2017). Access to safe blood in low-income and middle-income countries: lessons from India. BMJ Global Health. 2. E000167.

Kenward G. Jain TNM. Nicholson K. (2004). Mission Creep: An analysis of accident and emergency room activity in a military facility in Bosnia-Herzegovina. Journal of the Royal Army Medical Corps. 150. 20–23.

Kisat M. Zafar SN. Hashmi ZG *et al.* (2016). Experience of damage control trauma laparotomy in a limited resource healthcare setting. International Journal of Surgery. 28. 71–76. DOI: 10.1016/j.ijsu.2016.02.042.

Kushner AL. (2017). Preface. In: Kushner AL (ed). Operation crisis: surgical care in the developing world during conflict and disaster. Baltimore, MD: Johns Hopkins University Press.

Mbakile-Mahlanza L. Manderson L. Ponsford J. (2015). The experience of traumatic brain injury in Botswana. Neuro-psychological Rehabilitation. 25. 6. 936–958.

Meara JG. Leather AJ. Hagander L *et al.* (2016). Global surgery 2030: evidence and solutions for achieving health, welfare and economic development. International Journal of Obstetric Anesthesia. 25. 75–78.

Pearce P. (2015). Preparing to care for paediatric trauma patients. Journal of the Royal Army Medical Corps. 161. Suppl. 1. I52–I55.

Sae-Sia W. Songwathana P. Ingkavanich P. (2012). The development of clinical nursing practice guideline for initial assessment in multiple injury patients admitted to trauma ward. Australasian Emergency Nursing Journal. 15. 93–99.

Sands R. (2016). MSF seeks expert nurses. Nursing New Zealand. 22. 5. 4.

Sinclair M. (2017). Chapter 3: A surgeon's day in South Sudan. In: Kushner AL. Operation crisis: surgical care in the developing world during conflict and disaster. Baltimore, MD: Johns Hopkins University Press.

SPHERE. (2013). Humanitarian charter and minimum standards in humanitarian response. Available at: www.spherehandbook.org/.

Thomson CB. Greaves I. (2008). Missed injury and the tertiary trauma survey. Injury. 39. 1. 107–114.

Tomlinson J. Haac B. Kadyaudzu C *et al.* (2013). The burden of surgical disease on critical care services at a tertiary referral hospital in sub-Saharan Africa. Tropical Doctor. 43. 1. 27–29.

Turner L. (1998). An anthropological exploration of contemporary bioethics. Journal of Medical Ethics. 24. 127–133.

United Nations (2017). Sustainable Development Goal 3: Ensure healthy lives and promote well-being for all at all ages. Available at: https://sustainabledevelopment.un.org/sdg3.

Waweru-Siika W. Clement ME. Lukoko L *et al.* (2017). Brain death determination: the imperative for policy and legal initiatives in Sub-Saharan Africa. Global Public Health. 12. 5. 589–600.

World Health Organization (2004). Guidelines for essential trauma care. Available at: http://apps.who.int/iris/bitstream/10665/42565/1/9241546409_eng.pdf.

World Health Organization (2017). The WHO Trauma Care Checklist. Available at: www.who.int/emergencycare/publications/trauma-care-checklist.pdf?ua=1.

Wyldbore M. Aldington D. (2013). Trauma pain – a military perspective. British Journal of Pain. 7. 2. 74–78.

35

Burns care

The incidence of burns is particularly high in LICs and often affects the poorest communities in the world (Hashmi & Kamal, 2013; Olawoye *et al.*, 2014). While the focus is on the immediate care of burns, for the millions who are left disabled and disfigured this leaves long-term psychological, social and economic effects for both the survivor and their families (Van der Merwe & Steenkamp, 2012; Hashmi & Kamal, 2013; Grudziak *et al.*, 2017).

Burns prevention programmes in low-income settings are relatively new, with few NGOs focusing on burns prevention and management (Van der Merwe & Steenkamp, 2012). Indeed, first-aid practices remain sub-optimal with limited access and use of clean water to immediately cool the burn or reliance on traditional remedies which have no evidence base (Baker *et al.*, 2015; Fadeyibi *et al.*, 2015). In consequence, severe burns are a common reason for admission to critical care units. In addition, there may be no dedicated burns unit or team available, resulting in burns patients being managed in general critical care units, where mortality can be high (Hashmi & Kamal, 2013).

The principles of burns care involve resuscitation, early excision and skin grafting, infection control, wound care, pain management, nutrition and rehabilitation (Rogers *et al.*, 2014). The patient should be assessed using the <C>ABCDE approach and the mechanism of the burn should be noted: it may be thermal, blast, explosion, chemical or electrical (Mahoney *et al.*, 2017). The total body surface area (TBSA) should be assessed used an approved tool, e.g. Lund and Browder charts or the Rules of Nines. A major burn is classified as a TBSA >15% or 10% with associated inhalation injury.

The criteria for admission to critical care include (Hashmi & Kamal, 2013):

- adults with burns >15% TBSA;
- children with burns >10% TBSA;
- electrical burns;
- facial burns and suspected inhalation injury;
- perineal burns;
- patients with associated illnesses, e.g. ischemic heart disease, hypertension, diabetes.

Catastrophic haemorrhage

Control of any catastrophic haemorrhage was outlined in Chapter 34.

Airway

Upper airway burns may cause swelling to the larynx, epiglottis and glottis. Signs and symptoms may include stridor, changes in voice and swelling. Lower airway burns may result in hypersecretion of mucus, production of carbonaceous sputum and airway obstruction. Treatment involves securing the airway and use of adrenaline nebulisers.

GCS <8, hypoxia, hypercapnia and any evidence of airway burns are indications for early intubation. In adults it is recommended intubation should be with a large uncut ETT (>8.0mm). An uncut ETT may be required in cases of facial and airway swelling.

Breathing

Oxygen should be given to all patients since carboxyhaemoglobin levels may not be available. Take caution when using pulse oximetry as carbon monoxide poisoning may give a high (or normal reading).

Emergency escharotomies may be required with circumferential burns around the chest, as this may restrict ventilation.

Factors which predispose patients to pneumonia include (Rogers et al., 2014) include:

- intubation;
- cutaneous thermal injury, due to bacterial reservoir, systemic inflammation, immunosuppression;
- prolonged ventilation. Sustained micro-aspiration, inability to clear secretions, re-intubations;
- inhalation injury. Direct injury resulting in exudate formation, poor micro-ciliary clearance, reduced lung compliance, ARDS, prolonged ventilation;
- transfer. Risk of bacterial translocation;
- blood transfusions. Immunosuppression.

Rogers et al. (2014) reported that diagnosing a VAP in a burnt patient was challenging due to the respiratory dysfunction following inhalation injury, overwhelming systemic inflammatory response, pulmonary oedema and ARDS. In addition, fever, sputum, leucocytosis, deranged oxygenation and abnormal chest X-rays may also be present in a burns patient without pneumonia.

Circulation

Fluid resuscitation is an essential part of the management especially in the first few hours. The Parkland Formula is used to calculate the fluid requirements:

(4ml/kg/%TBSA burnt) = fluid requirements in first 24 hours.

Half in first 8 hours, remaining in next 16 hours.

For children, consider adding dextrose-containing fluid for the maintenance regimen. 4ml/kg for first 10kg, 2ml/kg for next 10kg and 1ml/kg >20kg.

Alternatively the Modified Parkland Formula may be used:

2ml/kg/hr × %TBSA

The Lund and Browder and Rules of Nines are guides to help guide fluid resuscitation particularly in the early stages. The amount of fluid should be in response to the patient's condition.

Fluids should be crystalloid and ideally they should be warmed. IV access may be difficult to establish due to the location of burns; intra-osseous access or central venous access may be the only route. However, Mahoney et al. (2016) identify there is no reason not to establish IV access through a burnt area if this is the only site available.

A urinary catheter should be passed and hourly urine recorded with the aim of an output of 1–2ml/kg/hr.

Attaching monitoring electrodes and blood pressure cuffs may be difficult due to the location of burns. In this case, monitoring may be limited, or alternative methods used, e.g. blood pressure cuff applied to a calf in a child.

Repeated debridement may lead to anaemia; patients may be able to tolerate this well until decompensation, therefore regular haemoglobin levels should be monitored and transfusion as indicated.

Pain management

Pain management can be complex. Analgesics may include ketamine, opioids, regional techniques and for neuropathic pain the use of amitriptyline (Mahoney et al., 2017) (Chapter 19).

Nutrition

Severe burns cause a hyper-metabolic response and hyper-catabolic state requiring an increased calorie requirement. Early enteral nutrition is recognised as important, as it not only prevents the catabolic state, but also reduces the incidence of ileus, preserves gut integrity and reduces stress ulceration. In many low resource settings, additional complications may include patients who are malnourished before admission to intensive care. Specialist dietician advice will be required before commencing any feeds. A naso- or orogastric tube should be inserted and enteral feeding commenced as soon as practicable. Access to commercial feeds is unlikely; the ICRC suggests the use of milk and egg mixes (Mahoney et al., 2017), which may be given as bolus feeds. Hyper-metabolic states can last up to one and a half years after injury.

Vijhuize et al. (2010) conducted a study in South Africa and found even with access to a dedicated dietician and supplements most burns patients did not receive sufficient daily calorie intake. This study demonstrates the importance of nutritional input but also the challenges in delivering enteral feeds. In a resource limited environment nursing several critically ill patients may result in patients not receiving nutrition regularly. If culturally appropriate, the bolus feeding via an NGT may be a role family members can undertake.

Wound care

All severely burnt patients should have their tetanus status confirmed and if required tetanus prophylaxis given. Early surgical debridement involves washing and debriding dead tissue and allows for accurate assessment of the burns and to reduce the chance of wound infection. Fasciotomies and escharotomies may be required for areas where there is a circumferential burn. This can lead to poor perfusion and cause compartment syndrome a surgical emergency. Surgical intervention is required to release the pressure; however, it provides another wound which could become infected. Dressings should be undertaken using a strict aseptic technique and ideally in the operating theatres. However, these may be undertaken on the unit due to a lack of theatre space.

Environmental

Prevent the patient from becoming become cold, especially during dressing changes, by aggressively managing hypothermia. Hypothermia leads to coagulopathy, infection and increased energy requirements. The ambient temperature of the room should be increased even in hot climates, IV fluids warmed and the patient's temperature recorded hourly.

The risk of infection is very high as immunosuppression is common after burns (Lam et al., 2008). Patients should be barrier nursed in a side room with access to a sink (or water supply) for hand hygiene. Observation for sources of sepsis may include VAP, urinary catheters, wounds, intravenous access. Prophylactic antibiotic administration is not recommended.

Paediatric patients

Burns and scalds result in a high mortality in children. Assessment of the child should follow the <C>ABCDE approach. The burn should be assessed to ascertain if the burn is full thickness or partial thickness. Full thickness burns can be black or white, have no sensation and do not blanch on pressure. This type of burn involves destruction of the skin and under entire sickness of the skin which will not regenerate. Partial thickness burns are pink or red, blistering, weeping or painful (WHO, 2013).

Assessment of the burn includes the following:

- Assessment using a body surface area chart which is appropriate to the age of the child.
- If not available, the child's palm can be used to estimate the burnt area. A child's palm represents approximately 1% of the total body surface area (TBSA).

Children with burns >10% of their BSA: those involving face, hands, feet, perineum, joints, circumferential and those that are complex should be admitted to hospital. Critical care input should be sought in case of deterioration, particularly if the patient is admitted to the ward. Challenges for ward staff include continually observing a patient with few staff, but this may be hindered if the child is admitted to a side room for barrier nursing.

If the child has smoke inhalation, oxygen must be given and the child closely observed. Severe facial burns and inhalation injuries may require early intubation or tracheostomy (WHO, 2013).

Fluid resuscitation is required for burns >10% total BSA. The WHO (2013) recommends the use of Ringer's lactate (Hartmann's Solution) or normal saline with 5% glucose. For maintenance Ringer's lactate with 5% glucose or half normal saline with 5% glucose. During the first 24, hours include the maintenance fluid to the additional emergency fluid requirements (4ml/kg for every 1% surface area burnt).

Half the total fluid should be administered in the first 8 hours, and the remaining in the next 16 hours. The second 24 hours give half to three-quarters of fluid required during the first day.

Blood may be used to correct anaemia or for deep burns to replace blood loss.

The child should be monitored closely for any signs of circulatory fluid overload.

Ongoing care involves the following:

- Nutrition. Enteral nutrition should be started within 24 hours of admission. The nutrition should be high calorie-including protein, vitamins and iron supplements (omit iron initially in severe malnutrition). Children with extensive burns require approximately one and a half times the normal calorie and two to three times the normal protein requirements (WHO, 2013).
- Prevention of contractures. Prevent contractures by passive mobilisation of the involved areas and by splinting flexor surfaces to keep them extended. Splints can be made of plaster of Paris and only worn at night (WHO, 2013). Early involvement of physiotherapist to start rehabilitation. Children should have access to toys and be encouraged to play.

References

Baker B. Amin K. Knor WS *et al.* (2015). Letter to the editor: practice of first aid in burn related injuries in developing countries. Burns. 41. 1891–1892.

Fadeyibi IO. Ibrahim NA. Mustafa IA *et al.* (2015). Practice of first aid in burn related injuries in developing countries. Burns. 41. 1322–1332.

Grudziak J. Snock C. Mjuwenui S *et al.* (2017). The effect of pre-existing malnutrition on paediatric burn mortality in sub-Saharan African burn unit. Burns 43. 1486–1492.

Hashmi M. Kamal R. (2013). Management of patients in a dedicated burns intensive care unit (BICU) in a developing country. Burns. 39. 3. 493–500.

Lam NN. Tien NG. Khoa CM. (2008). Early enteral feeding for burned patients – an effective method which should be encouraged in developing countries. Burns. 34. 192–196.

Mahoney PF. Jayanathan J. Wood P *et al.* (eds). (2017). Anaesthesia Handbook. Geneva: International Committee of the Red Cross.

Olawoye OA. Iyun AO. Ademola SA. Michael AI. Oluwatosin OM. (2014). Demographic characteristics and prognostic indicators of childhood burn in a developing country. Burns. 40. 1794–1798.

Rogers AD. Deal C. Argent AC. Hudson DA. Rode H. (2014). Ventilator associated pneumonia in major paediatric burns. Burns. 40, 1141–1148.

Van der Merwe AE. Steenkamp WC. (2012). Prevention of burns in developing countries. Annals of Burns and Fire Disasters. 25. 4. 188–191.

Vijhuize S. Verburg M. Marino L. van Dijk L. Rode H. (2010). An evaluation of nutritional practice in a paediatric burn unit. South African Medical Journal. 100. 6. 383–386.

World Health Organization. (2013). Pocket book of hospital care for children: guidelines for the management of common childhood illnesses. Geneva: World Health Organization.

36 Principles of post-operative care

In both military and resource limited environments critical care nurses may be required to nurse patients immediately post-operatively. While it is acknowledged recovery nursing is a highly specialist area, with few trained healthcare workers, critical care nurses may have the best experience and knowledge to undertake this role in the absence of a Recovery Nurse. Critical care nurses often receive critically ill patients immediately post-operative to the unit; however, recovering a patient who will be returned to the ward requires different skills.

Nurses must work in accordance with their professional code to protect and maintain the safety of any patient in their care. The International Council for Nurses (ICN) Code of Ethics (2012) states 'the nurse uses judgement regarding individual competence when accepting and delegating responsibility'. If you do not feel competent in recovering a patient, you must escalate your concerns and not undertake anything you are not competent to do. In a resource limited environment this may be difficult as you may be the only nurse. A solution may involve swapping with another experienced nurse and allowing them to recover the patient and you undertaking their duties. Many countries recognise recovery room nursing as part of the role of critical care nursing, therefore local nurses or other expatriates may have the experience to undertake this role (South African Nurses Council, 2014).

Working in recovery

Post-operative care and handover form part of the World Health Organization Safe Surgery Checklist (Figure 36.1). The Association of Surgeons of Great Britain and Ireland (ASGBI) have developed a skills resource for staff in poorly resourced country. Specific considerations nurses must understand when working in this environment include:

- what resources are available in the recovery room (including emergency equipment);
- the importance of close observation of the patient;
- awareness of anaesthetics used and the potential side effects;
- post-operative pain relief available.

(ASGBI, 2014; WHO, 2003)

Surgical Safety Checklist

World Health Organization | Patient Safety
A World Alliance for Safer Health Care

Before induction of anaesthesia ➤ **Before skin incision** ➤ **Before patient leaves operating room**

Before induction of anaesthesia

(with at least nurse and anaesthetist)

Has the patient confirmed his/her identity, site, procedure, and consent?
☐ Yes

Is the site marked?
☐ Yes
☐ Not applicable

Is the anaesthesia machine and medication check complete?
☐ Yes

Is the pulse oximeter on the patient and functioning?
☐ Yes

Does the patient have a:

Known allergy?
☐ No
☐ Yes

Difficult airway or aspiration risk?
☐ No
☐ Yes, and equipment/assistance available

Risk of >500ml blood loss (7ml/kg in children)?
☐ No
☐ Yes, and two IVs/central access and fluids planned

Before skin incision

(with nurse, anaesthetist and surgeon)

☐ Confirm all team members have introduced themselves by name and role.

☐ Confirm the patient's name, procedure, and where the incision will be made.

Has antibiotic prophylaxis been given within the last 60 minutes?
☐ Yes
☐ Not applicable

Anticipated Critical Events

To Surgeon:
☐ What are the critical or non-routine steps?
☐ How long will the case take?
☐ What is the anticipated blood loss?

To Anaesthetist:
☐ Are there any patient-specific concerns?

To Nursing Team:
☐ Has sterility (including indicator results) been confirmed?
☐ Are there equipment issues or any concerns?

Is essential imaging displayed?
☐ Yes
☐ Not applicable

Before patient leaves operating room

(with nurse, anaesthetist and surgeon)

Nurse Verbally Confirms:
☐ The name of the procedure
☐ Completion of instrument, sponge and needle counts
☐ Specimen labelling (read specimen labels aloud, including patient name)
☐ Whether there are any equipment problems to be addressed

To Surgeon, Anaesthetist and Nurse:
☐ What are the key concerns for recovery and management of this patient?

This checklist is not intended to be comprehensive. Additions and modifications to fit local practice are encouraged.

Revised 1 / 2009   © WHO, 2009

Figure 36.1 Surgical Safety Checklist

Reproduced with kind permission from the World Health Organisation, 2009a.

An additional challenge when working in the recovery area may include access to physician anaesthetists, particularly in remote and rural environments (Cherian *et al.*, 2010). In consequence nurses may not have the back-up of a skilled or experienced doctor when complications with the patient's airway or post-anaesthesia occur. In many low-income settings non-physician anaesthetists including clinical officers and nurse anaesthetists provide the majority of anaesthetic services. However, they may not be immediately available as they may be tending to other patients. To put this in perspective in Uganda, there are just 13 anaesthetists and 330 non-physician anaes-thetists, for a population of 27 million. In contrast the UK has an estimated 12,000 anaesthetists for a population of 60 million (Hodges *et al.*, 2007).

In practice, many anaesthetic practitioners have limited access to education, are often overwhelmed with the surgical workload and have limited time to review patients pre- or post-operatively (Cherian *et al.*, 2010; Chang *et al.*, 2015). Therefore, the recovery nurse needs to be able to manage a complex post-operative patient, with limited resources and immediate back-up in the event of any deterioration. This leads to 'task-shifting' where nurses are required to take on more responsibilities to void the gaps in services (Bisanzo *et al.*, 2012).

Considerations when recovering an adult patient

All stages of the surgical pathway are equally important and good nursing care in the immediate post-operative period can prevent early complications. The recovery room should be well staffed, warm and well-lit and have oxygen, suction and resuscitation equipment immediately available. This should not be shared with other departments or wards. Prior to the patient leaving the operating theatre, the surgeon, anaesthetist and nurse complete the following checks:

- The nurse verbally confirms the procedure as this may have changed or expanded during the operation.
- Completion of instruments, sponge and needle counts.
- Specimen labelling.
- Whether there any equipment issues.
- Identify any key concerns for the recovery and management of the patient focusing on any intraoperative or anaesthetic issues which might affect the patient (WHO, 2009a, 2009b).

This information must be verbally handed over, and the completed checklist and patient notes given to the recovery room nurse. The WHO (2003) propose the three most likely causes of post-operative mortality include the IV fluids not running, respiratory failure and post-operative hypotension.

Anaesthetic agents and drugs

Anaesthetic agents used in LICs may vary to those used in HICs. Modern fluorinated hydrocarbon anaesthetic agents (halothane, enflurane, isofluorane and sevoflurane) may not be used due to access in supply and cost. In Malawi, halothane accounted for a quarter of the entire anaesthetic department's budget (Totonidis, 2005). Anaesthetic agents used may vary and could include ether or halothane. Ether is an easy to manufacture, relatively safe and inexpensive anaesthesia; however, experience of using this inhalation drug is becoming less common. A significant problem with ether is it is highly flammable, especially in the presence of oxygen (Chang *et al.*, 2015).

Halothane is believed to be the most commonly used anaesthetic agent in low resource settings (Chang *et al.*, 2015). Complications includes cardiac arrhythmias and extreme bradycardia. There have also been reported cases of halothane hepatitis, which is why it is rarely used in HIC today (Mahboobi *et al.*, 2012).

Other methods of anaesthesia include spinal anaesthesia. Mgbakor and Adou (2012) reported this technique is often underutilised as a form of anaesthesia for surgical procedures below the umbilicus. In a study of 419 patients, they found although they had to adapt as they did not have the resources recommended to perform the procedure, many patients consented to this procedure (93.9%) and few adverse events were noted. Adverse events included hypotension and vomiting, which accounted for 1.67% of complications. Mgbakor and Adou (2012) concluded spinal anaesthesia is a 'simple, cheap and easy to learn'. Advantages of using this technique included reduced nursing workload, risk of aspiration and overall post-operative mortality and morbidity. The International Committee for the Red Cross (ICRC) recognise the use of regional anaesthesia (spinals, peripheral nerve blocks) and recommend their use in the conflict/disaster environment as they also have an advantage of having 'built-in' post-operative analgesia (Mahoney *et al.*, 2017).

The use of ketamine may be the anaesthetic choice when limited resources are available (Mahoney *et al.*, 2017). It is deemed a 'relatively safe drug' and can be administered intravenously or intramuscularly. Cardiovascular effects including increase in blood pressure, heart rate and cardiac output. Swallow, cough, sneeze and gag reflexes remain intact. Ketamine is a bronchodilator and can be used to treat asthma.

Disadvantages of ketamine include excessive salivation, vivid hallucinations requiring benzodiazepines, airway reflexes remain intact so laryngeal mask airways should not be used. Ketamine should be avoided in patients who are hyperthyroid or taking supplemental thyroxine as ketamine will worsen hypertension and those with schizophrenia. Careful administration is required in patients with ischaemic heart disease due to the hypertension and tachycardia effects. If used during a caesarean section ketamine crosses the placenta (Mahoney *et al.*, 2017).

Position

A post-operative patient should never be left unattended and should have one nurse to one patient during the immediate post-operative period.

The surgery performed will determine the position the patient will need to be recovered in and any specific nursing management required. To protect the patient's airway, patients may arrive in the left lateral, with the knees slightly bent and their hands placed comfortably beside the face. Patients post-abdominal, breast or orthopaedic surgery may be recovered in the supine position.

The position of the patient will determine where to position yourself to monitor the airway. In the lateral position you should sit at the patient's head, whereas in the supine position be at the patient's side.

Airway

On arrival a patient may still have an endotracheal tube or other airway device, e.g. a laryngeal mask airway, in place. Once the patient is fully conscious this will need to be removed. Post-extubation close monitoring of the patient is required to observe for any signs of airway obstruction and deterioration. The patient may be drowsy until all the effects of the anaesthesia have gone, therefore airway opening procedures including the head, tilt chin lift or jaw thrust may be required. If the patient has an ETT, self-extubation is not ideal as they may cause damage to the larynx as the cuff will have remained inflated and secretions around the pharynx may obstruct the airway.

Monitoring

Continuous cardiac and pulse oximetry should be monitored as well as non-invasive blood pressure, temperature and respiratory rate. The patient should also have a continuous pulse oximetry monitoring. A Cochrane Nursing Care Review (Lemanski, 2016) exploring the use of pulse oximetry in the immediate post-operative period reported pulse oximetry improved the recognition and reduced the incidence of hypoxaemia. Continuous observation of the patient and monitoring allowed healthcare workers to respond to deterioration and initiate appropriate interventions.

Observations should be recorded every 5 minutes for the first 20 minutes and recorded on the observation chart.

Temperature should be recorded. Keep the patient warm; just because the environmental temperature may be hot, the patient may still get cold. Although rare, both hypothermia and hyperthermia are post-operative complications.

The immediate risk post-surgery is haemorrhage. In addition to monitoring observations, check drains and dressings for any complications or deterioration.

Post-operative fluid management must take account of the following:

- Replacement of pre-operative deficit, e.g. the patient may have been dehydrated for several days, have a long history of illness before the operation. This may result in a significant positive fluid balance in the first 24 hours post-operatively.
- Replacement losses from the surgery and anaesthesia.
- Expected losses, e.g. naso-gastric tube drainage, drains.
- Hypothermic patients warming up will require more circulating volume as they peripherally dilate.
- Normal maintenance fluids.

The decision to give fluids is based on:

- the need to correct a deficit and may require a fluid challenge or bolus under your direct supervision;

- a maintenance schedule;
- monitoring for signs of improvement/deterioration (reducing tachycardia, increased urine output, increased blood pressure and return of skin turgor or sunken eyes returning).

Monitoring including recording and interpreting regular observations and maintaining a fluid balance chart are essential components of nursing the post-operative patient.

The WHO (2003) recommend post-operative maintenance fluids can be calculated as follows:

- Three litres a day to an adult (125ml/hr). With normal body electrolytes give normal saline followed by 5% dextrose (glucose), followed by Ringer's lactate (Hartmann's solution). These one-litre bags should be rotated over eight hours. 5% dextrose is suitable only as a replacement for water in patients who cannot drink.
- Replace other fluid losses with solutions containing sodium, normal saline or Hartmann's solution with added potassium 20mmol/litre only if necessary.
- Access to laboratory results for sodium and potassium will help guide and adjust treatment accordingly.

Post-operative pain

Post-operative pain is harmful to the patient. The type of anaesthetic given will determine the immediate pain management requirements, for example if halothane is used as the sole method for maintaining anaesthesia, when this has worn off the patient will be in pain, and must receive analgesia (WHO, 2003).

Pain should be assessed using the numerical rating scale (NRS) (Table 36.1) (Chapter 19). Factors which may affect the patient's post-operative management and recovery include delays in accessing surgical care or an inexperienced emergency and anaesthetic team, which may lead to the patient being poorly fluid resuscitated intra-operatively. If they remain in severe pain, this will cause adrenergic stimulation leading to hypertension, tachycardia, and increased oxygen consumption, peripheral and renal shutdown. When pain is relieved either through a bolus or continuous infusion of analgesia the 'true' blood pressure will be revealed, and the patient will become hypotensive (Boni, 2010). Pain can be identified as either surgical or non-surgical in origin (Gardner & Huddart, 2010).

Table 36.1 Pain assessment

0	No pain
1	Mild pain
2	Moderate pain
3	Severe pain

Surgical:

- Pain from surgery.
- Complications of the surgery (bleeding, infection, compartment syndrome).
- Nerve palsies secondary to surgery or intra-operative positioning.

Non-surgical:

- DVT (immobility or hypercoagulable state)
- Myocardial ischaemia.
- Pleuritic pain (PE, pneumonia).
- Pressure areas (especially immobile).
- Incidental pathology not related to surgery.

Depending on the drugs available, common opiates include pethidine and morphine. Morphine is ten times more potent and has a longer duration of action than pethidine (WHO, 2003). When administering analgesics the balance is to provide adequate pain relief while preventing respiratory depression. On the ward, opiate analgesia is likely to be given by intramuscular injection (WHO, 2003). Other drugs may include paracetamol or non-steroidal anti-inflammatory drugs (NSAIDs), e.g. diclofenac (1mg/kg) or ibuprofen (orally, intravenously or rectally) (WHO, 2003).

Common misconceptions can include the following (WHO, 2003):

- Sedations and analgesics are the same thing.
- Withholding analgesia to ensure the patient is fully awake to send them back to the ward.
- 'On demand' or 'as required' often means 'not given', therefore regular analgesia must be prescribed before the patient goes back to the ward.

If administering an opioid then a sedation score should be used (Table 36.2) and recorded with observations. In the event of an overdose (apnoeic, respiratory rate <8 or sedation score 3), you must do the following:

- Assess the patient using A–E approach.
- If the patient is apnoeic or has a respiratory rate <8 but has a pulse, immediately begin ventilating the patient via a bag, valve mask attached to oxygen. If no pulse begin CPR.
- Call for help.
- Administer naloxone (0.4mg per ampoule):

  o Adults: take one ampoule (0.4mg) and dilute to 8ml (= 0.05mg/ml). Inject IV 1ml incrementally until the patient responds. To a maximum dose of 4mg.
  o Children under 12 years of age: dose = 100μg/kg (diluted and incrementally dosed) repeated up to a maximum of 2mg.

- Naloxone is short acting; therefore, further doses may be required. In addition, naloxone will also reverse the analgesic effects, therefore the patient will be in pain.

(Mahoney *et al.*, 2017)

Table 36.2 Sedation scoring

0	None: patient awake and alert
1	Mild: occasionally drowsy but easy to rouse
2	Moderate: frequently drowsy, but easy to rouse
3	Severe: drowsy, difficult to rouse
S	Sleeping: normal sleep and easy to rouse

Post-operative nausea and vomiting

Causes of post-operative nausea and vomiting (PONV) are classified as patient, surgical or due to drugs (Gardner & Huddart, 2010). Patients identified as at increased risk for PONV include females, young patients, non-smokers, those with a history of travel sickness/PONV. Patients who have post-operative hypoxia, hypotension, electrolyte disturbance, uncontrolled pain. Surgical factors include type of surgery, e.g. ear, nose & throat (ENT), laparoscopic, laparotomy, gynaecological surgical. Gastric stasis due to ileus/obstruction and naso-gastric tube irritation, early resumption of oral intake. PONV due to drugs include anaesthetic agents (except propofol) and opioid drugs administration.

When to send to the ward

The recovering patient should be returned to the ward, when:

* conscious;
* extubated;
* observations are stable (blood pressure, pulse, respiratory rate, SpO2);
* no evidence of hypoxia;
* they can lift their head on command;
* appropriate analgesia has been prescribed and given (WHO, 2003).

A nurse should collect the patient and escort them back to the ward. During the handover key information includes the following:

* Surgery completed, including any complications.
* Patient's current conditions, including any medications given/running, e.g. IV fluids.
* Review of any drains, wounds.
* Any specific post-operative management.

The patient's notes (including X-rays, drug chart) should accompany the patient. In addition, all observations and fluid balance charts should be up to date and all care documented. Once the receiving nurse has assessed the patient and has no concerns, the patient should be transferred with a nurse escort to the ward area.

References

Association of Surgeons of Great Britain and Ireland. (2014). Theatre skills for staff in poorly resourced countries. Issues in Professional Practice. Available at: www.asgbi.org.uk/publications/issues-in-professional-practice?term=professional+practice.

Bisanzo M. Nicholas K. Hammerstedt H. (2012). Nurse-administration ketamine sedation in an emergency department in rural Uganda. Annals of Emergency Medicine. 59. 4. 268–275.

Boni F. (2010). Chapter 14: Pain management after major surgery. In: International Association for the Study of Pain. Guide to pain management in low-resource settings. Available at: www.iasp-pain.org/files/Content/ContentFolders/Publications2/FreeBooks/Guide_to_Pain_Management_in_Low-Resource_Settings.pdf.

Chang CY. Goldstein E. Agarwal N. Swan KG. (2015). Ether in the developing world: rethinking an abandoned agent. BMC Anaesthesiology. 15. 149. DOI: https://doi.org/10.1186/s12871-015-0128-3.

Cherian M. Choo S. Wilson I et al. (2010). Building and retaining the neglected anaesthesia health workforce: is it crucial for health systems strengthening through primary health care? Bulleting of the World Health Organization. 88. 637–639.

Gardner M. Huddart S. (2010). Chapter 1: post-operative pain. In: Leaper D. Whitaker I (eds). Post-operative complications. 2nd Edition. Oxford, Toronto: Oxford University Press.

Hodges SC. Mijumbi C. Okello M et al. (2007). Anaesthesia services in developing countries: defining the problems. Anaesthesia. 62. 1. 4–11.

International Council of Nurses. (2012). The ICN Code of Ethics for Nurses. Geneva: ICN.

Lemanski C. (2016). Pulse oximetry for perioperative monitoring. Cochrane Nursing Care Review. Journal of Peri-Anaesthesia Nursing. 31. 1. 86–88.

Mahboobi N. Esmaeili S. Habibollahi P et al. (2012). Halothane: how should it be used in a developing country? Eastern Mediterranean Health Journal. 18. 2. 159–164.

Mahoney PF. Jayanathan J. Wood P et al. (eds). (2017). Anaesthesia Handbook. International Committee of the Red Cross. Geneva: ICRC.

Mgbakor AC. Adou BE. (2012). Pleas for greater use of spinal anaesthesia in developing countries. Tropical Doctor. 1. 3. 49–51.

South African Nurses Council. (2014). Competencies for critical care nurse specialist (adult). Available at: http://sanc.co.za/pdf/Competencies/SANC%20Competencies-Critical%20Care%20Nurse%20Specialist%20(Adult)%202014-05.pdf.

Totonidis S. (2005). A role for trichloroethylene in developing nation anaesthesia. Kathmandu University Medical Journal. 3. 2. 181–190.

World Health Organization. (2003). Chapter 14.7: Post-Operative management. In: Surgical Care at the District Hospital. Geneva: World Health Organization.

World Health Organization. (2009a). Surgical Safety Checklist. Geneva: World Health Organization.

World Health Organization. (2009b). Implementation manual WHO Surgical Safety checklist 2009. Geneva: World Health Organization.

37 Wound care

Wound healing is a normal response to injury when the skin integrity has been damaged (Moore & O'Brien, 2014). Wounds can be classified as either acute or chronic. Acute wounds are caused by trauma or surgery and include incisions, lacerations (skin tears), burns, scalds, puncture, contusion, friction, pressure and shearing. A chronic wound is a prolonged or static wound for longer than six weeks; common chronic wounds include leg ulcers, diabetic foot ulcers, pressure ulcers, skin conditions, e.g. eczema, psoriasis, blistering (Peate & Glencross, 2015).

The aim of wound care is to 'prevent build-up of unwanted tissue types on the wound bed, while encouraging the growth of granulation and epithelial tissue to repair the wound' (Peate & Glencross, 2015, p. 41). Types of tissue found on the wound bed include the following:

- Necrotic tissue. Wet or dry tissue 'adhered' to the wound bed, consisting of red blood cells, skin cells, bacteria, foreign material, e.g. fibres from wound dressings, with varying amounts of exudate. The endotoxins and cell debris in the exudate causes wounds to remain in the inflammatory stages of wound healing. Necrotic tissue can also be gangrenous. This type of tissue is unwanted.
- Slough. Wet or dry tissue 'congealed' to the wound bed, consisting of wound exudate, debris, skin cells, bacteria and red blood cells. Colour can vary, for example grey exudate includes red blood cells, yellow contains white blood cells and green is likely to be infected with pseudomonas, although infection cannot be identified only by the colour of the slough. Slough is an unwanted tissue.
- Granulation. This occurs when new blood vessels (angiogenesis) needed for tissue repairs occur. The aim is to prevent build-up of unwanted tissue types while maintaining granulation.
- Epithelial. This is the final stage of wound healing and involves skin covering over the granulation tissue. Once the wound is entirely covered with epithelial tissue (skin) the wound is classed as being healed.

(Peate & Glencross, 2015; Rhodes & Carter, 2016; Shepherd *et al.*, 2010)

Specific challenges affecting wound healing in resource limited settings include anaemia, malnutrition, poor perfusion, immune-compromise due to infections including

HIV, wound care practices, overcrowding in clinical areas, understaffing, lack of equipment and laboratory support.

- Anaemia may be caused by chronic malaria, worm infestations, malnutrition, immune-compromise and poverty.
- Malnutrition, in addition to anaemia, is often related to poverty and results from patients eating or receiving foods with relatively little nutritional value, for example cassava flour or mashed plantain. Long-term malnutrition leads to a deficiency in amino acids, vitamins A and C, trace elements and low serum albumin level, which all affect wound healing.
- Poor perfusion may be caused by poorly controlled diabetes, sickle cell anaemia. Patients who are hypoxic will have limited oxygen supply to wound beds resulting in delayed healing.
- Overcrowding of ward areas, resulting in beds being close to each other. In malaria endemic areas, mosquito nets may not be available on the wards; with cramped, overcrowded wards mosquitoes may spread malaria between patients. Malaria leads to anaemia and directly affects wound healing. High humidity in the ward can add to the infection risk, and excessive wet and dry climates can affect wound healing.
- A lack of trained nurses providing care on the wards, resulting in dressings not being observed or changed when required. Healthcare staff with a lack of knowledge of the principles of asepsis and wound care. In many countries, families often provide day-to-day care to the patient. Patients and relative education can be difficult with few staff to conduct patient education and poor wound care by families and patients hinders the care provided.
- Wound care practices may involve inappropriate removal of dressings prior to ward rounds and appointments, resulting in the wound bed temperature dropping. Once the wound temperature drops below 28°C vasoconstriction occurs resulting in reduced oxygen supply to the wound bed. This may last for several hours, until the wound temperature improves. If the wound is left open to the air, the wound bed will dry out leading to increased scarring and delayed healing.
- Limited availability or a lack of sterile dressing packs and dressings on wards leads to difficulties in performing regular dressing changes and maintaining an aseptic technique.
- Limited or a lack of laboratory support for culturing of wound swabs results in delayed or an inability to process results in order to guide antibiotic use. Clinicians may use empirical knowledge to prescribe several antibiotics before the appropriate one is established. This leads to antimicrobial resistance and delayed healing.
- Access to antibiotics is variable, resulting in stronger antibiotics used initially due to a lack of availability or incomplete courses given due to a lack of supply; in consequence this leads to increased resistance.

(Carter & Mukonka, 2017; Rhodes & Carter, 2016;
Peate et al., 2012; Shepherd et al., 2010)

Common types of wounds encountered on critical care units may include both acute and chronic wounds. It is likely most wounds seen will be acute post-operative surgical wounds; however, patients may develop chronic wounds, e.g. pressure sores, during their admission. Infection is a significant risk for any patient with a wound and other complications of wound healing depend on the type of wound.

Infection

Any wound can become infected and this could be localised or systematic and lead to sepsis (Chapter 17). Signs of infection include (Woodrow *et al.*, 2013; Peate *et al.*, 2012; European Wound Management Association (EWMA), 2005):

- crepitus;
- increase in amount of exudate;
- pus;
- spreading erythema;
- viable tissues becoming sloughy;
- increasing pain in the wound;
- oedema;
- heat around the wound area;
- foul odour and purulent drainage;
- elevated white cell count;
- increased temperature;
- signs of cellulitis, osteomyelitis and sepsis;
- wound stops healing or continues to enlarge despite interventions;
- friable granulation tissue that bleeds easily.

Surgical wounds

Surgical wounds may heal by primary, secondary or tertiary (also termed 'delayed primary') intention. Complications of surgical wounds include surgical site infection (SSI) and dehiscence. The WHO (2016) identified SSI as the leading cause of surgical complication in low-income settings, affecting up to one-third of surgical patients, and is nine times higher than in HIC. In addition to the challenges outlined above, sterility during surgical procedures may also impact on SSI. Operating theatres often lack complete sterility such as laminar air flow. There may be a lack of sterile surgical drapes, gloves, gowns and consumables and during busy periods two operating tables may be used at the same time in the same room (Shepherd *et al.*, 2010).

To prevent surgical site infection best practice guidelines focusing on the care of a patient with a post-operative wound are outlined in Figure 37.1.

Dehiscence of the wound may occur due to the trauma and swelling caused by the surgical procedure, obesity, and too much tissue loss resulting in a greater tension on the wound closure and infection or underlying wound abscess. Once the wound has dehisced, healing occurs by secondary intention, but the wound is likely to be weak in tensile and scarring can be poorer than wounds that heal by primary intention (Peate & Glencross, 2015).

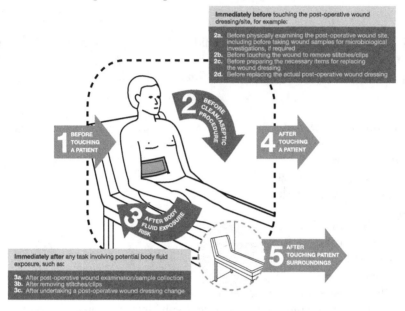

My 5 Moments for Hand Hygiene
Focus on caring for a patient with a post-operative wound

Immediately before touching the post-operative wound dressing/site, for example:

2a. Before physically examining the post-operative wound site, including before taking wound samples for microbiological investigations, if required
2b. Before touching the wound to remove stitches/clips
2c. Before preparing the necessary items for replacing the wound dressing
2d. Before replacing the actual post-operative wound dressing

1 BEFORE TOUCHING A PATIENT

2 BEFORE CLEAN/ASEPTIC PROCEDURE

4 AFTER TOUCHING A PATIENT

3 AFTER BODY FLUID EXPOSURE RISK

5 AFTER TOUCHING PATIENT SURROUNDINGS

Immediately after any task involving potential body fluid exposure, such as:

3a. After post-operative wound examination/sample collection
3b. After removing stitches/clips
3c. After undertaking a post-operative wound dressing change

Key additional considerations for post-operative wounds

- Avoid unnecessary touching of the post-operative wound site, including by the patient.
- Wear gloves if contact with body fluids is anticipated; the need for hand hygiene does not change even if gloves are worn, as per the WHO 5 Moments.
- Follow local procedures regarding use of aseptic non-touch technique for any required dressing changes/wound procedures.
- Don't touch dressings for at least 48 hours after surgery, unless leakage or other complications occur.
- Routine post-operative wound dressings should be basic dressing types (e.g. absorbent or low adherence dressings).
- When approaching a patient for the examination of a wound, the health worker may also perform other tasks (e.g. accessing a venous catheter, drawing blood samples, checking urinary catheter). Hand hygiene may be needed before and

- after these specific tasks, to once again fulfill Moments 2 and 3, for example (refer to WHO dedicated 5 Moments posters for line or catheter management).
- When indicated, pre-operative surgical antibiotic prophylaxis (SAP) should be administered as a single parenteral dose 2 hours or less before the surgical incision, while considering the half-life of the antibiotic. Do not prolong administration of SAP after completion of the operation.
- Antibiotic therapy for any proven surgical site infection should ideally be administered based on wound sample culture and sensitivity results.
- Common signs and symptoms of wound infection are: pain or tenderness; localized swelling; erythema; heat, or purulent drainage from the superficial incision.
- This guidance does not include information on *complicated* post-operative wound care, when specific treatments or therapies may be required.

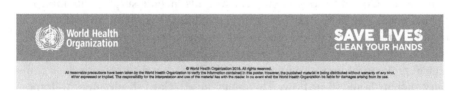

World Health Organization

SAVE LIVES
CLEAN YOUR HANDS

Figure 37.1 Considerations when managing a post-operative wound
Reproduced with kind permission from the World Health Organization.

Traumatic wounds and burns

Traumatic wounds are likely to be dirty and require irrigation and debridement. Infective wounds and clean wounds older than six hours should never be closed (WHO, 2018). Trauma patients are often haemodynamically compromised and cold; therefore treatment must include aggressive oxygenation, fluid resuscitation and warming in order to improve oxygenation and perfusion (WHO, 2018). Principles of trauma care are outlined in Chapter 34 and the care of burns is outlined in Chapter 35.

Diabetic wounds

Wounds caused by diabetes and cardiovascular disease are likely to be non-healing wounds. These types of wounds are occurring with increasing frequency and cause significant problems in low-income settings (WHO, 2011). Other complications associated with diabetic wounds include increased risk of developing pressure sores. Due to poor circulation and neuropathy, patients are unable to respond to the effects of pressure and change their position regularly (Peate & Glencross, 2015). Care of complex diabetic wounds in resource limited environments include:

- pressure relief;
- debridement of callus and de-sloughing where possible;
- antibiotics: consider broad spectrum antibiotics, e.g. metronidazole and Staph and Strep cover;
- dressings: should be non-adhesive (e.g. Vaseline-impregnated gauze) and/or natural dressings, e.g. honey, sugar paste, papaya;
- patient and family education.

(Gill & Mbanya, 2013)

Pressure sores

Critically ill patients are at considerable risk for developing pressure sores. The development of a pressure sore increases critical care and hospital stay, nursing workload, healthcare costs, pain and disability (Kaitani *et al.*, 2010; Mohajeri *et al.*, 2015). Additional challenges include poor nutrition and delayed presentation due to distance to healthcare facilities (Idowu *et al.*, 2011). With limited access to pressure relieving aids, healthcare workers may try innovative methods to relieve pressure; these include the following:

- Gloves filled with water and placed under heels (Picture 37.1);
- To prevent urinary catheterisation, IV fluid bags can be used to collect urine;
- Teaching patients and families to provide self-care, turning and encouraging a local diet which is high in protein (Nthumba, 2016).

Additional measures include the following:

- Checking pressure areas every shift. This should include checking the corners of the mouth as pressure sores may be caused by the ETT ties, top of the ears where oxygen mask straps may have caused rubbing or pressure damage.
- Use of pressure risk assessment tool, for example Waterlow Scoring Tool.

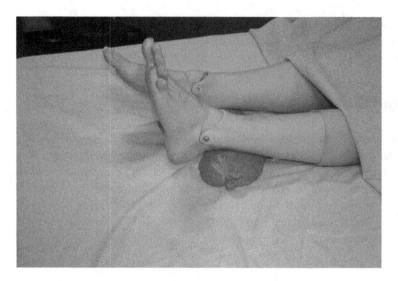

Picture 37.1 Gloves filled with water and placed under heels

- Avoid plastic draw sheets, incontinence pads and tightly tucked-in draw sheets (Waterlow, 2018).
- If a patient is using a wheelchair, they should sit on a cushion (Waterlow, 2018).
- Use of a turning chart.
- Provide good nutrition and pain relief.
- Use good manual handling techniques to prevent friction and shear forces.

Pressure sores should be graded using approved wound assessment criteria. The European Pressure Ulcer Advisory Panel (EPUAP) (2018) grades pressure sores as follows:

- Grade 1: Non-blanching erythema of intact skin. Discolouration of the skim, warmth, oedema, induration or hardness may be used as indicators, particularly with individuals with darker skin.
- Grade 2: Partial thickness of skin loss involving epidermis, dermis or both. The ulcer is superficial and may look like an abrasion or blister.
- Grade 3: Full thickness skin loss involving damage to or necrosis of subcutaneous tissue but not extending to the underlying fascia.
- Grade 4: Extensive destruction, tissue necrosis, or damage to muscle, bone or supporting structures with or without full thickness skin loss.

Wound assessment

Wound assessment should include the following (EPUAP, 2018; Woodrow *et al.*, 2013; EWMA, 2005):

- Location on body.
- Grade of pressure sore using an approved grading tool as outlined above.

- Size of wound (approximately in square centimetres) and document.
- Assess the wound bed (necrotic, sloughy, exudate, granulating).
  - Necrotic – debriding may be performed by:
    - use of specialist dressings if available by creating a moist wound environment to allow autolytic debriding;
    - surgical debridement by a surgeon or other specialist.
  - Signs of slough – colour, amount and whereabouts on wound bed.
  - Exudate – colour and consistency. If the wound appears infected, swab the wound for microscopy, culture and sensitivity.
  - Granulating.
- Pain.
- Assess status of surrounding skin:
  - healthy;
  - macerated;
  - inflamed;
  - localised erythema (if more than 2cm around the wound this may indicate spreading systemic infection).
- Mobility – is the patient mobile? Can they change their position?
- Any other complications which may affect wound healing, e.g. nutrition, malaria, diabetes or a smoker?
- Signs of infection as outlined above.

Ideally units and hospitals should have agreed wound assessment and care plans available, to ensure consistency in assessment and documentation.

Dressing choice

Choosing the right dressing may be challenging due to the limited dressing choice available and at times families may need to buy specialist dressings. This results in not using the best dressing due to cost and availability, and changes in treatment plans if the family cannot afford to continue treatment for chronic wounds. Delays may occur if the family needs to buy the dressing from a private pharmacy and when the wound leaks and causes strike through, the integrity of the dressing is no longer intact and will need to be changed. If there is no dressing available, then the delay may increase the risk of the patient developing an infection.

The use of traditional and 'home remedies' may be used within some communities as a way to provide affordable wound management choices (Benskin, 2013; Mohajeri *et al.*, 2015). Dressings may include:

- management of burns:
  - boiled potato peel;
  - banana leaf;
  - honey.

- methods of debridement:
  - papaya pulp;
  - sugar.
- chronic bedsore:
  - kiwi fruit.

While these treatments may be uncommon to nurses from HIC, Benskin (2013) conducted a literature review of the methods outlined above to manage burns and methods of debridement and found there is evidence to support their use (Benskin, 2013). Mohajeri *et al.* (2015) reported the use of kiwi fruit extract had antibacterial properties when used on chronic bedsores and concluded the application of kiwi fruit was a simple, applicable and effective way to treat bedsores. While these innovative methods to wound healing may not be used in HIC, and the studies are small scale making it difficult to replicate, with access to expensive dressings, alternatives including traditional methods may be the only dressings available.

Topical negative pressure

Topical negative pressure (TNP) is useful for managing heavily exudating wounds but devices are expensive and limited. In some hospitals TNP dressings and pumps are improvised. Although effective, without TNP, surgeons may result to the use of daily dressings of 0.9% saline-soaked gauzes, termed WET, and frequent surgical debridement. Perez *et al.* (2010) outline how to provide improvised TNP:

- Following surgical debridement. Povidone-iodine hand scrub brushes were trimmed and shaped to make close contact with the all surfaces of the wound. The number of sponges used was documented to avoid retention of sponges.
- Multiple holes were cut into a sterile suction catheter and this was placed in close contact with the brushes.
- The wound was then covered with an adhesive drape which extended at least two centimetres beyond the wound margins onto dry intact skin.
- The tube was then connected to a suction unit and a continuous negative pressure of 100mmHg was applied.
- The amount of fluid or blood drained was monitored every 30 minutes for the first 6 hours. In case of haemorrhage (>200ml per 30 minutes) the surgeon on call was informed.
- After six hours, the dressing and pump were checked every two hours and unless indicated dressings changed every four days under regional or general anaesthesia.

There are various other methods documented. For example, the application of TNP to a hand or foot is technically difficult to dress and create an airtight seal. Sreelesh and Bhandari (2017) outline the use of a collagen powder and a sterile surgical glove. Following surgical debridement and preparation of the wound bed, paraffin gauze and a sterilised sponge were placed over the wound. A suction tube made out of a sterile urobag or Ryles tube was placed into the sponge. The sterile glove was then stretched and placed over the dressing. An airtight seal was created using tincture benzoin and transparent adhesive tape. TNP was applied intermittently at −125mmHg for 15 minutes every 30 minutes for 3 days.

Positive results have been seen when using improvised TNP (Sreelesh & Bhandari, 2017; Perez et al., 2010) and its use has been documented in HIC and the military operations during operations in Afghanistan and Iraq (Nguyen et al., 2015; Taylor & Jeffrey, 2009). Concerns regarding patient safety when using equipment not intended for this purpose have been identified. The decision to perform this technique must be taken by the surgeon and the risk versus benefit justified (Perez et al., 2010). Other considerations include the nursing workload is increased when using TNP as they are required to monitor and adjust suction pressures to determine what is best. No alarms to alert healthcare workers when there is a problem means increased observation of the patient is required (Nguyen et al., 2015). Limitations to using both commercial and improvised TNP devices may limit or not allow patients to mobilise (Nguyen et al., 2015). Finally, the need for continuous electricity supply makes it difficult for many hospitals to use this technique (Benskin, 2013).

In summary, wound care is predominately the domain of the nurse. Critical care nurses may see both acute and chronic wounds; both types can be complex wounds and require innovative strategies to promote wound healing. In addition, many external factors are often not within the nurses' or patients' sphere of influence, including finances, overcrowding and limited resources. Intrinsic factors including malnutrition and malaria will add challenges to the management of wounds. With few experts in wound care available, often nurses rely on a combination of experience and local remedies to manage complex wounds.

References

Benskin LLL. (2013). A review of the literature informing affordable, available wound management choices for rural areas of tropical developing countries. Ostomy/Wound Management. 59. 10. 20–41.

Carter C. Mukonka P. (2017). Malaria: diagnosis, treatment and management of a critically ill patient. British Journal of Nursing. 26. 13. 762–767.

European Pressure Ulcer Advisory Panel. (2018). European Pressure Ulcer Advisory Panel: Pressure Ulcer Treatment Guidelines. Available at: www.epuap.org/.

European Wound Management Association. (2005). Position document: identifying criteria for wound infection. London: Medical Education Partnership.

Gill G. Mbanya JC. (2013). Chapter 58: Diabetes mellitus. In: Mabey D. Gill G. Parry E. Weber MW. Whitty CJM (eds). Principles of Medicine in Africa. 4th Edition. Cambridge: Cambridge University Press.

Idowu OK. Yinusa W. Gbadegesin SA. Adebule GT. (2011). Risk factors for pressure ulceration in a resource constrained spinal injury service. Spinal Cord. 49. 643–647.

Kaitani T. Tokunaga K. Matsui N. Sanada H. (2010). Risk factors related to the development of pressure ulcers in the critical care setting. Journal of Clinical Nursing. 19. 414–421.

Mohajeri G. Safaee M. Sanei MH. (2015). Effects of topical kiwifruit on healing of chronic bedsores. Indian Journal of Surgery. 77. Suppl. 2. S442–446.

Moore Z. O'Brien JJ. (2014). Chapter 11: Nursing care of conditions related to the skin. In: Brady AM. McCabe C. McCann M (eds). Fundamentals of medical-surgical nursing: a systems approach. Chichester, West Sussex: Wiley Blackwell.

Nguyen TQ. Franczyk M. Lee JC et al. (2015). Prospective randomized controlled trial comparing two methods of securing skin grafts using negative pressure wound therapy: vacuum assisted closure and gauze suction. Journal of Burn Care & Research. 324–328. DOI: 10.1097/BCR.0000000000000089.

Nthumba PN. (2016). Chapter 17: Pressure ulcers. In: Carter LL. Nthumba PM (eds). Principles of reconstructive surgery. Available at: www.paacs.net/wp-content/uploads/2012/09/PAACS-Reconstructive-Surgery-Text-v.-2-072516.pdf.

Peate I. Glencross W. (2015). Wound care at a glance. Chichester, West Sussex; Malden, MA: Wiley Blackwell.

Peate I. Nair M. Hemming L et al. (2012). Chapter 5: Caring for people with altered skin function. In: LeMone P. Peate I. Nair M et al. (eds). LeMone and Burke's Adult nursing: acute and ongoing care. Harlow, UK: Pearson.

Perez D. Bramkamp M. Exe C, von Ruden C. Ziegler A. (2010). Modern wound care for the poor: a randomized control trial comparing the vacuum system with conventional saline-soaked gauze dressings. The American Journal of Surgery. 199. 14–20.

Rhodes B. Carter L. (2016). Chapter 1: Wound healing and care: hypertrophic scars and keloids. In: Carter LL. Nthumba PM (eds). Principles of reconstructive surgery. Available at: http://paacs.net/wp-content/uploads/downloads/2013/03/1_Title-Page-Editors-and-Authors.pdf.

Shepherd P. Shepherd H. Mueller S. (2010). Treating surgical wounds in rural South-western Uganda. Wounds International. 1. 4. 11–14.

Sreelesh LS. Bhandari PL. (2017). An easy technique for negative pressure wound therapy for extremities using collagen powder and sterile gloves. Indian Journal of Surgery. 79. 1. 81–83.

Taylor C. Jeffrey S. (2009). Management of military wounds in the modern era. Wounds UK. 5. 4. 50–58.

Waterlow J. (2018). Waterlow Score Card. Available at: www.judy-waterlow.co.uk/waterlow_downloads.htm.

Woodrow P. Elliott J. Beldon P. (2013). Chapter 12: Assessment and care of tissue viability, and mouth and eye hygiene needs. In: Mallett J. Albarran JW. Richardson A (eds). Critical care manual of clinical procedures and competencies. Chichester, West Sussex: Wiley Blackwell.

World Health Organization. (2011). Noncommunicable diseases major health threats. Available at: http://apps.who.int/iris/bitstream/10665/128038/1/9789241507509_eng.pdf.

World Health Organization. (2016). Global guidelines on the prevention of surgical site infection. Available at: www.who.int/gpsc/ssi-guidelines/en/.

World Health Organization. (2018). Prevention and management of wound infection. Available at: www.who.int/hac/techguidance/tools/guidelines_prevention_and_management_wound_infection.pdf.

38 Paediatrics

The UN Convention on the Rights of the Child (UNICEF, 2017) requires the care to sick and injured children to be delivered or supervised by someone with paediatric training. The World Federation of Paediatric Intensive and Critical Care (Kissoon et al., 2009) defined critical care as 'the treatment of a child with a life-threatening illness or injury in its broadest sense, without regard for the location and including pre-hospital and emergency and intensive care'. These mandates and definitions provide significant challenges for nurses working in resource limited environments who may not have access to specialist children's nurses or paediatricians. In consequence, you may be involved in resuscitating and stabilising critically ill patients in a variety of settings. This chapter provides practical insight into providing care to children for nurses who have varying paediatric experiences.

Nursing a critically ill patient is stressful, especially when dealing with children that may have different conditions and challenges not normally seen in HIC. Gaining appropriate experience and confidence to nurse an acutely and critically ill child has specific challenges which are unlikely to be gained in HIC. Practical challenges may include the following (Bowen et al., 2016; Wright et al., 2015; Pearce, 2015; Kenward et al., 2004):

- Weighing scales may be broken, not calibrated or not available.
- Using formulae, e.g. Advanced Life Support Group/European Resuscitation Council, based on US or Western children and may not reflect malnourished children.
- Children may be more independent than their Western counterparts.
- Communication challenges if they do not speak English, when assessing patients and gaining consent.
- Parents may not accompany children, which may pose issues with consent.
- Ethical challenges when dealing with child soldiers.
- Challenges in gaining consent if the child is unaccompanied.
- Delays in accessing healthcare due to geographical distance to healthcare facilities, or limited critical care units meaning patients need to be transferred considerable distances.
- Access to equipment, drugs and disposable materials.
- Not all ventilators will be able to ventilate children under 1 year or a certain weight.

- Local or district hospitals may not have 24-hour physician staffing on wards. Meaning nurses may be the only staff immediately available to respond to an emergency.
- Nursing staff are not trained specifically in paediatric nursing, resulting in a lack of confidence and delays in initiating treatment.

With limited pre-hospital emergency medical services, patients may present in late stages and arrive with minimal to no interventions (Khilnani & Chhabra, 2008). On arrival in a medical treatment facility the child will need to be assessed and stabilised. Drugs and treatments, e.g. endotracheal tubes, are based on the child's weight. There are several ways to estimate the weight of a child, including formulas (Box 38.1) and measuring tapes. Bowen *et al.* (2016) reported that formulas tended to either under- or overestimate children's weights, and measuring tapes, e.g. Broselow, Oakley or Mercy tapes, appeared to be more accurate, but were not always available when evaluating paediatric weight estimation in Zambia. Bowen *et al.* (2016) suggested given children from high-income countries are more obese, perhaps calculations used in the 1970s would be better for estimation. While the gold standard remains to weigh a child when possible, there appears to be no universal tool that rivals this method (Bowen *et al.*, 2016). When calculating the risk of error due to stress is high, this should be checked by another practitioner (Bowen *et al.*, 2016). With additional training, the following considerations will help practitioners who are not familiar with nursing children to respond.

Box 38.1 Emergency paediatric calculations (WETFLAG)

Weight:

The following calculation is used to approximate the weight of a child between 1 and 10 years.

$$(\text{Age} + 4) \times 2 = \text{body weight (in kg)}$$

Energy (defibrillation):

4joules/kg

Tube (endotracheal tube) sizes:

Size internal diameter (uncuffed tube) = (age/4) + 4
Length (oral) = age/2 + 12
6 months – size 3.5 tube
Term infant – 3.0 tube
Premature – 2.5 tube

Fluid bolus:

10–20ml × weight (kg) = ml

Adrenaline cardiac arrest:

10mcg/kg of 1 in 10000 solution = 0.1ml kg

Glucose:

2ml/kg (10% dextrose)

(Resuscitation Council (UK), 2016)

With limited resources it is possible to assess and monitor seriously ill children by using fundamental assessment skills including pulses, pulse pressure, oxygen saturations, respiratory rate, blood pressure, capillary refill, peripheral temperature, urine output and coma scoring. Simple and effective serial measurements will help identify and monitor response to treatment (Molyneux & Maitland, 2005). Children must be closely observed and monitored, as an estimated 50% of in-hospital deaths in children occur within the first 24 hours of admission (Robertson & Molyneux, 2001). With limited access to paediatric trained staff, many children will be initially managed by healthcare workers with varying paediatric skills and experiences (Goh *et al.*, 2003. Wright *et al.*, 2015).

Wright *et al.* (2015) describe the delivery of healthcare workers' characteristics and hospital resources when delivering a resuscitation training programme in Botswana. Wright *et al.* (2015) reported 100% of healthcare workers had immediate access to oxygen, intravenous fluids and initial antibiotics for pneumonia, yet only 50% had received any training in how to give these in an emergency. This study demonstrates the importance of ensuring healthcare workers have the knowledge and experience to use the resources that are available, otherwise the preventable deaths will continue.

Airway

Infants have large heads in relation to the rest of their body. Combined with a prominent occiput, this means the head tends to flex on the neck when the infant is in the supine position. This could lead to potential airway obstruction when the level of consciousness is reduced.

The infant's face is small therefore appropriately sized face masks need to be used to provide an effective seal and protect the infant's eyes. Inside the small mouth the tongue is relatively large. The mouth is easily compressible and the soft tissues could become compressed causing an airway obstruction when performing airway manoeuvres. Infants are predominately nasal breathers for the first six months of life.

Choking may be caused by a complete or partial obstruction. Choking tends to be sudden, or there is a sudden onset of stridor or respiratory distress. An airway obstruction is a medical emergency (Figure 38.1).

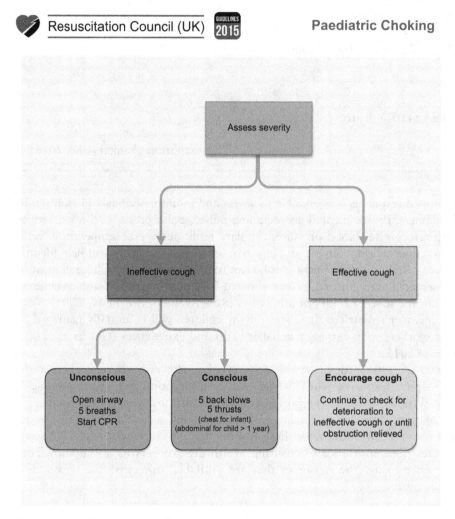

Figure 38.1 Choking algorithm

Reproduced with kind permission from the Resuscitation Council (UK).

Choking infant (conscious with an ineffective cough) (WHO, 2013; Resuscitation Council (UK), 2016) (<1 year old):

- Lay the infant on your arm or thigh, in a head-down position.
- Give up to five back blows on the infant's back using the heel of your hand.
- If obstruction persists, try up to five chest thrusts, using two fingers on the lower half of the sternum.
- Repeat back slaps/chest thrusts until the obstruction is cleared.
- If the infant becomes unconscious, start cardio-pulmonary resuscitation (CPR). You are doing this to remove the obstruction; once the obstruction has been cleared, reassess the infant and act on what you find.

Choking child (conscious with ineffective cough) (>1 year old):

- Lean the child forward, sitting, kneeling or lying, and give up to five back blows in the middle of the back with the heel of your hand.
- If unsuccessful from behind, pass your hands around the child's body, form a fist and with one hand immediately below the sternum. Place your other hand over the fist and pull upwards into the sternum. Repeat this up to five times. This is termed an abdominal thrust or Heimlich manoeuvre.
- Repeat back slaps/abdominal thrusts until the obstruction is cleared.
- If the child becomes unconscious, start CPR. Once the obstruction has been cleared, reassess and act on what you find.

To open an infant's airway, the head should be in a neutral position, and the neck not hyperextended.

A child's airway is opened by moving the head into a 'sniffing the morning air' position. If the child is unconscious and you are concerned about neck trauma, a jaw thrust technique should be used. The child should be kept lying on their back with C-spine immobilisation. This includes taping the child's forehead and chin to the sides of a firm board to secure this position. Blocks or bags of IV fluids should support the child's head to stop it moving. If the child vomits, turn them onto their side keeping the head in line with the body (WHO, 2013).

Airway complications may include stridor, wheeze, drooling. If suction is required, care should be taken and an appropriately sized rigid suction catheter (Yankeur) should be used. Only suction what you can see.

The epiglottis in infants is larger and floppier than adults, which makes it vulnerable to damage by airway devices. Up until 8 years old the child's airway is funnel shaped with the narrowest segment at the level of the cricoid cartilage. When intubating an infant a straight blade is used and in both infants and children uncuffed endotracheal tubes are used. To secure ETTs, tape tends to be used (Melbourne Strapping) instead of ties.

Breathing

Examination of the child includes the following:

- Assess the child's cough and what the quality of their cough is. If the child has a chronic cough, this may be indicative of TB, asthma, pertussis, HIV, bronchiectasis, lung abscess.
- Assess the child's work of breathing by:
  - counting a respiratory rate (Table 38.1);
  - looking for signs of recession, use of accessory muscles, 'see-saw' respiration, nostril flaring and position;
  - listening for inspiratory or expiratory noises (stridor, wheeze). Grunting is a sign of severe respiratory compromise. Any reduced air entry, crepitations?
  - looking for signs of cyanosis;
  - looking for any swelling of the neck.

Table 38.1 Respiratory rate

Age (years)	Respiratory rate (per minute)
<1	30–40
1–2	26–34
2–5	24–30
5–12	20–24
>12	12–20

Assess the child's efficacy of breathing by:

- observing chest movement;
- palpation;
- percussion;
- chest auscultation;
- pulse oximetry.

Potential differential diagnosis in a child presenting with an airway or severe breathing problem include the following (WHO, 2013):

- Pneumonia: cough, tachypnoea, pyrexia, grunting or difficulty in breathing, development over days, crepitations and signs of consolidation or effusion.
- Asthma: history of recurrent wheeze, prolonged expiration, wheezing or reduced air entry, respond to bronchodilators.
- Retropharyngeal abscess: slow deterioration over days, inability to swallow and pyrexia.
- Croup: barking cough, hoarse voice, associated with an upper respiratory tract infection, stridor on inspiration and respiratory distress.
- Diphtheria: 'bull neck' appearance due to raised lymph nodes, signs of airway obstruction, stridor, recession, grey pharyngeal membrane, history of no DPT vaccination.
- Epiglottitis: stridor, child with sepsis, little or no cough, drooling of saliva, inability to drink.
- Burns: swollen lips, smoke inhalation.
- Anaphylaxis: history of allergen exposure, wheeze, shock, urticaria and swelling of lips and face.
- Bronchiolitis: first wheeze in a child aged <2 years, wheeze episode at a time of seasonal bronchiolitis, hyperinflation of the chest, prolonged expiration, reduced airway entry, no/little response to bronchodilators, apnoea in young infants.

Treatment involves identifying and treating the cause. Pneumonia is common and can be either viral or bacterial. This may be complicated by TB and/or HIV (WHO, 2013).

If wheeze is present, a bronchodilator should be given. To give a bronchodilator, e.g. salbutamol, you may not have immediate access to a nebuliser in a self-ventilating child. An inhaler can be used with a spacer; if no commercial spacer is available, use a plastic cup or a 1-litre plastic bottle.

Oxygen may be provided using a non-re-breath mask, nasal prongs or a nasal catheter (WHO, 2013).

- If using a non-re-breath mask this is very drying, ensure the oxygen does not go directly into the child's eyes.
- Place the nasal prongs inside the child's nostrils and secure with tape. Nurses should check the nasal prongs a minimum of every three hours to check they are not blocked with mucus and are in the correct position.
- Using an 8Fr gauge catheter, measure the distance from the side of the nostril to the inner eyebrow with the catheter. Insert the catheter and tape in place.
- Commence oxygen at 1–2 litres/min; aim for oxygen saturation >90%.

Regardless of the method used, monitoring including respiratory rate and pulse oximetry must be performed and any concerns escalated.

If the child is not apnoeic, has a respiratory rate <8/min or not breathing adequately, you will need to ventilate the child using a bag-valve mask.

- Use an appropriately sized self-inflating bag. Use just enough pressure to see the chest rise. This should have a reservoir bag and high flow oxygen applied.
- Check you use an appropriately sized face mask.
- Check ventilators can ventilate the child weight and set to paediatric mode.

Circulation

Circulating volume of the newborn is 80ml/kg and decreases with age to 60–70/kg in adulthood. This means relatively small losses of volume can be a significant percentage of their circulating volume. Normal heart rates (Table 38.2) and blood pressure (Table 38.3) vary with age. Central capillary refill time may provide a better assessment of perfusion than blood pressure. Children can compensate, and hypotension tends to a terminal sign; in consequence, shock may be present with a normal blood pressure (WHO, 2013; Resuscitation Council (UK), 2011). When measuring blood pressure ensure you use an appropriate sized cuff (Ralston et al., 2013).

Table 38.2 Heart rates

Age	Mean	Awake	Deep sleep
Newborn–3 months	140	85–205	80–140
3 months–2 years	130	100–180	75–160
2–10 years	80	60–140	60–90
>10 years	75	60–100	50–90

Table 38.3 Blood pressure

70 + (age in years × 2) = lower systolic BP limit (in mmHg)

Age	Systolic blood pressure	
	Normal	Lower limit
0–1 month	>60	50–60
1–12 months	80	70
1–10 years	90 + 2 × age in years	70 + 2 × age in years
>10 years	120	90

Assess for:

- restlessness or irritability;
- lethargy;
- sunken eyes;
- decreased skin turgor;
- thirsty or drinks eagerly;
- abdominal distension;
- blood in stools;
- signs of volume loss, e.g. diarrhoea. Diarrhoea is a common cause of volume loss; assess:

    o frequency of stools;
    o number of days of diarrhoea;
    o any signs of blood in the stool;
    o report of cholera outbreak in the area;
    o recent antibiotic or other treatment.

In the presence of poor perfusion/hypotension, give aliquots of 10ml/kg and reassess. Expert input must be sought when dealing with a shocked child. Fluid regimens may vary in the following situations (Ralston *et al.*, 2013; Reynolds & Wallis, 2013):

- The use of bolus fluids in malaria remains controversial, especially with severe anaemia. However, the restoration of perfusion in the shocked child is essential.
- In septic shock if >60ml/kg of fluid is required, consider blood transfusion.
- If concerned about heart failure, use 5–10ml/kg aliquots and reassess.
- In trauma divide boluses into 10ml/kg and reassess.
- Burns follow the Parkland Formula (Chapter 35).
- Head injury or recent surgery, avoid hypotonic intravenous fluids.
- Caution with aggressive, rapid rehydration, in infants <3 months, severe, acute malnutrition, cardio-respiratory or neurological co-morbidity or hypernatraemia, which could have adverse effects.

- The treatment of shock in a malnourished child differs from a well-nourished child, because dehydration and sepsis may co-exist. Refer to local or international guidelines (e.g. pocket book of hospital care for children) for guidance on fluid regimes.
- When fluid resuscitating a child, always assess every five to ten minutes to identify if they are improving or deteriorating.

Establishing intravenous access may by peripheral or central venous access, intra-osseous or venous cut down (Chapter 18). Common sites for cannulation include scalp veins, external jugular vein, antecubital fossa vein, dorsum of the hands, femoral or ankle veins. In children <2 years the scalp vein is most suitable. However, in emergency situations, e.g. resuscitation, care should be taken when using scalp veins as there is a risk of extravasation and potential tissue necrosis (Resuscitation Council (UK), 2011).

The total daily fluid requirement for a child is calculated using the following formula:

100mg/kg for the first 10kg, then 50ml/kg for the next 10kg, thereafter 25ml/kg for each subsequent kg.

If the child has fever, increase the amount of fluid by 10% for every 1°C of fever (WHO, 2013).

When giving fluids, in the absence of infusion pumps, burettes may be used to provide maintenance fluids or blood transfusions (WHO, 2013).

In the event of pyrexia (>39°C or >102.2°F) and the child is in distress paracetamol should be given.

In low-income settings, children are at significant risk of AKI due to single disease insults, e.g. diarrhoeal disease, malaria, haemolytic uremic syndrome and acute glomerulonephritis, and carry significant mortality (Esezobor et al., 2012). Esezobor et al. (2012) identified that the incidence of AKI in hospitalised children is high and rising, with primary kidney disease and sepsis as the commonest causes. Maintaining a fluid balance chart to help assess hydration is an important aspect of nursing care. In catheterised children, normal urine outputs:

- infants >2ml/kg/hr;
- children >1ml/kg/hr;
- alternatively, weigh the baby's nappies or pads to measure urine output.

A good urine output suggests an adequate response to fluid resuscitation.

Disability (neurological)

Infants and children have limited communication, which needs to be considered when assessing neurological status and pain. They may not understand you, be frightened of a stranger or being in a strange environment. Assessing pain is difficult and the child may not behave the way you expect them to. They may be more independent, scared or culturally it may not be appropriate to complain.

Pain management varies between countries, institutions and cultures (Mathew *et al.*, 2011). An understanding of these factors will allow you to provide appropriate pain management strategies which are not only realistic and achievable within the environment you are working in, but will also be continued by other nurses when you are not on duty. In critical care many painful procedures are undertaken by nurses, and studies have shown if nurses have appropriate education in pain management this directly impacts on decision-making regarding pain management. A survey exploring the knowledge, attitude and practices of paediatric critical care nurses found the commonest method used when undertaking painful procedures was restraint and distraction, and the use of sedatives and local anaesthetics were least used (Mathew *et al.*, 2011). Only one-third of nurses had received formal training in pain management and experience and knowledge was gained from peers (Mathew *et al.*, 2011). If available, analgesia must be given and restraint avoided as this will cause distress for both the child and mother. Analgesia may include (WHO, 2013):

- mild pain: paracetamol 10–15mg/kg every four to six hours, orally or rectally. Ibuprofen 5–10mg/kg every six to eight hours;
- moderate to severe pain: morphine sulphate 0.05–0.1mg/kg IV every four to six hours.

When giving analgesics titrate the response to the patient, as each patient will respond differently. The route of administration is also important. Giving analgesics via intra-muscular (IM) injection can be painful and in a shocked patient can delay the effect, therefore this route should be avoided.

Sedation prior to procedures may include:

- diazepam 0.1–0.2mg/kg IV;
- ketamine 2–4mg/kg IM.

When giving analgesics and sedations ensure emergency airway equipment including a self-inflating bag is immediately available. Never leave a child unattended as they may roll off the bed.

Assess the neurological status of the child either using the Alert, Voice, Pain or Unresponsive (AVPU) approach or modified Glasgow Coma Scale (Table 38.4). Both methods should include assessment of pupil size and reaction. The frequency of neurological observations should be determined by the patient's current and underlying condition.

Table 38.4 Modified Glasgow Coma Scale

Eyes	4	Spontaneous eyes opening.
	3	Eyes opening to speech (speak to child using appropriate language and familiar names. If appropriate involve family to encourage the child to respond to verbal stimuli).
	2	Eyes opening to painful stimuli.

Table 38.4 Continued

	1	No eyes opening to painful stimulus. If the child is unable to open eyes due to swelling, it is important this is documented by recording 'C' in the appropriate space on the assessment tool.
Verbal	5	Infant/pre-verbal child – smiling or contented infant who may coo or babble. Orientated, verbal. Involve the family to use appropriate familiar words to encourage the child to verbalise.
	4	Infant/pre-verbal child – crying. Disorientated verbal.
	3	Consider cognitive status when assessing verbal score. Infant/pre-verbal child – inappropriate crying. The pitch of the cry is important. A high-pitched cry should be recorded within significant events. Child – verbal, monosyllabic responses.
	2	Infant/pre-verbal child – occasional whimper. Child – incomprehensible sounds.
	1	Infant/pre-verbal child – no verbal response to both verbal and painful stimuli.
Motor response	6	An infant moves the arms spontaneously. The child is able to obey commands.
	5	Central painful stimuli to evoke localised response will need to be applied when: • an infant does not move limbs spontaneously; • a child does not obey commands.
	4	Normal flexion: Infant – best motor response to stimulation in an infant up to six months is flexion. Child – not localising to central painful stimulus but can bend their arm towards the source of the pain. • The arm bends at the elbow and wrist extends rapidly in response to pain, but does not attempt to remove the source of the painful stimulus.
	3	Abnormal flexion: • Decorticate posturing describes abnormal flexion of the upper limbs and extension of the lower libs, the arms are flexed over the chest.
	2	Extension to painful stimulus: Decerebrate posturing describes abnormal extension of all four limbs.
	1	No response to painful stimulus

Source: Great Ormond Street Hospital for Children, 2017

The posture of the child is also an important part of the neurological assessment. A floppy child or stiff posturing child identifies neurological derangement and brain dysfunction.

Don't forget to check the child's blood glucose level, as hypoglycaemia is common. Potential causes may include hypoglycaemia (blood glucose level <2.5mmol/l (<45mg/dl) or <3.0mmol/l (<54mg/dl) in a malnourished child, meningitis, malaria, Japanese encephalitis, dengue haemorrhagic fever, measles encephalitis, typhoid, relapsing fever, diabetic ketoacidosis.

If a child presents fitting, consider:

- temperature – does the child have fever?
- head injury;
- drug overdose;
- how long have the convulsions lasted?
- what is the child's blood glucose level?

If meningitis is suspected, a lumbar puncture needs to be performed. If malaria is suspected, a rapid diagnosis test or blood smear should be performed. Hypoglycaemia can also be associated with severe malaria and a known side effect of quinine.

Exposure

When examining the child for any injuries, rashes or sources of fluid loss avoid heat loss, with a large surface area to volume ratio, they can become hypothermic fast. The child's core temperature should be taken and the use of warming blankets to actively manage hypothermia should be used.

A systematic assessment will allow you to check for petechial rash, neck stiffness, abnormal posture, e.g. opisthotonos (arched back), which may be indicative of meningitis. In newborns check the fontanelle for signs of a 'bulging fontanelle' and umbilicus for signs of infection (WHO, 2013).

Family

The child may be accompanied by the mother or other family members as cultural and situations allows. This not only provides a reassuring figure for the child and can help with the delivery of care but also helps you to understand how the child might behave. Families will also need to be reassured and provision for them to stay at the hospital or bedside arranged.

Resuscitation

It is widely recognised there is a need to develop culturally appropriate paediatric advanced life support (PALS) guidelines for use in resource limited environments, due to the different challenges and conditions seen (Wright *et al.*, 2015; Ralston *et al.*, 2013). The current delivery of PALS is most relevant in hospitals where there is a full range of paediatric services (Opiyo & English, 2010) (Figure 38.2). Cardio-respiratory arrest in children tends to occur following a prolonged period of deterioration and causes tend to be due to hypoxia or shock. Overall outcome following cardio-respiratory arrest is poor, even when witnessed and monitored in hospital; respiratory arrest when

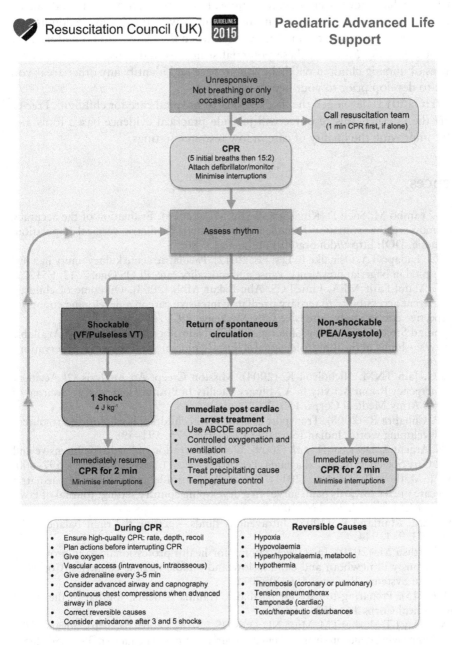

Figure 38.2 Advanced life support algorithm

Reproduced with kind permission from the Resuscitation Council (UK).

there is still a cardiac output has better outcome with long-term survival (Resuscitation Council, (UK) 2011).

In this chapter, the principles of caring for a critically ill child have been outlined. Children require access to specialist staff trained in paediatrics. The types of conditions requiring admission will pose unique challenges for both general and paediatric HIC nurses who may have never seen these conditions. Further complications include a lack of specialist units to refer patients to, meaning nurses who trained in predominately adult specialities are required to care for children when they have had limited training and experience. Being aware of these potential scenarios and considering your own experiences of nursing children will help you prepare and identify any other areas you may want to develop prior to your departure.

The WHO (2013) developed the 'Pocketbook of hospital care for children'. Free to access via the internet, this resource will provide practical evidence-based tools and advice for improving the quality of care in low resource settings.

References

Bowen L. Zyambo M. Snell D. Kinnear J. Bould MD. (2016). Evaluation of the accuracy of common weight estimation formulae in a Zambian paediatric surgical population. Anaesthesia. DOI: https://doi.org/10.1111/anae.13780.

Esezobor CI. Ladapo TA. Osinaike B. Lesi FE. (2012). Paediatric acute kidney injury in a tertiary hospital in Nigeria: prevalence, cause and mortality rate. PLOS One. 7. 12. E51229.

Goh AYT. Abdul-Latif MEA. Lum LCS. Abu-Bakar MN. (2003). Outcome of children with different accessibility to tertiary paediatric intensive care in a developing country – a prospective cohort study. Intensive Care Medicine. 29. 97–102.

Great Ormond Street Hospital for Children. (2017). Neurological observations. Available at: www.gosh.nhs.uk/health-professionals/clinical-guidelines/neurological-observations #References.

Kenward G. Jain TNM. Nicholson K. (2004). Mission Creep: An Analysis Of Accident And Emergency Room Activity In A Military Facility In Bosnia-Herzegovina. Journal of the Royal Army Medical Corps. 150. 20–23.

Khilnani P. Chhabra R. (2008). Transport of critically ill children: how to utilize resources in the developing world. Indian Journal of Paediatrics. 75. 591–598.

Kissoon N. Argent A. Devictor D et al. (2009). World Federation of Paediatric Intensive and Critical Care Societies: its global agenda. Pediatric Critical Care Medicine. 10. 597–600.

Mathew PJ. Mathew JL. Singh S. (2011). Knowledge, attitude and practice of paediatric critical care nurses towards pain: survey in a developing country setting. Journal of Post-Graduate Medicine. 57. 11. 196–200.

Molyneux EM. Maitland K. (2005). Intravenous fluids – getting the right balance. The Lancet. 353. 941–944.

Opiyo N. English M. (2010). In-service training for health professionals to improve care of the seriously ill newborn and child in low and middle-income countries. Cochrane Database of Systemic Reviews. 4. CD007071.

Pearce P. (2015). Preparing to care for paediatric trauma patients. Journal of the Royal Army Medical Corps 161. i52–i55.

Ralston ME. Day LT. Slusher TM. Musa NL. Doss HS. (2013). Global paediatric advanced life support: improving child survival in limited-resource settings. The Lancet. 381. 256–265.

Resuscitation Council (UK). (2011). Paediatric immediate life support. 2nd Edition. London: Resuscitation Council (UK).

Resuscitation Council (UK). (2016). Paediatric Life Support. Available at: www.resus.org. uk/faqs/faqs-paediatric-life-support/.

Reynolds TA. Wallis LA. (2013). Chapter 4: Volume resuscitation in children. In: Wallis LA. Reynolds TA (eds). AFEM Handbook of acute and emergency care. Oxford: Oxford University Press.

Robertson MA. Molyneux EM. (2001). Description of cause of serious illness and outcome in patients identified using ETAT guidelines in urban Malawi. Archives of Disease in Childhood. 85. 3. 214–217.

UNICEF. (2017). United Nations convention on the rights of the child. Available at: www. unicef.org.uk/Documents/Publication-pdfs/UNCRC_PRESS200910web.pdf.

World Health Organization. (2013). Pocket book of hospital care for children: guidelines for the management of common childhood illnesses. 2nd Edition. Geneva: World Health Organization.

Wright SW. Steenhoff AP. Elci O *et al.* (2015). Impact of contextualized paediatric resuscitation training on paediatric healthcare providers in Botswana. Resuscitation. 88. 57–62.

39 | Women's and maternal emergencies

The UN Sustainable Development Goals (2015) has set an ambitious aim to empower gender equality and empower all women and girls, which includes access to healthcare. Women's healthcare needs are often neglected in low resource settings, for a variety of reasons including their status, cultural issues or lack of healthcare planning (Nour, 2008; Bricknell & Cameron, 2013). While maternal health has rightly attracted significant resources to prevent death or complication during pregnancy, childbirth and six weeks post-partum, this is a very narrow period of a woman's life and only focuses on the woman if she is pregnant. Mortality and reduction in life expectancy for chronic and non-communicable diseases are now higher than maternal complications (Knaul et al., 2012; Bustreo et al., 2012). Conditions or situations which may require a woman to be admitted to a critical care unit include:

- rise of non-communicable disease;
- unsafe/illegal abortions;
- cancers;
- Poor sexual health exposing women to HIV/AIDS and other sexually transmitted diseases;
- gender-based violence;
- complications from female genital mutilation;
- maternal emergencies.

Non-communicable diseases

Within LICs and LMICs there is a perception that non-communicable diseases including cardiovascular disease, diabetes, obesity only affect men; however, these conditions and their associated problems also affect women. Harmful use of alcohol, drugs and substances and tobacco all contribute to this. Mental health, depression and self-inflicted injuries and road injuries are a significant cause of death amongst adult women (20–59 years) globally (WHO, 2013). Women suffer significantly more fire-related injuries and deaths, due to cooking accidents or as the result of intimate partner and family violence (WHO, 2013).

Child marriage

Girls are more likely to suffer sexual abuse than boys. Pregnant adolescents are more likely to have unsafe abortions. An estimated 3 million unsafe abortions occur globally every year amongst girls aged 15–19 years (WHO, 2013). This may lead to sepsis or other complications.

Cancer

Breast and cervical cancers are a significant cause of mortality. Breast cancer is the leading cause of mortality in women aged 20–59 worldwide (WHO, 2013) and cervical cancer is the second most common cause of cancer in women in low-income settings (WHO, 2017a). Cervical cancer is also associated with sexually transmitted genital infection with the human papilloma virus (HPV) (WHO, 2013). With limited screening services, patients may present late with advanced diseases and over 90% of deaths occur (WHO, 2013).

Sexual health

Limited access to healthcare services and unequal power in relationships can expose women (particularly young women) to HIV and AIDS, leading to other infections, e.g. TB.

Gender-based violence

An estimated 35% of women worldwide have experienced either intimate partner violence or non-partner sexual violence. Globally, as many as 38% of murders of women are committed by an intimate partner (WHO, 2013). Women who have been physically or sexually abused can have:

- higher incidence of mental health illness including depression, use of alcohol;
- unintended pregnancies;
- abortions;
- increased exposure to HIV and other sexually transmitted infections.

(WHO, 2013)

Female genital mutilation

Female genital mutilation (FGM), also known as female genital cutting (FGC) or Female circumcision (FC), is defined by the WHO (2017b) as 'all procedures that involve partial or total removal of the external female genitalia, or other injury to the female genital organs for non-medical reasons'. FGM may be practised in certain countries in which you work. An estimated 200 million girls and women globally have

Table 39.1 Categories of FGM

Stage 1	Clitoridectomy. The partial or total removal of the clitoris or the removal of the prepuce.
Stage 2	Excision. The partial or total removal of the clitoris and the labia minora, with or without excision of the labia majora.
Stage 3	Infibulation. The narrowing of the vaginal opening through the creation of a covering seal.
Stage 4	Other. All other harmful procedures to the female genitalia for non-medical purposes, e.g. piercing, incising, scraping the genital area.

undergone this procedure and are living with its consequences. Four categories have been identified to outline the type of FGM performed (WHO, 2017b) (Table 39.1).

Acute and chronic complications of FGM are outlined in Table 39.2. The presentation, e.g. obstructed labour, septic shock post-FGM, will determine the treatment; however, principles may include:

- assessment using A–E approach;
- wound debridement, saline irrigation, removal of all foreign material;
- removal of minimal tissue, drain abscess;
- antibiotics for infected wounds, cellulitis, abscess;
- catheterisation of bladder;
- tetanus toxoid if non-immune;
- excision of epidermal tissue, if present, to permit urinary flow and sexual intercourse.

(WHO, 2017b; RCN, 2016)

While the short-term consequences of FGM may require admission to critical care, e.g. obstructed labour or sepsis due to urological complications, the long-term mental consequences should not be underestimated (Momoh et al., 2016). The role of the nurse is to provide supportive care but gaining information and how to deal with this subject may be limited in both the country you are working in and where you are from. It is recognised specialist training is required to deal with this sensitive and personal issue, and organisations that work in areas with FGM must provide training prior to departure to adequately prepare you for your role (Momoh et al., 2016).

Maternal physiology

The WHO estimated 289,000 maternal deaths occurred in 2010, with 99% occurring in low- and middle-income countries (WHO, 2014). There are a variety of maternal conditions which may require admission to critical care. Within LICs and LMICs, maternal mortality remains high (UN, 2015). During pregnancy, the following physiological changes occur to the woman's body:

Table 39.2 Acute, delayed and long-term complications of FGM

Acute and immediate complications	Delayed complications	Long-term complications
• Pain • Haemorrhage • Shock • Urinary retention • Damage to urethra, anus • Vaginal fistula • Ulceration of the genital region • Cellulitis • Abscess formation • Sepsis • Tetanus • Bacterial or viral infections including hepatitis and HIV due to use of unsterilised instruments • Death	• Delayed healing • Abscesses • Scarring/keloid formation, dysmennorrhoea and haematocolpus – obstruction to menstrual flow • Pelvic infections • Obstruction to urinary flow • Urinary tract infection	• Psychosocial trauma and flashbacks, post-traumatic stress disorder • Lack of trust in carers • Vaginal closure due to scarring • Epidermal cyst formation • Neuromata – benign tumours of nerve tissue that may arise from cut nerve endings and cause pain • Pain and chronic infection from obstruction to menstrual flow • Recurrent urinary tract infection and renal damage • Painful intercourse • Infertility from pelvic inflammatory disease and obstructed genital tract • Risk of HIV through traumatic intercourse • Childbirth trauma – perineal tears and vaginal fistulae • Post-natal wound infection • Prolonged or obstructed labour from tough scarred perineum, uterine inertia or rupture, and death of infant and mother • Vaginal fistulae as consequence of obstructed labour • Sexual dysfunction, dyspareunia • Psychological disturbance • Urinary obstruction • Keloids • Large epidermal inclusion cysts • Difficult urination • Vaginal stenosis; may cause obstructed labour, often complicated by vesico- or recto-vaginal fistulae

Sources: WHO, 2017b; RCN, 2016

- Cardiac output, circulatory volume, minute ventilation and oxygen consumption all increase.
- In the supine position, the gravid uterus can compress the iliac and abdominal vessels, leading to reduced cardiac output and hypotension.

Women may be admitted to critical care due to complications during pregnancy, including the following:

- Severe bleeding (particularly after childbirth).
- Infections (after childbirth).
- Hypertensive disorders during pregnancy (pre-eclampsia and eclampsia).
- Complications from delivery.
- Unsafe abortion.
- Pulmonary or amniotic embolism.
- Ectopic pregnancy.
- Psychiatric disorders.
- Chronic anaemia. In many low resource settings, girls aged between 15 and 19 years old are anaemic, most commonly caused by iron-deficiency. Anaemia increases the risk of haemorrhage and sepsis during childbirth.
- Pregnant women infected with syphilis could lead to adverse birth outcomes including stillbirth.

(WHO, 2013, 2014, 2016; Nolan *et al.*, 2011)

Non-obstetric disorders requiring admission to critical care include:

- maternal cardiac disease;
- trauma;
- anaesthetic complications;
- anaphylaxis;
- cerebrovascular accidents;
- drug overdose;
- diabetes;
- malaria or other infection.

Severe bleeding

Severe haemorrhage may occur in either the ante-partum or post-partum periods. Ante-partum haemorrhage could be caused by placental abruption, placental previa or placental accrete. Post-partum haemorrhage includes retained placenta, failure of uterine contraction, trauma and coagulopathy. Treatment includes the following:

- Aggressive co-ordinated teamwork from obstetricians, midwives, anaesthetists, blood bank and critical care.
- Initial management will depend on the cause and whether the patient has been delivered.

- Monitoring including haematological and hourly physiological observations.
- Urinary catheter and fluid balance monitoring.
- Check mother's rhesus status.
- Confirm the patient is cross-matched and administer warmed blood products as required.
- Hourly urine measurements and fluid balance charting.
- Keep the patient warm.

Pregnancy induced hypertension

Pregnancy induced hypertension (PIH) is defined as 'gestational hypertension with proteinuria developing during pregnancy or labour' (Leach, 2009). Hypertensive disorders during pregnancy may be a sign of life-threatening pre-eclampsia. Eclampsia is diagnosed if convulsions occur (Leach, 2009). Pre-eclampsia is defined by:

- hypertension:
  - systolic blood pressure >140mmHg or diastolic BP >90mmHg on two occasions, six hours to seven days apart;
  - *or* one BP >160/110mmHg.

- proteinuria:
  - 24–hour urine specimen >0.3g protein;
  - *or* >+2 dipstick;
  - *or* >100mg/l on two random urine samples collected at least four hours apart.

Other signs of pre-eclampsia include:

- hypertension;
- proteinuria;
- headaches;
- visual changes;
- seizures;
- reduced level of consciousness;
- epigastric pain;
- vomiting;
- generalised oedema;
- bruising;
- oliguria;
- disseminating intravascular coagulopathy;
- HELLP syndrome (haemolysis, elevated liver enzymes and low platelets);
- platelets <100,000, altered liver and renal function tests.

The presence of proteinuria changes the diagnosis from pregnancy-induced hypertension to pre-eclampsia. Other conditions which may cause proteinuria or a false positive include severe urinary infection, severe anaemia, heart failure, difficult labour, blood in the urine due to traumatic catheterisation, schistosomiasis, contamination from vaginal blood and vaginal secretions or amniotic fluid containing urine specimens (WHO, 2003).

Management of pre-eclampsia includes:

- specialist obstetric input, to deliver baby, either vaginally or via caesarean section in an emergency. Delivery is the only cure for pre-eclampsia and eclampsia;
- organ optimisation, e.g. oxygen, cardiac and blood pressure monitoring, observation for pulmonary oedema. Invasive monitoring may be required if oliguria persists;
- IV access;
- vital signs monitoring;
- acute blood pressure control to reduce blood pressure but not affect uterine perfusion:

  o 1st line: hydralazine;
  o 2nd line: nifedipine or labetalol.

- urinary catheter;
- fluid balance monitoring;
- observation for signs of fluid overload and/or pulmonary oedema;
- observation for signs of convulsions.

(Nolan et al., 2011; Rouhani & Waji, 2016; Leach, 2009)

Eclampsia

Immediate management of a pregnant women with eclampsia includes the following:

- Rapid assessment of ABC.
- Position the woman on the left lateral side.
- Administer high flow oxygen.
- Check for neck rigidity and temperature.
- Call for help.
- Consider securing the airway and assisting with ventilations if required.
- If the woman is convulsing:

  o protect her from injury, but do not restrain;
  o position her on her side to reduce the risk of aspiration.

- Give magnesium sulphate. Magnesium is the drug of choice due to the central nervous system depression, cerebral vasodilation and mild-anti-hypertensive effects. If convulsions continue, consider diazepam 10mg.
- If diastolic blood pressure >110mmHg, give antihypertensive drugs.
- Start IV fluids and strict fluid balance charting.
- Observe/prevent fluid overload including pulmonary oedema.
- Urinary catheterisation to monitor urine output and proteinuria.
- Delivery must occur within 12 hours of the onset of convulsions in eclampsia (WHO, 2004).

Magnesium sulphate for pre-eclampsia and eclampsia

Loading dose:

- Magnesium sulphate 20% solution, 4g IV over five minutes.
- Followed by 10g of 50% magnesium sulphate (5g in each buttock as deep IM injection with 1.0ml of 2% lidocaine in same syringe).
- If convulsions continue after 15 minutes, give 2g magnesium sulphate (50% solution) IV over 5 minutes.

Maintenance dose:

- 5g magnesium sulphate (50% solution) + 1ml lidocaine 2% IM every four hours into alternate buttocks.
- Continue treatment with magnesium sulphate for 24 hours after delivery of last convulsion, whichever occurs last.
- Before repeat administration, check:

  o respiratory rate >16/min;
  o patellar reflexes are present;
  o urine output >30ml/hr over last four hours.

- Withhold or delay administration if any of the above signs are not meet.
- In case of respiratory arrest, assist ventilation and give calcium gluconate 1gm (10ml or 10% solution) IV slowly.

Diazepam for severe pre-eclampsia and eclampsia:
  Loading dose:

- Diazepam 10mg IV slowly over two minutes.
- If convulsions continue, repeat loading dose.

Maintenance dose:

- Diazepam 40mg in 500ml IV fluids (normal saline or Ringer's lactate) titrated to keep patient sedated by rousable.
- Do not give more than 100mg in 24 hours.

(WHO, 2004)

Sepsis

Common causes of maternal sepsis include:

- genital tract infections, including endometritis, retained products of conception, or infected peritoneal wound;

- urinary tract infections, for example acute pyelonephritis;
- mastitis. Untreated mastitis can be complicated by breast abscess, necrotising fasciitis and septic shock;
- respiratory tract infections;
- gastro-intestinal tract infections;
- skin and soft tissue infections due to intravenous cannulas, spinal abscesses due to obstetric spinal anaesthesia.

(Patil *et al.*, 2016)

Risk factors for maternal sepsis includes obesity, diabetes, anaemia, sickle cell disease, history of pelvic infection of group B streptococcal infection (Patil *et al.*, 2015). Recognition of sepsis in pregnancy may be difficult as clinical signs including tachycardia or tachypnoea may be mistaken for normal physiological changes associated with pregnancy, instead of a sign of deterioration (Patil *et al.*, 2016). Monitoring and observation for trends in observations will help detect abnormal physiology, assessing the mother holistically and not focusing on one physiological sign will assist in early detection. Standard treatment of sepsis should be followed as outlined in Chapter 17.

Critical care considerations

A multi-disciplinary team approach to the women's care, including obstetric and midwifery input and support, is essential, to avoid conflict between healthcare professionals over the needs of the mother and the foetus (Mushambi & Jaladi, 2016). Critical care interventions focus on the reason for admission; considerations for nursing a critically ill maternal patient may include:

Airway

- In an emergency, women should be placed in the left lateral position. This will help with airway management and postural drainage if the patient vomits. Rapid sequence induction and cricoid pressure should be performed when securing the airway. Prophylactic H2 antagonists and antacids should be used if available.
- There is an increased risk of pulmonary aspiration of gastric contents, therefore early tracheal intubation decreases the risk.
- Difficult airway is more likely in pregnancy due to poor positioning, obesity, large breasts and laryngeal oedema. Difficult airway equipment must be available in the event of failed intubation. The consequences for mother and baby can be catastrophic.
- Nasal intubation should be avoided.

Breathing

- Supplementary oxygen should be given to keep oxygen saturations >95%.
- Positioning may be difficult if the patient is full term.

- High risk for hypoxia due to altered lung function, diaphragmatic splitting by the large uterus and increased oxygen consumption.

Circulation

- In an emergency the woman is placed in the left lateral position or manual displacement of the uterus can reduce compression on the inferior vena cava.
- Increased cardiac output means large volumes can be lost quickly, especially from the uterus, which receives 10% of blood volume on term.
- Wide bore IV access must be established, and fluid boluses should be given in the evidence of hypotension or hypovolaemia.
- Bloods (full blood count, urea and electrolytes, coagulation and any other appropriate tests, e.g. cross-match, blood cultures) should be taken.
- Hypercoagulability results in an increased risk of VTE.
- Careful fluid balance monitoring particularly in eclampsia.
- Urinary catheterisation and one-hourly urine measurements.
- Cardiac monitoring particularly when using magnesium.

Emergency caesarean section

If appropriate, an emergency caesarean section, should be performed in maternal resuscitation, within 5 minutes (if >20–week gestation) if there no response to correctly performed CPR. Once the foetus has been delivered, resuscitation of the newborn child can commence.

Other considerations

- Critical care units that admit maternal patients must have immediate availability of obstetric drugs including hydralazine, magnesium, oxytocin, ergometrine, carboprost, labetolol, eclampsia pack, and post-partum haemorrhage packs.
- Specialist dietician input.
- Specialist pharmacist involvement during the ante-natal and post-natal period.

(Patil *et al.*, 2016; Nolan *et al.*, 2011;
Patil *et al.*, 2015; Mushambi & Jaladi, 2016)

Cardiac arrest in pregnancy

In cardiac arrest, all the principles of basic and advanced life support (Chapter 12) apply. In addition to an adult cardiac arrest team, expert help including an obstetrician, anaesthetist, and neonatologist to facilitate resuscitation of both the mother and foetus are required. The following adaptations to standard resuscitation are as follows:

- In advanced pregnancy hand position may be slightly higher on the sternum when performing chest compressions.
- After 20 weeks gestation, the woman's uterus can partially occlude the inferior vena-cava (IVC) and aorta. IV/IO access should be established above the IVC to ensure fluids and drugs given reach the circulating volume and are delayed by IVC pressure.
- Manual displacement of the uterus should also be undertaken to reduce IVC depression.
- Positioning on the left lateral position may only be possible if a firm, flat surface is available. The use of pillows and wedges are not effective. The optimal angle is 15–20°.
- Emergency caesarean section should be attempted in gestation over 20 weeks.
- Defibrillation should follow standard energy doses. Left lateral positioning and large breasts can make it difficult to place defibrillator pads/paddles.
- Potential causes of cardiac arrest include:

  o haemorrhage:

    o rapid transfusion;
    o tranexamic acid and correction of coagulopathy;
    o oxytocin, ergometrine, prostaglandins and uterine massage to correct urine atony;
    o uterine compressions sutures, uterine packs and intrauterine balloon devices;
    o interventional radiology to identify and control bleeding;
    o surgical control including aortic cross clamping/compression and hysterectomy.

  o drugs;
  o cardiovascular disease;
  o pre-eclampsia and eclampsia;
  o amniotic fluid embolism;
  o pulmonary embolus.

(Nolan *et al.*, 2011)

References

Bricknell MCM. Cameron E. (2013). Military medical engagement with the civilian health sector. MCIF. 4. 34–37.

Bustreo F. Knaul F. Bhadelia A *et al.* (2012). Women's health beyond reproduction: meeting the challenges. Bulletin of the World Health Organization. 90. 478–478A. DOI: 10.2471/BLT.12.103549.

Knaul F. Bhadelia A. Gralow J *et al.* (2012). Meeting the emerging challenge of breast and cervical cancer in low and middle income countries. International Journal of Gynaecology and Obstetrics. 119 Suppl. 1. S85–88.

Leach R. (2009). Acute and Critical Care Medicine at a Glance. 2nd Edition. New York: John Wiley & Sons.

Momoh C. Olufade O. Redman-Pinard P. (2016). What nurses need to know about female genital mutilation. British Journal of Nursing. 25. 9. S30–S34.

Mushambi MC. Jaladi S. (2016). Airway management and training in obstetric anaesthesia. Current Opinion in Anaesthesiology. 29. 3. 261–267.

Nolan J. Soar J. Lockley A *et al.* (2011). Advanced Life Support. 6th Edition. London: Resuscitation Council (UK).

Nour NM. (2008). An Introduction to Global Women's Health. Reviews in Obstetrics and Gynecology. 1. 1. 33–37.

Patil V. Jigajinni S. Wijayatilake DS. (2015). Maternal critical care: 'one small step for woman one giant leap for womankind'. Current Opinion in Anaesthesiology. 28. 3. 290–299.

Patil V. Wong M. Wijayatilake DS. (2016). Clinical 'pearls' of maternal critical care: part 1. Current Opinion in Anaesthesiology. 29. 3. 304–316.

Rouhani S. Waji ST. (2016). Chapter 183: Hypertensive disorders during pregnancy. In: Wallis LA. Reynolds TA (eds). African Federation of Emergency Medicine: Handbook of Acute and Emergency Care. Oxford: Oxford University Press.

Royal College of Nursing. (2016). Female Genital Mutilation: An RCN resource for nursing and midwifery practice. 3rd Edition. Available at: www.rcn.org.uk/professional-development/publications/pub-005447.

United Nations. (2015). Sustainable Development Goals. Available at: www.un.org/sustainabledevelopment/gender-equality/.

World Health Organization. (2003). Surgical care at the District Hospital – The WHO Manual. Available at: www.who.int/surgery/publications/scdh_manual/en/.

World Health Organization. (2004). Surgical care at the district hospital. Geneva: World Health Organization.

World Health Organization. (2013). Women's Health. Available at: www.who.int/topics/womens_health/en/.

World Health Organization. (2014). Trends in maternal mortality: 1990 to 2013. Available at: www.who.int/reproductivehealth/publications/monitoring/maternal-mortality-2013/en/.

World Health Organization. (2016). Sexually transmitted infections (STIs). Available at: www.who.int/mediacentre/factsheets/fs110/en/.

World Health Organization. (2017a). Improving access to health products for people co-infected with HIV and HPV: Unitaid board passes resolution. Available at: www.who.int/reproductivehealth/topics/cancers/co-infection-hpv-hiv/en/.

World Health Organization. (2017b). Female genital mutilation: fact sheet No.241 (updated 2014). Geneva: World Health Organization. Available at: https://apps.who.int/iris/bitstream/handle/10665/112328/WHO_RHR_14.12_eng.pdf;jsessionid=7529F135FDB185D24CB2CF2E1161DF9D?sequence=1.

Index

Printed in the United States
by Baker & Taylor Publisher Services